Psychopharmacology: Current Trends

Editors

Daniel E. Casey   A. Vibeke Christensen

With 18 Figures

Springer-Verlag Berlin Heidelberg New York
London Paris Tokyo

Daniel E. Casey, MD
Chief, Psychiatry Research
V.A. Medical Center, and
Professor of Psychiatry
Oregon Health Sciences University
Veterans Hospital Road
Portland, OR 97207, USA

A. Vibeke Christensen, D. Sc.
Sct. Hans Hospital
Department E
DK-4000 Roskilde, Denmark

Vols. 1 and 2 of this series appeared under the title "Psychopharmacology Supplementum"

The figure on the front cover was prepared by Lisa Leong.

ISBN 3-540-18693-X Springer-Verlag Berlin Heidelberg New York
ISBN 0-387-18693-X Springer-Verlag New York Berlin Heidelberg

Library of Congress Cataloging-in-Publication Data
Psychopharmacology: current trends / editors, Daniel E. Casey, A. Vibeke Christensen. (Psychopharmacolgy series: 5) Based on a symposium held in Denmark in 1987, arranged in honor of Povl V. Petersen and sponsored by the Lundbeck Foundation. Includes bibliographies and index.
ISBN 0-387-18693-X (U.S.)
1. Psychopharmacology – Congresses. 2. Schizophrenia – Chemotherapy – Congresses. 3. Affective disorders – Chemotherapy – Congresses. 4. Petersen, P. V. – Congresses. I. Casey, Daniel E., II. Christensen, A. Vibeke, III. Petersen, P. V. IV. Lundbeck Foundation. V. Series. [DNLM: 1. Affective Disorders – drug therapy – congresses. 2. Anxiety Disorders – drug therapy – congresses. 3. Dementia – drug therapy – congresses. 5. Schizophrenia – drug therapy – congresses.
W1 PS773J v. 5 / OV 77 P97211 1987] RM315.P7533 1988 615'.78 – dc19 DNLM/DLC

Typesetting, printing and bookbinding: Brühlsche Universitätsdruckerei, Giessen
2125/3145-543210

Preface

The landmark description by Delay and Deniker in 1952 of chlorpromazine's effect in psychosis suddenly eclipsed all other progress in psychopharmacology over the previous centuries. Since this report 35 years ago, a vast amount of research has contributed to the major advances in treatment that have improved the lives of millions of patients who would otherwise be incapacitated by their psychiatric disorders. This research has also led to valuable new insights into the causes of mental illnesses and the mechanisms of action of therapeutic drugs.

However, there is much more work to be done. Thus, it is of great value periodically to assess the present state of knowledge as a first step to charting future directions. This symposium held in Denmark in 1987 covered many critical issues in psychopharmacology. The etiology, pathogenetic mechanisms, clinical aspects, and future directions of research in schizophrenia, affective disorders, anxiety, and dementia are addressed. Several of the problems with current therapeutic agents, such as side effects and limited efficacy, are also reviewed. Preclinical strategies with existing and new animal and computer models are discussed to point the way for developing better psychopharmacologic treatments of all psychiatric disorders.

The symposium was arranged in honor of Povl V. Petersen, the chemist whose scientific works forms the basis of H. Lundbeck's international business. Among the achievements in his career are the development of chlorprothixene, clopenthixol, flupentixol, amitriptyline, and ketobemidone. Having served the company for 44 years with the highest standards of science and ethics, Povl V. Petersen retired in 1987.

We gratefully acknowledge the support provided by the Lundbeck Foundation which sponsored this symposium.

Bymose Hegn, Denmark, April 1988

Daniel E. Casey
A. Vibeke Christensen

Table of Contents

Schizophrenia

Affective Disorders

Anxiety, Dementia, and Other Special Topics

List of Contributors

You will find the addresses at the beginning of the respective contribution

Schizophrenia

Reflections on the History of Psychopharmacology

A. CARLSSON

It is a distinct honour and a great pleasure for me to have the opportunity of speaking on this occasion. I have accepted the kind invitation of the organizing committee to talk about the history of psychopharmacology. This topic is obviously appropriate for the occasion – as we just heard, this meeting is dedicated to my old, dear friend P. V. PETERSEN. However, I feel a certain inadequacy since I have not had the opportunity to study the history of pharmacology systematically. It is left for me to go by my personal recollections and, needless to say, this involves a lot of bias and necessitates some important omissions. I hope that in the discussion and later in the course of this meeting some of those in this audience who were actively engaged in the early developments in the 1950s can share with us some of their experience and feelings of when, for example, the neuroleptics were introduced and the first clinical results were reported. That was before my time as an active investigator in this field.

The natural starting point for this presentation is to try to trace back to the first formulations of the basic concept in psychopharmacology, i.e., the use of drugs as scientific probes to understand the mind and mental disorders and to create a rational basis for their treatment.

MOREAU DE TOURS (1845), a famous French psychiatrist, seems to have been the first to formulate the concept of using a drug for understanding mental functions and mental disorders. MOREAU was a member of a hashish club in Paris, a club whose membership included several other famous names such as CHARLES BAUDELAIRE, HONORÉ DE BALZAC, and ALEXANDRE DUMAS. These people came together and used hashish and I understand that the doses they used were substantial. They had some very striking experiences and MOREAU (1845) wrote a book that has been translated into English, *Hashish and Mental Illness.* He pointed out some striking similarities between the experiences that one may have under the influence of hashish and the various deviations that occur in the course of mental illness. He also suggested that normal feelings and enjoyment arising from experiences in life may actually be the same as what one can experience when these processes are brought into play by the use of hashish. Another person to be mentioned in this context is the famous German psychiatrist, EMIL KRAEPELIN (1892). He was the first to use the term "psychopharmacology" even though he turned it around, calling it "pharmacopsychology." His ideas were very much the same as those of MOREAU. The reason for such a discipline would be to use drugs

---

Department of Pharmacology, University of Göteborg, P.O. Box 33031, S-40033 Göteborg, Sweden.

to achieve an understanding of the mechanisms underlying mental functions. KRAEPELIN, however, had an entirely different personality from MOREAU. He was a teetotaller and did not go as much by personal experience as MOREAU had done. In terms of personal experience he would probably hardly have gone beyond caffeine, but still, he had something to play on and he published some papers dealing with the mental effects of caffeine and alcohol.

SIGMUND FREUD was another early prophet of psychopharmacology. In a famous letter to MARIA BONAPARTE he predicted that organic chemistry, or access to it through endocrinology, would show the way towards understanding psychosis and to chemical therapy. Interestingly, this future was still believed to be far distant. He wrote the letter in 1930, and at about the same time two Indian psychiatrists, SEN and BOSE (1931), described the antipsychotic action of rauwolfia in a paper published and also made available to Western medicine; unfortunately, nobody paid much attention to this action of rauwolfia which, of course, had been utilized to some extent in Indian folk medicine for a long time. In other words, at the time of Freud's prediction, things were underway, although further progress took some time and we had to wait until the 1950s until things really started to happen. However, I would like to draw attention to an earlier, perhaps even more unfortunate, oversight. In the first textbook of neurology published in America by WILLIAM A. HAMMOND (1871) the author indicated that lithium had a specific effect in mania. It was very clear that he distinguished between lithium bromide and sodium bromide, stating that to treat mania, lithium bromide should be used. For other mental disturbances sodium bromide was recommended. It seems clear that he had made a significant discovery. It is amazing and inexplicable to me that no attention was paid to this observation. It is really unfortunate if we consider the large number of patients whose suffering could have been alleviated if HAMMOND'S recommendations had been followed. We had to wait for CADE (1949) to rediscover this effect, and in fact it was not until Mogens Schou started to investigate this problem thoroughly that lithium finally could be introduced as a psychotropic agent (see SCHOU 1983).

I am now coming to the 1950s, to the discovery of chlorpromazine. I will not go into details of the synthesis of the compound by CHARPENTIER, the important role of LABORIT in conceptualizing this new type of action and, finally, the actual observations by DELAY and DENIKER (see DENIKER 1983). We have to look upon this as a classic example of serendipity. But serendipity, of course, has to be followed by systematic inquiry and one of the first fundamental questions dealt with the medicinal chemistry of chlorpromazine and the structure–activity relations. For example, was the phenothiazine nucleus essential for this newly discovered effect? This was where PETERSEN came in, at a very early stage. He was then a young chemist employed by LUNDBECK and started to look into the matter. He and his collaborators, among them the pharmacologist IVAR MØLLER-NIELSEN, soon found out that the phenothiazine nucleus was not essential for the action. The nitrogen of this tricyclic nucleus can be replaced by a carbon atom provided that this is linked by means of a double bond to the carbon side chain. This in turn led to some interesting stereochemistry that was elegantly elucidated by PETERSEN and his colleagues and led to the introduction of a new series of important neuroleptic agents (see PETERSEN and MØLLER-NIELSEN 1964).

These discoveries, together with others such as the discovery of the butyrophenones by JANSSEN (see JANSSEN and TOLLENAERE 1983), considerably increased our understanding of the structure-activity relations and not only gave us a large number of valuable drugs, but also formed the basis for studying the mechanism of action of the neuroleptic drugs. With only the phenothiazines, it would have been much more difficult to investigate the problem of the mode of action of the drugs. PETERSEN and his colleagues were also able to demonstrate that the corresponding modification of the tricyclic nucleus of imipramine could be made without loss of therapeutic efficacy and this led to the discovery of amitriptyline, another significant achievement. All this was done in competition with the giants of the pharmaceutical industry, and it is remarkable and interesting to see how this team – including, in addition to PETERSEN and MØLLER-NIELSEN, JØRGEN RAVN, the clinician who started to investigate and to demonstrate the efficacy of the new neuroleptics and antidepressants – could compete so successfully and make such important contributions. This is basically thanks to PETERSEN's creativity. I think one can say that what LUNDBECK is today – a drug company with very high ethical and scientific standards – is largely the result of PETERSEN's remarkable creativity.

As mentioned, it was necessary to have a broad basis in terms of known chemical entities in order to go into the problem of mechanism and action of the recently discovered psychotropic drugs. An important breakthrough came from the work of BRODIE, SHORE, and their colleagues who demonstrated that reserpine is capable of depleting serotonin stores in the body tissues, including the brain (PLETSCHER et al. 1955). This was preceded by other important discoveries, e.g. that LSD is a remarkable hallucinogenic agent, that serotonin is a compound occurring naturally in the brain, and that serotonin receptors could be blocked by LSD, which in turn led to speculation about the role of serotonin in mental functions (for references, see CARLSSON 1987).

I had the privilege of working with BRODIE and his colleagues shortly after this discovery, and after returning home I thought it might also be worthwhile to look at the effect of reserpine on the catecholamines. BRODIE and his colleagues did not find this terribly exciting as they were convinced that serotonin was the compound to focus on at this time, this being the general feeling among the scientific community in the mid 1950s. After returning to Lund, HILLARP and I looked at this problem, and found that catecholamines are also depleted (CARLSSON and HILLARP 1956). Moreover, when we stimulated adrenergic nerves, they no longer responded (BERTLER et al. 1956; CARLSSON et al. 1957b), so it appeared more like a deficiency condition, which was not what BRODIE and his colleagues had in mind. They rather thought that this would be a release phenomenon so the reserpine syndrome could be due to continued release of serotonin onto the receptors. In any event, we felt it might be the other way round and that catecholamines also had to be taken into account. We treated animals with reserpine and then with dopa. The idea was that if the reserves of catecholamines were restored, then function might also be restored; indeed these animals, first made akinetic by reserpine, started to run around quite a lot and we were also very excited. We quickly published a paper in *Nature* (CARLSSON et al. 1957a) and then analysed the brains for catecholamines. The implication, of course, was that now we could refill the store of norepinephrine and that would restore the function. Much to our disappointment, despite this very striking effect of dopa, the brains of these rabbits were still depleted of noradrenaline. We were then forced to look into dopamine, which at that time was known as a not very interesting intermediate compound in the synthesis of noradrenaline; we found that dopamine also occurs in the brain, just as VOGT (1954) had found that noradrenaline and adrenaline do, and that reserpine also causes depletion of dopamine (CARLSSON et al. 1958).

When we looked at the effect of dopa and dopamine levels in the brain, we found that the behavioral effect of dopa was closely related to the accumulation of dopamine in the brain. We then found the peculiar distribution of dopamine, with high levels in the basal ganglia (BERTLER and ROSENGREN 1959; CARLSSON 1959), and that led to speculation about the role of dopamine not only in alertness, but also in extrapyramidal functions. That in turn led EHRINGER and HORNYKIEWICZ (1960) to investigate brains of parkinsonian patients. They discovered the depletion of dopamine in these brains and this formed the basis of the introduction of L-dopa by BIRKMAYER and HORNYKIEWICZ (1962) into the treatment of Parkinson's disease.

All this was very exciting and we felt that we had more than ample evidence to demonstrate that monoamines were indeed very important agonists in their own right in the brain and that presumably they worked as neurotransmitters; however, we were very disappointed in finding quite a lot of resistance to these ideas. Among other things, it was felt that they might not be neurotransmitters and might not be that important. I remember in particular a meeting on adrenergic mechanisms in London in 1960 when these critical views were expressed (VANE et al. 1960).

Therefore, when the amines could be visualized in the fluorescence microscope by means of histochemical fluorescence techniques, that was a very important discovery. I was privileged to be able to follow this development very closely. I had been working with HILLARP for a number of years, and when I moved to the chair of pharmacology in Gothenburg, I was delighted to hear that HILLARP would join me, bringing GEORG THIEME, his very clever engineer, with him. One of the projects we had in mind was to develop a method for visualization of monoamines in the fluorescence microscope. Some very clever model experiments, using formaldehyde, were done in our department of pharmacology in Gothenburg and finally, in collaboration with FALCK (a former student of HILLARP who was still in Lund), it became possible to visualize the monoamines (for review, see DAHLSTRÖM and CARLSSON 1986).

This achievement dramatically changed the attitude of the scientific community. There was no longer any need to argue that these compounds had a role as neurotransmitters. Rather, the discussions moved to the problem of whether one should consider these compounds in terms of neurotransmitters or neuromodulators. Of course, one can always argue about that. The various monoaminergic pathways were mapped out using this technique, and in addition the synaptology of the monoaminergic systems could be worked out.

We had a problem with the neuroleptics. We thought we could understand the action of reserpine resonably well in terms of catecholamines depletion, but how about the major neuroleptic drugs, chlorpromazine and the others? They did not cause depletion and, therefore, many felt that the effect of reserpine on the monoamines was actually some sort of epiphenomenon unrelated to its therapeutic actions. So we looked into this and found that chlorpromazine and haloperidol did in fact have a specific effect on the catecholamines, showing up as a stimulation of turnover as could be indicated by means of metabolites (CARLSSON and LINDQVIST 1963).

In view of the close similarity in pharmacological profile between reserpine and these neuroleptic agents, it became rather obvious what was going on here. These compounds were proposed as receptor blocking agents, and what we see here is the result of feedback control of the system. As a consequence of the blockade of the receptors, the activity of the catecholamine neurones is stimulated, leading to increased synthesis, release and metabolism. It took until the early 1970s for this concept to become generally accepted, even though it was rather quickly confirmed.

An important advance was the discovery that one can record the electrical activity from identified monoaminergic neurones, and thus it could be seen that apomorphine, which is a dopaminergic agonist, can silence dopaminergic neurones entirely, and that this can be blocked, for example, haloperidol and other dopamine-receptor antagonists (AGHAJANIAN and BUNNEY 1974, 1977). Biochemically, a similar antagonism in the area of the nerve terminals had already been found and could be shown not to be due to a feedback loop, but to be a local phenomenon (FARNEBO and HAMBERGER 1971; KEHR et al. 1972). These were the various observations that led to the autoreceptor concept. Apparently, autoreceptors occur both in the terminal area and in the somatodendritic region. The autoreceptor concept has opened up new strategies for selective manipulation of dopaminergic activity which are now being pursued.

A real challenge came when SEEMAN and LEE (1975) found that there was a significant correlation between the biological activity of a large number of neuroleptic compounds in terms of clinical dosage and blockade of dopamine release from striatal slices. In other words, according to these results the therapeutic action of these compounds appeared to be mediated by blocking the release of dopamine; this was exactly the opposite of what we had found, so we wondered very much how it could be explained.

Fortunately, shortly afterwards, SEEMAN and his colleagues (for review, see SEEMAN 1980) and SNYDER et al. (1976) independently published the same kind of results, but now showing something entirely different, namely a correlation between clinical potency and the ability of these compounds to combine with dopamine receptors and to displace a dopamine receptor ligand. The only difference between the earlier and the later results was that the concentrations necessary to induce the blockade of dopamine receptors were considerably lower.

Since then, not much attention has been paid to the earlier results, but they are still there, and I think they are interesting. I wonder about the mechanism of this opposite action, this blockade of release showing such a good correlation to clinical potency. What can it be? Perhaps it is related to the observation of BUNNEY and his colleagues (see CHIODO and BUNNEY 1984) that during treatment with neuroleptic drugs the increased firing of dopaminergic neurons, seen initially in animal experiments, is followed after several days by a so-called depolarization block. Whether the two phenomena are related remains to be proved, however.

It has become clear that there exist at least two dopamine receptors, D_1 and D_2, as originally proposed by KEBABIAN and CALNE (1979). The D_1 receptor is related to adenylcyclase. The D_2 is to some extent related to inhibition of the cyclase, but this is still unclear.

We also have to consider how complicated the situation is becoming. According to classical concepts, neuronal transfer of information is a one-way process. However, it has been found recently that release also occurs from the dendrites. These are in touch with other neurones, so the neurones "speak with two different tongues," and apparently the two release mechanisms are not always coordinated (see NISSBRANDT et al. 1985).

A recent beautiful demonstration of the mode of action of the neuroleptic drugs has been made in man, using the positron camera. Following injection of carbon-11-labelled raclopride or spiperone (D_2 antagonists) into a normal subject the dopamine-receptor ligand accumulates in the basal ganglia. One cannot detect any uptake of raclopride in the cerebral cortex, which I think is an interesting observation. Apparently, the density of D_2 receptors in human cortex is extremely low. In patients treated with different neuroleptic drugs much less accumulation of raclopride is detected, simply because the receptors are now occupied by the therapeutic agent (FARDE et al. 1987b). The receptors demonstrated in this way are presumed to be predominantly postsynaptic. It is also possible by means of positron emission tomography (PET) to demonstrate the D_1 receptors using a ligand that is relatively specific for D_1 receptors, namely SCH 23390 (FARDE et al. 1987a).

It would be nice to be able to demonstrate the autoreceptors (which, incidentally, are D_2 receptors) in a similar way, although this has not yet been possible. But in rat experiments the autoreceptors of the substantia nigra have been visualized by means of autoradiography, using radioactive sulpiride, which is a D_2 selective ligand. After degeneration of the nigral dopamine neurons on one side by means of local 6-hydroxydopamine treatment there is a marked decrease in the accumulation of sulpiride, indicating a loss of D_2 receptors on the side of the lesion (MORELLI et al. 1987). This is a final demonstration of dopamine D_2 autoreceptors. In future we hope to have selective compounds that can be used as ligands for autoreceptors.

A few words are needed about the much-debated dopamine hypothesis of schizophrenia. There is solid pharmacological evidence in favour of the role of dopamine in psychotic behaviour. The chemical pathology of schizophrenia has been for a long time and still is a controversial area. In post-mortem studies an increased density of D_2 receptors in schizophrenic brains has been found. The problem with these results is that there is divergence of opinion as to whether this increase is related to the disease as such, or induced by the drug treatment. PET data are now beginning to emerge. In one American study by WONG et al. (1986) an increased density of D_2 receptors was found in schizophrenic, drug-naive patients. However, FARDE et al. (1987c), using a somewhat different PET procedure, found no difference between schizophrenics and controls. These powerful new techniques are obviously at a very early stage. We must wait for the techniques to be further refined and for more data to come in from a larger number of centers before we can decide whether there is an increase in the D_2 density of schizophrenic brains that is disease-related rather than drug-related (even though a drug-related increase probably occurs as well).

Another interesting development in this area concerns the D_1 receptors. According to one American study (CREESE and HESS 1986), the D_1 receptors are reduced in density in schizophrenic brains analysed post-mortem. If this can be confirmed, it can hardly be a drug-induced effect because drugs, if anything, would have the opposite action. Paradoxically, at the same time there seems to be an increase in the function of this receptor in the sense that the agonist-induced activation of adenylcyclase is elevated in schizophrenic brains, so there is a reduction in density and an increase in function. In this context, we cannot tell for the time being if we are dealing with some sort of compensatory phenomenon.

There is, of course, a lot more to be said about developments in many different areas of psychopharmacology. The field has virtually exploded, leading to many ongoing fascinating extensions, for example into molecular biology. Obviously, psychopharmacology has a tremendous future.

References

Aghajanian GK, Bunney BS (1974) Pre- and postsynaptic feedback mechanisms in central dopaminergic neurons. In: Seeman P, Brown GM (eds) Frontiers of neurology and neuroscience research. University of Toronto Press, Toronto, pp 4–11

Aghajanian GK, Bunney BS (1977) Dopamine autoreceptors: pharmacological characterization by microiontophoretic single cell recording studies. Naunyn Schmiedebergs Arch Pharmacol 297:1–8

Bertler Å, Rosengren E (1959) Occurrence and distribution of dopamine in brain and other tissues. Experientia 15:10

Bertler Å, Carlsson A, Rosengren E (1956) Release by reserpine of catecholamines from rabbits' hearts. Naturwissenschaften 22:521

Birkmayer W, Hornykiewicz O (1962) Der 1-Dioxyphenylalanin (=L-DOPA)-Effekt beim Parkinson-Syndrom des Menschen: Zur Pathogenese und Behandlung der Parkinson-Akinese. Arch Psychiatr Nervenkr 203:560–574

Cade JFJ (1949) Lithium salts in the treatment of psychotic excitation. Med J Aust 36:349–352

Carlsson A (1959) The occurrence, distribution and physiological role of catecholamines in the nervous system. Pharmacol Rev 11:490–493

Carlsson A (1983) Antipsychotic agents: elucidation of their mode of action. In: Parnham MJ, Bruinvels J (eds) Psycho- and neuro-pharmacology. Elsevier, Amsterdam (Discoveries in pharmacology, vol 1), pp 197–206

Carlsson A (1987) Perspectives on the discovery of central monoaminergic neurotransmission. Annu Rev Neurosci 10:19–40

Carlsson A, Hillarp N-Å (1956) Release of adrenaline from the adrenal medulla of rabbits produced by reserpine. K Fysiogr Sällsk Förhandl 26(8)

Carlsson A, Lindqvist M (1963) Effect of chlorpromazine and haloperidol on the formation of 3-methoxytyramine and normetanephrine in mouse brain. Acta Pharmacol (Copenh) 20:140–144

Carlsson A, Lindqvist M, Magnusson T (1957a) 3,4-Dihydroxyphenylalanine and 5-hydroxytryptophan as reserpine antagonists. Nature 180:1200

Carlsson A, Rosengren E, Bertler Å, Nilsson J (1957b) Effect of reserpine on the metabolism of catecholamines. In: Garattini S, Ghetti V (eds) Psychotropic drugs. Elsevier, Amsterdam, pp 363–372

Carlsson A, Lindqvist M, Magnusson T, Waldeck B (1958) On the presence of 3-hydroxytyramine in brain. Science 127:471

Chiodo LA, Bunney BS (1984) Effects of dopamine antagonists on midbrain dopamine cell acticity. In: Usdin E, Carlsson A, Dahlström A, Engel J (eds) Catecholamines: neuropharmacology and central nervous system – theoretical aspects. Liss, New York, pp 369–391
Creese I, Hess EJ (1986) Biochemical characteristics of D1 dopamine receptors: relationship to behavior and schizophrenia. Clin Neuropharmacol [Suppl 4] 9:14–16
Dahlström A, Carlsson A (1986) Making visible the invisible. Recollections of the first experiences with the histochemical fluorescence method for visualization of tissue monoamines. In: Parnham MJ, Bruinvels J (eds) Chemical pharmacology and chemotherapy. Elsevier, Amsterdam, pp 97–125 (Discoveries in pharmacology, vol 3)
Deniker P (1983) Discovery of the clinical use of neuroleptics. In: Parnham MJ, Bruinvels J (eds) Psycho- and neuro-pharmacology. Elsevier, Amsterdam, pp 163–180 (Discoveries in pharmacology, vol 1)
Ehringer H, Hornykiewicz O (1960) Verteilung von Noradrenalin und Dopamin (3-Hydroxytyramin) im Gehirn des Menschen und ihr Verhalten bei Erkrankungen des extrapyramidalen Systems. Klin Wochenschr 38:1236–1239
Farde L, Halldin C, Stone-Elander S, Sedvall G (1987a) PET analysis of human dopamine receptor subtypes using ^{11}C-SCH 23390 and ^{11}C-raclopride. Psychopharmacology, (in press)
Farde L, Wiesel F-A, Halldin C, Sedvall G (1987b) Central D2 dopamine-receptor occupancy in schizophrenic patients treated with antipsychotic drugs. Arch Gen Psychiat, (in press)
Farde L, Wiesel F-A, Hall H, Halldin C, Stone-Elander S, Sedvall G (1987c) No D-2 receptor increase in PET study of schizophrenia. Arch Gen Psychiatry, 44:671–672
Farnebo L-O, Hamberger B (1971) Drug-induced changes in the release of ^{3}H-monoamines from field stimulated rat brain slices. Acta Physiol Scand [Suppl] 371:35–44
Freud S (1957) Letter to Maria Bonaparte, 15 January 1930. In: Jones E (ed) The life and work of Sigmund Freud, vol 3. Basic, New York, pp 449
Hammond WA (1871) A treatise on diseases of the nervous system. Appleton, New York, pp 381
Janssen PAJ, Tollenaere JP (1983) The discovery of the butyrophenone type neuroleptics. In: Parnham MJ, Bruinvels J (eds) Psycho- and neuro-pharmacology. Elsevier, Amsterdam, pp 163–180 (Discoveries in pharmacology, vol 1)
Kebabian JW, Calne DB (1979) Multiple receptors for dopamine. Nature 277:93–96
Kehr W, Carlsson A, Lindqvist M, Magnusson T, Atack C (1972) Evidence for a receptor-mediated feedback control of striatal tyrosine hydroxylase. J Pharm Pharmacol 24:744–747
Kraepelin E, (1892) Über die Einflussung einfacher psychischer Vorgänge durch einige Arzneimittel Fischer, Jena, S. 227
Moreau de Tours JJ (1845) Du hachisch et de l'aliénation mentale. Masson, Paris (Translation 1973: Hashish and mental illness. Raven, New York)
Morelli M, Carboni E, Devoto S, di Chiara G (1987) 6-Hydroxydopamine lesions reduce specific 3-H-sulpiride binding in the rat substantia nigra: direct evidence for the existence of nigral D-2 autoreceptors. Eur J Pharmacol, (in press)
Nissbrandt H, Pileblad E, Carlsson A (1985) Evidence for dopamine release and metabolism beyond the control of nerve impulses and dopamine receptors in rat substantia nigra. J Pharm Pharmacol 37:884–889
Petersen PV, Möller-Nielsen I (1964) Thiaxanthene derivatives. In: Gordon M (ed) Psychopharmacological agents, vol 1. Academic, New York, pp 301–324
Pletscher A, Shore PA, Brodie BB (1955) Serotonin release as a possible mechanism of reserpine action. Science 122:374–375
Schou M (1983) Lithium perspectives. Neuropsychobiology 10:7–12
Seeman P (1980) Brain dopamine receptors. Pharmacol Rev 32:229–313
Seeman P, Lee T (1975) Antipsychotic drugs: direct correlation between clinical potency and presynaptic action of dopamine neurones. Science 188:1217–1219
Sen G, Bose KC (1931) *Rauwolfia serpentina*, a new Indian drug for insanity and high blood pressure. Indian Med World 2:194–201
Snyder SH, Burt DR, Creese I (1976) The dopamine receptor of the mammalian brain: direct demonstration of binding to agonist and antagonist states. Science 192:481–483
Vane JR, Wolstenholme GEW, O'Connor M (eds) (1960) Ciba Foundation symposium on adrenergic mechanisms. Churchill, London

Vogt M (1954) The concentration of sympathin in different parts of the central nervous system under normal conditions and after the administration of drugs. J Physiol (Lond) 123:451–481

Wong DF, Wagner HN Jr, Tune LE, Dannals RF, Pearlson GD, Links JM, Tamminga CA, Broussolle EP, Ravert HT, Wilson AA, Thomas Toung JK, Malat J, Williams JA, O'Tuama LA, Snyder SH, Kuhar MJ, Gjedde A (1986) Positron emission tomography reveals elevated D2 dopamine receptors in drug-naive schizophrenics. Science 234:1558–1563

Receptor Interactions of Dopamine and Serotonin Antagonists: Binding In Vitro and In Vivo and Receptor Regulation

J. E. LEYSEN, W. GOMMEREN, P. F. M. JANSSEN, P. VAN GOMPEL, and P. A. J. JANSSEN

Abstract

The advent of receptor binding techniques has provided new ways of studying the mechanism of action of drugs. In vitro radioligand binding is now currently applied to investigate the specificity or multiple action of compounds. By using the same technique, the binding affinity of a drug can be measured for a variety of neurotransmitter, drug, peptide and ion channel receptor binding sites, providing the drug's receptor binding profile (LEYSEN et al. 1981; LEYSEN 1984). However, in vitro receptor binding is only the initial step in the investigation of drug-receptor interactions. Investigations in vivo are required to allow evaluation of how and where a drug acts. In fact, the study of drug-receptor interactions comprises three main stages: (a) in vitro radioligand receptor binding; (b) in vivo receptor binding, providing information on the accessibility of the drugs to the receptors localized in various central and peripheral tissues, on the drug potency for occupying various receptors, on the duration of receptor occupation and on the relationship between the degree of receptor occupation and pharmacological effects; and (c) the study of receptor regulation: the effect of chronic drug treatment on receptor alterations compared with alterations in functional responses in vivo.

In this article, we will illustrate the three stages of investigation of receptor interactions and discuss the relevance and importance of the findings, using as examples three drugs known in psychopharmacological research: (a) the neuroleptic haloperidol, a prototype of a dopamine D_2 antagonist: (b) Setoperone, a potential antipsychotic agent with very potent serotonin S_2 and moderate D_2 antagonistic activity (CEULEMANS et al. 1985; LEYSEN et al. 1986); and (c) ritanserin, a potent and long-acting S_2 antagonist (LEYSEN et al. 1985), which has revealed therapeutic activity in dysthymia and negative symptoms of schizophrenia (REYNTJENS et al. 1986; GELDERS et al. 1986). Particular attention will be paid to the problem of receptor regulation. We challenge the general applicability of the receptor regulation theory, which states that persistent receptor stimulation causes desensitisation and receptor downregulation, whereas chronic deprivation of receptor stimulation leads to supersensitivity and receptor upregulation. Recent research has revealed that the theory does not hold for S_2 receptor alterations, which were found to downregulate following chronic receptor blockade.

1 Drug-Receptor Interactions in Vitro

Various neurotransmitter receptors and neurotransmitter receptor subtypes have been identified in radioligand binding studies; models are presented in Table 1. For haloperidol, setoperone and ritanserin, the equilibrium inhibition constants (K_i value: the drug concentration producing 50% occupation of the receptor) for a series of neurotransmitter receptor site subtypes and the IC_{50} values for inhibition of neurotransmitter uptake in synaptosomes are reported. Less frequently investigated is the drug-receptor dissociation rate. The drug-receptor dissociation

Department of Biochemical pharmacology, Janssen Research Foundation, B-2340 Beerse, Belgium.

Table 1. Receptor binding properties (binding affinity, K_i in nM; half-time of drug-receptor dissociation, $t_{1/2}$ in min) and potencies for inhibition of neurotransmitter uptake in vitro (IC_{50} in nM)

		Mean values ± SD (n): a, K_i (nM); b, $t_{1/2}$ (min)		
		Haloperidol	Setoperone	Ritanserin
A. Receptor binding models				
D_2	*a*	1.2±0.3 (4)	20±4 (3)	22±3 (3)
[^{3}H]Haloperidol, striatum	*b*	5.6±1.4 (4)	4.8±0.04 (6)	11±3 (3)
D_1	*a*	185±24 (3)	2630±120 (2)	600±170 (3)
[^{3}H]SCH 23390, striatum	*b*	–	–	–
S_2	*a*	22±7 (3)	0.4±0.1 (3)	0.20±0.04 (4)
[^{3}H]Ketanserin, frontal cortex	*b*	6.6±0.8 (2)	6.8±0.7 (6)	160±20 (10)
S_{1A}	*a*	2680±430 (2)	2520±170 (3)	1800±540 (4)
[^{3}H]8-OHDPAT, hippocampus	*b*	–	–	–
α_1-Adrenergic	*a*	10±2 (3)	10±2 (3)	35±9 (4)
[^{3}H]WB4101, forebrain	*b*	3.3±3.0 (4)	4.3±0.6 (4)	18±1 (10)
α_2-Adrenergic	*a*	>10000	17±2 (3)	70±20 (3)
[^{3}H]Clonidine, cortex	*b*	–	4±1 (2)	26±3 (7)
β-Adrenergic	*a*	>10000	>10000	>10000
[^{3}H]Dihydroalprenolol, cortex	*b*	–	–	–
H_1[a]	*a*	1250 (2)	13±4 (4)	2.2±1.8 (4)
[^{3}H]Pyrilamine, cerebellum	*b*	–	5.1±0.3 (5)	77±4 (7)
Cholinergic muscarinic	*a*	2650±1150 (3)	>10000	>10000
[^{3}H]Dexetimide, striatal	*b*	–	–	–
μ-Opiate	*a*	980±160 (2)	>10000	2150 (1)
[^{3}H]Sufentanil, forebrain	*b*	–	–	–
Ca-channel sites	*a*	660±230 (3)	>10000	360±40 (3)
[^{3}H]Nitrendipine, cortex	*b*	–	–	–
B. Neurotransmitter uptake			IC_{50} (nM)	
[^{3}H]Noradrenaline, hypothalamus		815±260 (2)	6000±2800 (2)	540±310 (3)
[^{3}H]Serotonin, cortex		840± 70 (2)	2410± 250 (2)	650±210 (2)
[^{3}H]Dopamine, striatum		1560±210 (2)	9000±1500 (2)	240± 20 (2)
[^{3}H]GABA, cortex		>10000	>10000	2000

For methodology and references see Leysen and Gommeren (1986); Leysen (1987); Leysen and Janssen (1987).

[a] For H_1 receptor binding guinea pig cerebellum was used; for all other assays rat brain tissue was used.

rate used to be readily measurable for the radioactive ligands only. Recently, we developed a new technique for measuring the drug-receptor dissociation rate of unlabelled drugs (Leysen and Gommeren 1984, 1986). It was found that the drug-receptor dissociation rate varies considerably amongst drugs, and for a particular drug it may differ widely for various receptors. Knowledge of the drug-receptor dissociation rate appears to be essential for the interpretation of findings in receptor studies in vitro and in vivo, as well as in pharmacological and pharmacokinetic studies (Leysen and Gommeren 1984, 1986). The half-life of dissociation of haloperidol, setoperone and ritanserin from various receptors is also shown in Table 1. The primary activity of haloperidol is high-affinity binding to dopamine D_2 receptor sites; the drug binds with moderate affinity to α_1-adrenergic and serotonin S_2 receptor sites. The interaction with other listed receptor and neurotransmitter uptake sites is negligible compared with the high D_2 receptor binding affinity. Haloperidol dissociates rapidly from D_2, α_1-adrenergic and S_2 receptor sites. The binding of haloperidol to the receptor is readily reversible and hence of a competitive nature. The drug is not likely to persist at receptor sites following acute or chronic treatment. The duration of action of the drug in vivo is determined by the drug metabolism and elimination of the drug from the tissues (LEYSEN and GOMMEREN (1984). Both setoperone and ritanserin have as primary activity high-affinity binding to S_2 receptors. They have the same moderate binding affinity in vitro for D_2 receptor sites. Both drugs interact with α_1- and α_2-adrenergic receptor sites and with histamine H_1 receptor sites, setoperone being somewhat more potent than ritanserin at the adrenergic receptor sites, and ritanserin being more potent at the H_1 receptor sites. The most marked distinction between both drugs resides in the very slow dissociation of ritanserin, in particular from the S_2 receptor sites. The dissociation of ritanserin from H_1 and adrenergic receptor sites is also relatively slow, but the drug dissociates rapidly from the D_2 receptor. Setoperone dissociates rapidly from the various receptors. In contrast to setoperone, ritanserin is likely to persist for a prolonged time at S_2 receptors; its binding to these sites is of a noncompetitive nature (LEYSEN et al. 1985), and in functional tests the S_2 receptor blockade produced by ritanserin is insurmountable (DE CHAFFOY DE COURCELLES et al. 1986).

In this article, we report an extensive list of in vitro receptor binding and neurotransmitter uptake models. Although the drugs which are presently discussed only interact with a limited number of these sites, it is of interest to investigate drugs in the widest possible variety of biochemical tests in vitro. Because of the simplicity and uniformity of the technique in vitro, various assays can be readily performed; it can reveal properties of the drugs which are not directly apparent from the usual in vivo pharmacological studies. Binding studies in vitro have revealed the interaction of certain neuroleptics and antidepressants with α_2-adrenergic receptor sites. Besides the presently reported setoperone and ritanserin, piflutalixol, methitepine and mianserin were also found to bind potently to these sites. Neuroleptics of the diphenylbutylpiperidine class bind potently to the nitrendipine binding sites, which are associated with Ca^{2+} entry into cells. Chlorpromazine and chlorprothixene were found at nanomolar concentration to inhibit the uptake of noradrenaline in synaptosomes (see LEYSEN and JANSSEN 1987). These are not commonly known properties of these drugs, yet they may have importance for interpreting certain clinical or pharmacological observations. Otherwise, demonstration of the absence of a given activity may be helpful for ruling out certain hypotheses on drug action. For instance, it has recently appeared that akathisia caused by neuroleptics can be treated with the β-adrenergic receptor blocker propranolol (LIPINSKI et al. 1984). In a series of 31 clinically used neuroleptics belonging to six different chemical classes, none of the drugs showed binding to β-adrenergic receptors up to the highest concentration tested of 10^{-5} M (LEYSEN and JANSSEN 1987). This makes it unlikely that akathisia is produced by direct stimulation of β-adrenergic receptors by the neuroleptics. If β-adrenergic receptors are involved, it is more likely to be the consequence of an indirect effect, such as enhanced neurotransmitter turnover. Alternatively, the possibility must be considered that propranolol may have other properties besides blocking β-adrenergic receptors.

2 In Vivo Receptor Binding

2.1 Labelling of D_2 and S_2 Receptors In Vivo

Although the in vitro receptor binding profile of drugs gives indications of the possible primary and specific or multiple action of drugs, the possible activities need to be confirmed by in vivo tests. Functional tests are required for assessing agonistic or antagonistic action of drugs; this cannot be inferred from receptor binding studies. Nor is there any guarantee that all the receptors which can be occupied in vitro will be reached by the drug in vivo following systemic administration; moreover, the accessibility of the drug to the receptors in different tissues may differ. In order to study whether a drug can occupy receptors in vivo, we developed an in vivo receptor binding technique (LADURON et al. 1978; LEYSEN et al. 1987). In these studies, laboratory animals are treated systemically with the drug. After a certain time, a small dose of a highly labelled radioactive ligand (usually 5 µCi/animal, corresponding to 0.1–0.2 µg/kg) is given i.v. The animal is

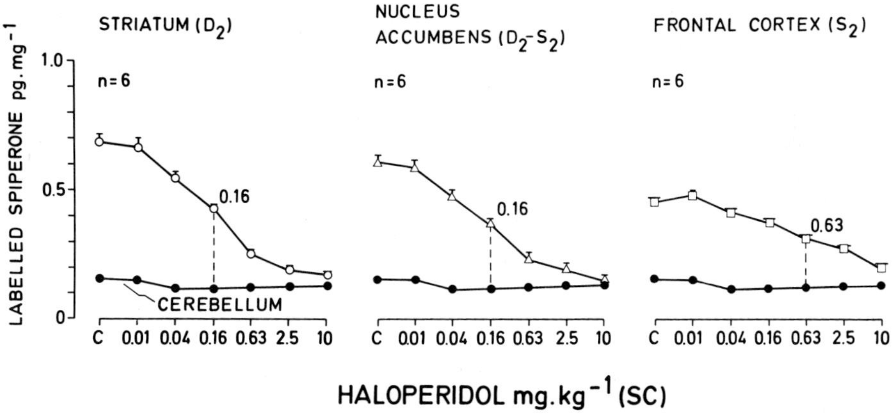

Fig. 1. Receptor binding in vivo. Labelling of D_2 receptors in the striatum, S_2 receptors in the frontal cortex and D_2 and S_2 receptors in the nucleus accumbens by [^{3}H]spiperone in control rats (*C*) and in rats treated with various doses of haloperidol. Labelling in the cerebellum represents nonspecifically retained radioactivity in the tissue. [^{3}H]Spiperone (5 µCi/kg, i.v.) was given 1 h after the haloperidol administration, and rats were killed 1 h later. Brain areas were rapidly dissected, weighed and dissolved in liquid scintillation cocktail. Radioactivity in the tissue was measured in a liquid scintillation counter equipped to calculate disintegrations per minute. The doses of haloperidol producing 50% inhibition of receptor labelling are indicated next to the *curves*

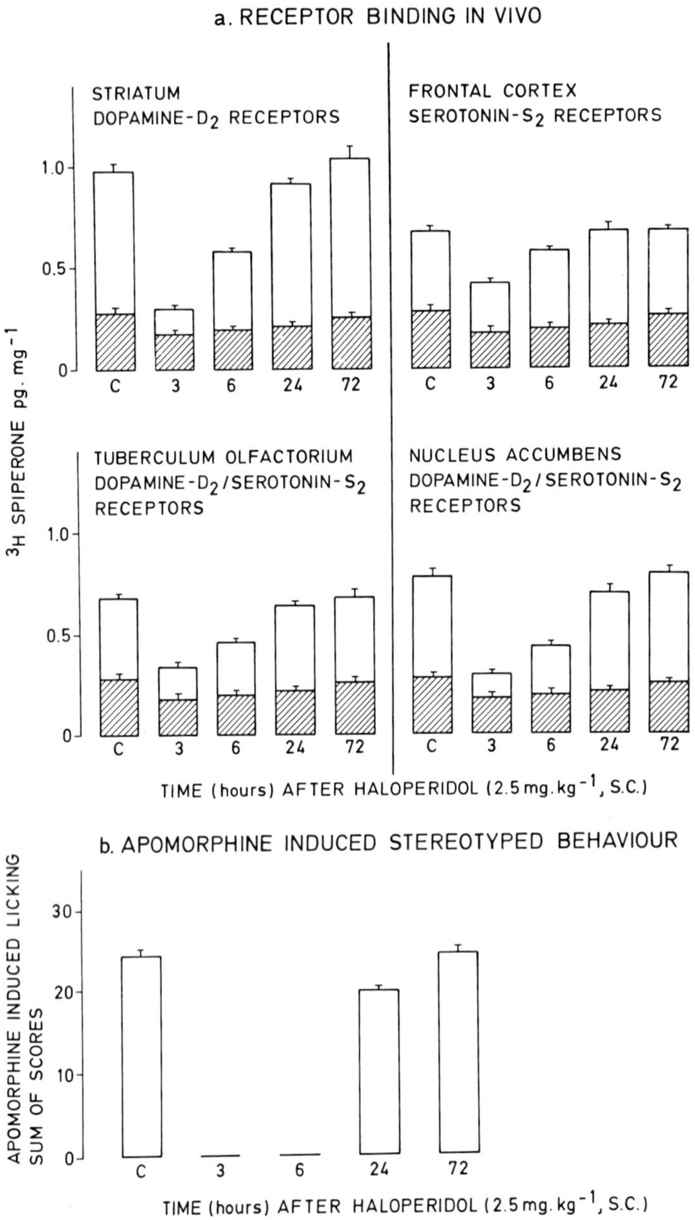

Fig. 2. a Receptor binding in vivo. Rats were treated with haloperidol (2.5 mg/kg, s.c.). At 2 h, 5 h, 23 h or 71 h after haloperidol, [^{3}H]spiperone was administered (5 µg/kg, i.v.); 1 h later, the rats were killed and radioactivity counted as described in the legend to Fig. 1. Mean values $\pm$SD, $n=6$. *Hatched parts* of the bars indicate labelling in the cerebellum, i.e. nonspecifically retained radioactivity. **b** Apomorphine-induced stereotyped behaviour. Rats were treated with haloperidol (2.5 mg/kg, s.c.). At 3 h, 6 h, 24 h or 72 h after haloperidol, apomorphine was administered (1.25 mg/kg, i.v.). Stereotyped behaviour (sniffing and licking) and agitation was scored (scale 0–3) every 5 min for 1 h (after 1 h, scores were 0 in all animals). The sum of scores of licking observed over 1 h is presented, mean values $\pm$SD, $n=5$. Similar findings were made for agitation

killed 1 h after the administration of the radioactive drug. Various tissues are dissected, and the tissues are dissolved in liquid scintillation cocktail. This is followed by estimation of the amount of radioactivity in the tissues.

[^{3}H]Spiperone was found to display the required properties for in vivo labelling of both D_2 receptors, which are particularly enriched in the striatum, and S_2 receptors, which are predominantly found in the frontal cortex (LEYSEN et al. 1978). It was found that systemically administered dopamine antagonists with central activity specifically and dose-dependently prevent the labelling by [^{3}H]spiperone of D_2 receptors in the striatum, whereas centrally acting serotonin antagonists selectively prevent the labelling of S_2 receptors in the frontal cortex. Hence, the technique provides a means of concomitantly evaluating the ability of drugs to occupy striatal D_2 and frontal cortical S_2 receptor sites. In Fig. 1, the prevention by haloperidol of the labelling in vivo of D_2 receptors in the striatum and of S_2 receptors in the frontal cortex is shown. From these curves, the ID_{50} values, i.e. the doses producing 50% inhibition of receptor labelling, are derived. The nucleus accumbens is known to contain approximately equal amounts of D_2 and S_2 receptors; however, using the low i.v. dose of [^{3}H]spiperone, the labelling of D_2 receptors appears to predominate in this brain area. This is probably due to the over tenfold higher affinity of [^{3}H]spiperone for D_2 than for S_2 receptors (K_D values in vitro: 0.07 nM and 1 nM respectively). Figure 1 reveals a similar ID_{50} value of 0.16 mg/kg for occupation by haloperidol of D_2 receptors in the striatum and the nucleus accumbens, and an ID_{50} of 0.63 mg/kg for occupation of S_2 receptors in the frontal cortex. This corresponds to a higher affinity of haloperidol for D_2 than for S_2 receptors, although the difference in potency for interacting with both receptors is smaller in vivo than in vitro.

Recently, CAMPBELL et al. (1985) reported prolonged inhibition (up to 30 days) of apomorphine-induced behavioural effects in rats following a single low dose of haloperidol. We could not confirm these findings either in the apomorphine behavioural test or in the duration of occupation in vivo of D_2 receptors in rat brain. Figure 2 shows that following a high dose of haloperidol (2.5 mg/kg s.c., i.e. 150 times higher than the lowest active pharmacological dose), D_2 and S_2 receptors are markedly occupied at 3 and 6 h. There is still a very slight occupation at 24 h, but at 72 h, occupation of the receptors is no longer observed. The time course of receptor occupation in vivo was found to be parallel to the time course of antagonism of apomorphine-induced behavioural effects. At 3 and 6 h after haloperidol, there was complete antagonism of apomorphine-induced effects. At 24 h after haloperidol, an inhibition by 15% of apomorphine-induced stereotyped behaviour and agitation was still observed, but 72 h after haloperidol, apomorphine-induced effects were at control levels.

2.2 Relationship Between Drug-Receptor Binding In Vitro and In Vivo and Pharmacological Responses

Table 2 shows for haloperidol, setoperone and ritanserin the potencies for in vitro and in vivo occupation of D_2 and S_2 receptors, and also the potencies of the drugs to antagonise apomorphine-induced stereotyped behaviour, a D_2 receptor-medi-

Table 2. Potencies of drugs for in vitro and in vivo occupation of D_2 and S_2 receptors and for antagonising apomorphine- and tryptamine-induced behaviour in rats

		Receptor binding				Behaviour: minimal ED_{50} [c]	
		In vitro [a] K_i (nM)		In vivo [b] ID_{50} (mg kg^{-1}) (s.c.)		(mg kg^{-1}) (s.c.)	
Haloperidol	D_2	1.2	Ratio 0.055	0.16	Ratio 0.25	0.016	Ratio 0.12
	S_2	22		0.63		0.13	
Setoperone	D_2	20	Ratio 50	0.4	Ratio 13	0.11	Ratio 6.9
	S_2	0.4		0.03		0.016	
Ritanserin	D_2	22	Ratio 110	>40	Ratio >500	>40	Ratio >400
	S_2	0.2		0.08		0.097	

[a] K_i values for receptor binding in vitro using [^{3}H]haloperidol and rat striatum for D_2 receptor and [^{3}H]ketanserin and rat frontal cortex for S_2 receptors.
[b] ID_{50} values for prevention of labelling in vivo by [^{3}H]spiperone of D_2 receptors in the striatum and of S_2 receptors in the frontal cortex, measured as described in the legend to Fig. 1.
[c] Minimal ED_{50} value for antagonism in rats of apomorphine-induced stereotypy (mediated by central D_2 receptors) and tryptamine-induced clonic seizures (mediated by central S_2 receptors). Minimal ED_{50} value: minimal dose producing a significant antagonistic effect in 50% of the animals at the time of peak effect (NIEMEGEERS, personal communication).

ated response, and to antagonise tryptamine-induced clonic seizures, a central S_2 receptor-mediated effect. The data in Table 2 illustrate the necessity of the evaluation of drug action and potency in vivo. For the S_2 receptors, there is a fair relationship between the drugs' receptor binding affinity in vitro and their potencies for receptor occupation and antagonism of the tryptamine-induced behavioural effects in vivo. For the D_2 receptor, it appears that haloperidol and setoperone can occupy the striatal D_2 receptors at low dose. The dose for antagonising apomorphine-induced behaviour is still ten and four times lower respectively than the dose for producing 50% receptor occupation. Hence, the pharmacological response appears to require only a low degree of receptor occupation. In vitro, setoperone is 17-fold less potent than haloperidol for binding to D_2 receptors, but in the in vivo tests, the potency difference is only 2.5-fold for the receptor occupation and 6.8-fold for antagonising the behavioural effect. This indicates that setoperone reaches the striatal D_2-receptors more easily than haloperidol. A big anomaly is observed for ritanserin. Ritanserin and setoperone revealed the same D_2 receptor binding affinity in vitro, but ritanserin fails to occupy the striatal D_2-receptors in vivo up to doses of 40 mg/kg. The same high dose did not antagonise apomorphine-induced behaviour. It appears that ritanserin cannot reach the striatal D_2 receptors in vivo, although the drug penetrates into the brain and at low dose occupies the S_2 receptors in the frontal cortex. In contrast to the common assumption, the penetration of a drug into the brain is not directly proportionate to its lipophilicity. For ritanserin, the apparent octanol-water partition coefficients, log P values at pH 7.4, and the percentage ionisation at pH 7.4 are 3.34 and 86.3%; for setoperone, 1.42 and 90.1%; and for haloperidol, 2.80 and 94.8%. Hence, setoperone is the least lipophilic, yet it penetrates most easily into the different brain areas. Moreover, drugs do not penetrate equally well into different brain areas or do not reach certain receptors in different brain areas equally well.

From our findings, we hypothesise that D_2 receptors in the striatum are probably localised at a greater distance from the blood capillaries than those in other brain areas, in such a way that more cell membrane barriers have to be crossed in order to reach these receptor sites. Optimal physicochemical properties – in terms of lipophilicity, ionisation and dipole moment – are required for membrane barrier penetration. Certain very lipophilic agents tend to stick to membranes and appear to be unable to cross several barriers. At the moment, we have insufficient knowledge of the parameters involved, and neither in vitro receptor binding data nor the structural and physicochemical properties of the drugs allow one to make predictions on the accessibility of receptors for drugs in various areas. Therefore, experimental verification is required.

2.3 Differences in Accessibility of Receptors for Drugs in Vivo: Implications for Drug Actions

The group of neuroleptics consists of several classes of compounds, which are heterogeneous in terms of chemical structure, physicochemical properties, biochemical and pharmacological profile (LEYSEN 1984; LEYSEN and NIEMEGEERS 1985). Except for the amine-depleting drugs, such as reserpine and tetrabenazine, the common property of all neuroleptics appears to be dopamine antagonism mediated through binding to D_2 receptors. Significant correlations have been found between the in vitro D_2 receptor binding affinity of drugs and the average clinical dose used in schizophrenic patients (SEEMAN 1980), on one hand, and the neuroleptic threshold dose assessed in the handwriting test described by HAASE (1978), on the other (VAN WIELINK and LEYSEN 1983). This indicates that both the therapeutic effect and the extrapyramidal side effect of the drugs are mediated by blockade of D_2 receptors.

Nevertheless, it has been amply reported and discussed that neuroleptics differ in their propensity to induce extrapyramidal side effects at therapeutically active doses. To explain these differences, several hypotheses have been put forward. Preferential action in mesolimbic areas has been claimed for the so-called atypical neuroleptics, such as sulpiride and clozapine. The existence of different subtypes of dopamine receptors has been suggested. Differences in the balance of occupation of D_2 and D_1 receptors have been proposed to play a role (SEEMAN 1980; SEEMAN and GRIGORIADIS 1987; STRANGE 1987). However, firm evidence for these hypotheses is lacking.

Based on our observations with in vivo receptor binding, we believe that differential accessibility of receptors in different brain areas and resulting differences in degree of receptor occupation produced by drugs may be an important, if not the predominant, factor. Since neuroleptics are a very heterogeneous group of compounds with regard to chemical structure and physicochemical properties, they are expected to have different abilities for reaching receptors in different brain areas. Weak dopamine antagonists or drugs which penetrate poorly into the brain or which reach the dopamine receptors in the basal ganglia with difficulty will probably elicit fewer extrapyramidal side effects. Indeed, such drugs are unlikely to produce readily a high degree of striatal D_2 receptor occupation, which probably accounts for many of the side effects. In contrast, D_2 receptors in mesolimbic or cortical brain areas, presumably related to the control of psychosis or agitation, may be reached more easily. One goal may be to aim for drugs with differential distribution in the brain; however, it seems likely that with a careful dosing of available drugs, therapeutic activity can be achieved with minimal risk of extrapyramidal symptoms.

Of course, differences between neuroleptics exist with regard to their profile for interaction with various neurotransmitter receptors; this will affect their action. A built-in anticholinergic muscarinic activity, a property of thioridazine, clozapine, chlorprothixene and chlorpromazine, can mask extrapyramidal symptoms but may concomitantly attenuate the antipsychotic activity. Drugs with antihistaminic and α-lytic properties are likely to be more sedative. Recently, beneficial effects have been claimed for S_2 receptor blockade: the S_2 antagonist, ritanserin, was reported to alleviate negative symptoms of schizophrenia and to attenuate certain extrapyramidal symptoms (REYNTJENS et al. 1986; GELDERS et al. 1986). However, the precise role of S_2 receptors in these observations remains to be elucidated.

3 Receptor Regulation Following Chronic Drug Treatment

3.1 The Receptor Regulation Theory and Anomalies in S_2 Receptor Regulation

The phenomenon of desensitisation of tissue responses following persistent agonist stimulation was observed in early pharmacological and physiological studies (KATZ and THESLEFF 1957). Subsequent behavioural and clinical studies, in particular of dopamine-mediated functions, revealed the development of supersensitivity to agonist stimulation following chronic receptor denervation, achieved either by neuronal lesions or by chronic receptor blockade by drugs (UNGERSTEDT 1971; TARSY and BALDESSARINI 1974). In radioligand receptor binding studies, it was found that chronic denervation of the dopaminergic system caused an increase in the number of D_2 receptor sites (CREESE et al. 1977; CREESE and SNYDER 1980). The increase in the number of D_2 receptor sites was thought to correlate with observed behavioural supersensitivity to dopamine agonists (FLEMINGER et al. 1983). All these observations eventually gave rise to the earlier-mentioned receptor regulation theory. In this article, we challenge the general applicability of that theory; in particular, S_2 receptors have been found to be differently regulated.

S_2 receptors, like β-adrenergic receptors, were reported to be downregulated in rat brain following chronic treatment with the antidepressant amitriptyline (PEROUTKA and SNYDER 1980). The findings were interpreted according to the receptor regulation theory: the downregulation was ascribed to enhanced receptor stimulation as a consequence of the inhibition of amine uptake by the drug. The 3 weeks' time required for the establishment of the effect has been related to the time course for the development of therapeutic activity with the antidepressants. Hence, it was hypothesised that supersensitive S_2 and β-adrenergic receptor sites may be involved in the etiology of depressive illnesses (PEROUTKA and SNYDER 1980; VETULANI et al. 1976). Following the original observations, S_2 and β-adrenergic receptor downregulation was observed with various purported antidepressant drugs, with different biochemical profiles (GANDOLFI et al. 1984; HALL et al. 1984; SNYDER and PEROUTKA 1982). However, the explanation of the mechanisms of S_2 receptor downregulation has been challenged by several findings. Chronic treatment with selective and potent serotonin uptake inhibitors, not belonging to the class of tricyclic antidepressants (zimelidine, alaproclate, citalopram), did not reduce S_2 receptor numbers. Lesioning or depletion of serotonergic neurones by themselves did not cause alterations in S_2 receptor binding (LEYSEN et al. 1983) and appeared not to abolish the S_2 receptor downregulation produced by tricyclic antidepressants (GANDOLFI et al. 1984; HALL et al. 1984; HYTTEL et al. 1984). Moreover, drugs known as potent serotonin antagonists, such as cyproheptadine, pizotifen, mianserin and ketanserin, also produced a decrease in S_2 receptor numbers (BLACKSHEAR et al. 1983; GANDOLFI et al. 1985). These observations indicated that the S_2 receptor regulation is not in accordance with the current theory.

3.2 Differences in Regulation of S_2, D_2, and α_1- and α_2-Adrenergic Receptors

We investigated alterations in neurotransmitter receptor binding sites and alterations in behavioural responses in rats following chronic treatment with ritanserin and setoperone. Treatment of rats with ritanserin, 10 mg/kg orally for 3 weeks, resulted in a downregulation of the S_2 receptors. The numbers of S_2 receptors in the frontal cortex remained significantly reduced for 8 days after stopping treatment. Cortical α_1-, α_2-, and β-adrenergic receptors, substance P and benzodiazepine receptors, and striatal D_2 receptors were not affected by the treatment. There were several indications that the observed reduction in S_2 receptor numbers was not due to persistence of the drug at the receptor sites; however, the interpretation of the findings following ritanserin treatment remained ambiguous because of the demonstrated slow dissociation of ritanserin from the S_2 receptors. Therefore, studies were performed using setoperone, which was shown to be readily washed off the receptors. Moreover, since binding studies in vivo had revealed occupation by setoperone of both S_2 and D_2 receptors in the brain, alterations in both receptors and changes in dopaminergic and serotoninergic behavioural responses could be concomitantly studied.

Figure 3 shows the time course of development and extinction of decreased behavioural responses to tryptamine along with a decrease in the number of frontal cortical S_2 receptor sites. Both were significantly reduced following 7 days' treatment, and following 21 days' treatment, the reduction in both parameters was

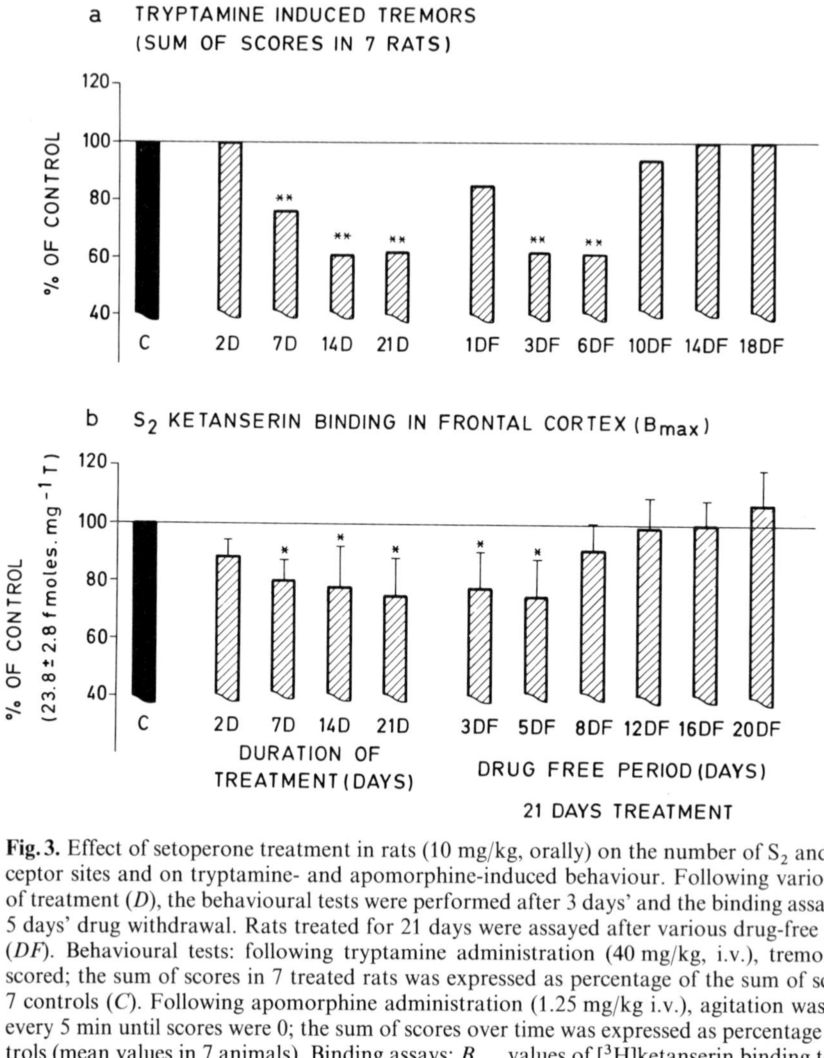

Fig. 3. Effect of setoperone treatment in rats (10 mg/kg, orally) on the number of S_2 and D_2 receptor sites and on tryptamine- and apomorphine-induced behaviour. Following various days of treatment (*D*), the behavioural tests were performed after 3 days' and the binding assays after 5 days' drug withdrawal. Rats treated for 21 days were assayed after various drug-free periods (*DF*). Behavioural tests: following tryptamine administration (40 mg/kg, i.v.), tremors were scored; the sum of scores in 7 treated rats was expressed as percentage of the sum of scores in 7 controls (*C*). Following apomorphine administration (1.25 mg/kg i.v.), agitation was scored every 5 min until scores were 0; the sum of scores over time was expressed as percentage of controls (mean values in 7 animals). Binding assays: B_{max} values of [^{3}H]ketanserin binding to S_2 receptors and of [^{3}H]spiperone binding to D_2 receptors were derived from Scatchard plots (LEYSEN et al. 1986; mean values $\pm$SD of 4 independent determinations). K_D values were similar in tissues from control and treated animals – [^{3}H]ketanserin, K_D = 0.38 n*M*; [^{3}H]spiperone, K_D = 0.041 n*M*. Significant difference from controls according to Student's *t* test: *$p < 0.05$; **$p < 0.01$, ***$p < 0.001$

slowly reversed over an 8- to 10-day drug-free period. The tryptamine-induced cyanosis was also abolished in rats chronically treated with setoperone, and the effect similarly persisted for 8 days after stopping treatment. This indicated that peripheral S_2 receptors in vessel walls were also desensitised. Whereas B_{max} values of [^{3}]ketanserin binding in frontal cortical tissue were significantly reduced, no changes in the binding affinity (K_D values) were observed. These observations pointed to a real, but transient, downregulation of S_2 receptors following chronic

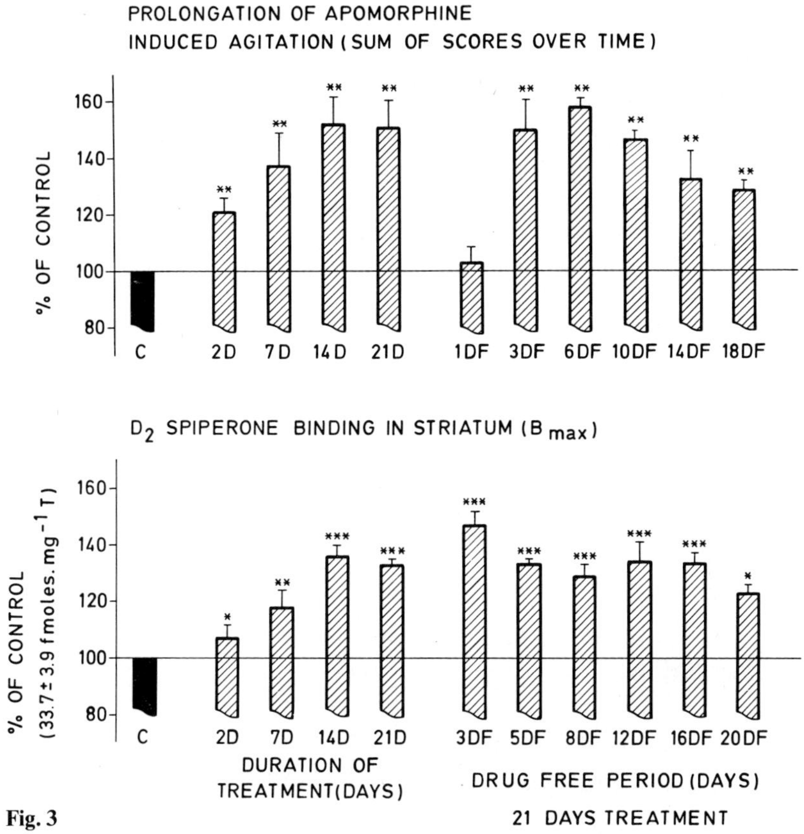

Fig. 3

receptor blockade, the effect being accompanied by a reduction in sensitivity to serotonin agonists.

It is unlikely that the S_2 receptor downregulation would be a consequence of a partial serotonin agonistic effect of the drugs. No agonistic effects of either ritanserin or setoperone were ever observed in functional studies of S_2-mediated effects in platelets (serotonin-induced aggregation and phospholipid turnover), in isolated vascular and tracheal tissue (serotonin-induced contraction) and in behavioural studies (discriminative stimulus).

The same groups of setoperone-treated animals were found to be supersensitive to apomorphine. This was measured as a significant prolongation of apomorphine-induced stereotyped behaviour and agitation. It was also seen in a significant response of the animals to a low dose of apomorphine (0.04 mg/kg), which was inactive in all control rats. The supersensitivity to apomorphine was accompanied by an increase in the number of striatal D_2 receptor sites, whereas there were no changes in binding affinity of [^{3}]-spiperone for these sites. The effects were already apparent after 2 days' treatment, and following 21 days' treatment, enhanced behavioural responses and elevated D_2-receptor sites persisted for a further 20 days (Fig. 3). Hence D_2 and S_2 receptors were regulated in opposite ways by treatment with setoperone.

Cortical tissues of the same rats were analysed for α_1- and α_2-adrenergic receptor binding. Only in two groups was a significant increase in the B_{max} value of [^{3}H]WB4101 binding to α_1-adrenergic receptors observed, i.e. in rats treated for 21 days, at 3 days after stopping treatment ($B_{max} \simeq 146 \pm 14\%$) and at 5 days after stopping treatment ($B_{max} \simeq 123 \pm 9\%$, $n = 4$). K_D values of [^{3}H]WB4101 binding remained unchanged. No significant changes were observed in the B_{max} or K_D values of [^{3}H]clonidine binding to α_2-adrenergic receptors. Hence, achievement of an increase in α_1-adrenergic receptors required longer treatment and was much more rapidly reversed than elevations in D_2 receptors. In vitro, setoperone shows a similar binding affinity for D_2 and α_2-adrenergic receptor sites. Because of the ready penetration of setoperone in various brain areas, it can be assumed that cortical α_2-adrenergic receptors become occupied by treatment with the drugs. It thus appears that α_2-adrenergic receptors are not prone to alterations following chronic receptor blockade. It can be concluded that treatment with setoperone, which in vivo blocks S_2, D_2, and α_1- and α_2-adrenergic receptors, revealed marked differences in the regulation of these receptors. Only one of these, the D_2 receptor, was clearly regulated according to the theory.

4 Conclusions

Our studies on in vitro and in vivo receptor interactions of haloperidol, ritanserin and setoperone and on receptor regulation have illustrated the following:

1. In vitro receptor binding profiles of drugs provide indications of possible selective versus multiple actions of drugs. Because of the relative simplicity of in vitro assays, they allow one to investigate properties which are not readily apparent from current pharmacological studies.
2. In vivo receptor binding is required to investigate the accessibility of receptors for the drugs in various tissues. Marked differences have been observed in the drugs' ability to reach D_2 receptors in the striatum. The accessibility of receptors for drugs in various brain regions appeared not to be predictable from the structural and physicochemical properties of the drugs. Variations in the ability of neuroleptics to reach D_2 receptors in different brain areas are probably important to explain or make distinctions in therapeutic and extrapyramidal effects. In vivo binding further allows one to relate degree of receptor occupation and pharmacological effects and to study the duration of receptor occupation in relation to that of pharmacological action.
3. The current theory on receptor regulation appears not to be generally applicable to all receptor systems. This has been revealed by a concomitant study of alterations in S_2, D_2, and α_1- and α_2-adrenergic receptors, along with alterations in functional effects in rats chronically treated with setoperone. In particular, the demonstrated downregulation of S_2 receptors following chronic receptor blockade is not in accordance with the theory. The differential regulation of S_2 receptors may have beneficial implications for the clinical applica-

tion of serotonin antagonists. Induction of adverse supersensitivity is not to be feared with these drugs. On the contrary, receptor downregulation may be part of the therapeutic action of the drugs in certain depressive disorders.

References

Blackshear MA, Friedman RL, Sanders-Bush E (1983) Acute and chronic effects of serotonin (5HT) antagonists on serotonin binding sites. Naunyn Schmiedebergs Arch Pharmacol 324:125–129

Campbell A, Baldessarini RJ, Teicher MH, Kula NS (1985) Prolonged antidopaminergic actions of single doses of butyrophenones in the rat. Psychopharmacology 87:161–166

Ceulemans DLS, Gelders YG, Hoppenbrouwers M-LJA, Reyntjens ASM, Janssen PAJ (1985) Effect of serotonin antagonism in schizophrenia: a pilot study with setoperone. Psychopharmacology 85:329–339

Creese I, Snyder SH (1980) Chronic neuroleptic treatment and dopamine receptor regulation. Adv Biochem Psychopharmacol 24:89–94

Creese I, Burt DR, Snyder SH (1977) Dopamine receptor binding enhancement accompanies lesion-induced behavioral supersensitivity. Science 197:596–598

De Chaffoy de Courcelles D, Leysen JE, Roevens P, van Belle H (1986) The serotonin-S_2 receptor: a receptor-transducer coupling model to explain insurmountable antagonist effects: Drug Dev Res 8:173–178

Fleminger S, Rupniak NMJ, Hall MD, Jenner P, Marsden CD (1983) Changes in apomorphine-induced stereotypy as a result of subacute neuroleptic treatment correlates with increased D-2 receptors, but not with increase in D-1 receptors. Biochem Pharmacol 32:2921–2927

Gandolfi O, Barbaccia ML, Costa E (1984) Comparison of iprindole, imipramine and mianserin action on brain serotonergic and beta adrenergic receptors. J Pharmacol Exp Ther 229:782–786

Gandolfi O, Barbaccia ML, Costa E (1985) Different effects of serotonin antagonists on ^{3}H-mianserin and ^{3}H-ketanserin recognition sites. Life Sci 36:713–721

Gelders Y, Vanden Bussche G, Reyntjens A, Janssen P (1986) Serotonin-S_2 receptor blockers in the treatment of chronic schizophrenia. Clin Neuropharmacol [Suppl 4] 9:325–327

Haase HJ (1978) The purely neuroleptic effects and its relation to the "neuroleptic threshold". Acta Psychiatr Belg 78:19–36

Hall H, Ross SB, Sällemark M (1984) Effect of destruction of central noradrenergic and serotonergic nerve terminals by systemic neurotoxins on the long-term effects of antidepressants on β-adrenoceptors and 5-HT_2 binding sites in the rat cerebral cortex. J Neural Transm 59:9–23

Hyttel J, Fredericson Overø K, Arnt J (1984) Biochemical effects and drug levels in rats after long-term treatment with the specific 5-HT-uptake inhibitor, citalopram. Psychopharmacology 83:20–27

Katz B, Thesleff S (1957) A study of the "desensitization" produced by acetylcholine at the motor end plate. J Physiol (Lond) 138:63–80

Laduron PM, Janssen PFM, Leysen JE (1978) Spiperone: a ligand of choice for neuroleptic receptors. 2. Regional distribution and in vivo displacement of neuroleptic drugs. Biochem Pharmacol 27:317–321

Leysen JE (1984) Receptors for neuroleptic drugs. In: Burrows GD, Werry JS (eds) Advances in human psychopharmacology 3. Jai, London, pp 315–356

Leysen JE (1987) The use of 5-HT receptor agonists and antagonists for the characterization of their respective receptor sites. In: Boulton AA, Blake GB, Juorio AV (eds) Drugs as tools in neurotransmitter research. Humana, Clifton (Neuromethods, neuropharmacology, vol 2) (in press)

Leysen JE, Gommeren W (1984) The dissociation rate of unlabelled dopamine antagonists and agonists from the dopamine-D_2 receptor, application of an original filter method. J Recept Res 4:817–845

Leysen JE, Gommeren W (1986) Drug-receptor dissociation time, new tool for drug research: receptor binding affinity and drug-receptor dissociation profiles of serotonin-S_2, dopamine-D_2, histamine-H_1 antagonists, and opiates. Drug Dev Res 8:119–131

Leysen JE, Janssen PAJ (1987) Specificity of ligands used in psychiatric research. In: Sen AK, Lee T (eds) Receptors and ligands in psychiatry and neurology, vol 1. Cambridge University Press, Cambridge (in press)

Leysen JE, Niemegeers CJE (1985) Neuroleptics. In: Lajtha A (ed) Handbook of neurochemistry. Plenum, New York, pp 331–361

Leysen JE, Niemegeers CJE, Tollenaere JP, Laduron PM (1978) Serotonergic component of neuroleptic receptors. Nature 272:168–171

Leysen JE, Awouters F, Kennis L, Laduron PM, Vandenberk J, Janssen PAJ (1981) Receptor binding profile of R 41 468, a novel antagonist at 5-HT_2 receptors. Life Sci 28:1015–1022

Leysen JE, Van Gompel P, Verwimp M, Niemegeers CJE (1983) Role and localization of serotonin$_2$ (S_2)-receptor-binding sites: effects of neuronal lesions. In: Mandel P, DeFeudis FV (eds) CNS receptors – From molecular pharmacology to behavior. Raven, New Yor, pp 373–383

Leysen JE, Gommeren W, Van Gompel P, Wynants J, Janssen PFM, Laduron PM (1985) Receptor-binding properties in vitro and in vivo of ritanserin. A very potent and long-acting serotonin-S_2 antagonist. Mol Pharmacol 27:600–611

Leysen JE, Van Gompel P, Gommeren W, Woestenborghs R, Janssen PAJ (1986) Down regulation of serotonin-S_2 receptor sites in rat brain by chronic treatment with the serotonin-S_2 antagonists: ritanserin and setoperone. Psychopharmacology 88:434–444

Leysen JE, Van Gompel P, Gommeren W, Laduron PM (1987) Differential regulation of dopamine-D_2 and serotonin-S_2 receptors by chronic treatment with the serotonin-S_2 antagonists, ritanserin, and setoperone. In: Dahl SG, Gram LF, Paul SM, Potter WZ (eds) Clinical pharmacology in psychiatry. Springer, Berlin Heidelberg New York, pp 214–224 (Psychopharmacology series, vol 3)

Lipinski JF, Zubenko GS, Cohen BM, Barreira PJ (1984) Propranolol in the treatment of neuroleptic induced akathisia. Am J Psychiatry 141:412–415

Peroutka SJ, Snyder SH (1980) Regulation of serotonin$_2$ (5-HT_2) receptors labeled with [^{3}H]spiroperidol by chronic treatment with the antidepressant amitriptyline. J Pharmacol Exp Ther 215:582–587

Reyntjens A, Gelder YG, Hoppenbrouwers M-LJA, Vanden Bussche G (1986) Thymosthenic effects of ritanserin (R 55 667), a centrally acting serotonin-S_2 receptor blocker. Drug Dev Res 8:205–211

Seeman P (1980) Brain dopamine receptors. Pharmacol Rev 32:229–313

Seeman P, Grigoriadis D (1987) Dopamine receptors in brain and periphery. Neurochem Int 10:1–25

Snyder SH, Peroutka SJ (1982) A possible role of serotonin receptors in antidepressant drug action. Pharmacopsychiatry 15:131–134

Strange PG (1987) Dopamine receptors in the brain and periphery: "state of the art". Neurochem Int 10:27–33

Tarsy D, Baldessarini RJ (1974) Behavioural supersensitivity to apomorphine following chronic treatment with drugs which interfere with the synaptic function of catecholamines. Neuropharmacology 13:927–940

Ungerstedt U (1971) Postsynaptic supersensitivity after 6-hydroxydopamine induced degeneration of the nigro-striatal dopamine system in the rat brain. Acta Physiol Scand [Suppl 367] 82:69–93

Van Wielink PS, Leysen JE (1983) Farmacologische keuzecriteria voor neuroleptica. Tijdschr Geneesmiddelenonderz 8:1984–1997

Vetulani J, Starwarz RJ, Dingell JV, Sulser F (1976) A possible common mechanism of action of antidepressant treatments. Arch Pharmacol 239:109^{1}14

PET Scanning – A New Tool in Clinical Psychopharmacology

G. SEDVALL [1], L. FARDE [1], H. HALL [2], S. PAULI [1], A. PERSSON [1], and F. A. WIESEL [1]

Abstract

Quantitative methods were developed for the determination of dopamine and benzodiazepine receptor characteristics in the living human brain by positron emission tomography (PET). As ligands, the ^{11}C-labelled analogues of the selective antagonists of dopamine receptor subtypes, SCH 23390 and raclopride, and the benzodiazepine antagonist, Ro 15-1788, were used. Tracer amounts of the ligands were injected intravenously into healthy volunteers and schizophrenic patients. The distribution of ligand indicated high densities of D_1 as well as D_2 dopamine receptors in the basal ganglia. Binding of [^{11}C]-SCH 23390 was also significant in the neocortex where it was shown to represent binding to D_1 as well as to 5-HT_2 serotonin receptors. High densities of specific benzodiazepine receptor binding were obtained in most neocortical brain areas and in the cerebellum.

Using saturation procedures, B_{max} and K_d values could be obtained for D_2 and benzodiazepine receptors. A comparison of D_2 receptor densities in drug-naive schizophrenic patients and healthy volunteers demonstrated similar receptor characteristics in the major basal ganglia in these groups of subjects. Different chemical classes of conventional and unconventional antipsychotic drugs produced a 65%–85% occupancy of D_2 receptors when given in clinical doses to schizophrenic patients. High doses of diazepam produced a marked occupancy of benzodiazepine receptors during the first hours after oral administration to healthy volunteers.

These in vivo methods should be valuable tools for the further analysis of the effects of drug on neuroreceptors in the living brain of neuropsychiatric patients.

1 Introduction

Most psychopharmacological agents have been shown to induce their effects by interfering with specific neurotransmitter receptors in the central nervous system. This holds true for antipsychotic, anxiolytic, and analgesic drugs of the opiate type. Until recently little has been known concerning the quantitative aspects of the receptor interference required for inducing various psychological effects in human subjects. Developments in the field of positron emission tomography (PET) have now offered a possibility of studying the effects of these types of drugs on neuroreceptor binding directly in the living brain of human subjects.

[1] Department of Psychiatry and Psychology, Karolinska Institute, S-10401 Stockholm, Sweden.

[2] Astra Alab AB, S-12585 Södertälje, Sweden.

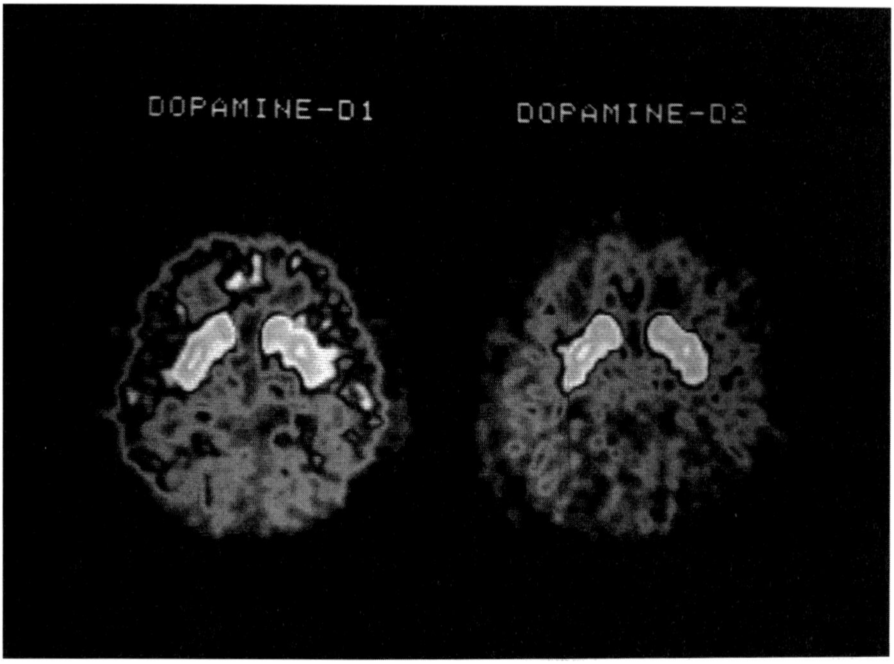

Fig. 1. PET images showing the distribution of radioactivity in a section through the brain of a healthy man after intravenous injection of [^{11}C]-SCH 23390 (*left*) and [^{11}C]-raclopride (*right*). Note marked accumulation of radioactivity in the basal ganglia from both ligands indicating high densities of D_1 as well as D_2 receptors in these brain regions. Note also the difference in accumulation of radioactivity in the neocortex where [^{11}C]-SCH 23390 shows a significant accumulation resulting from binding to D_1 as well as to 5-HT_2 receptors

Such achievements were accomplished by the combined use of PET and in vivo ligand binding to receptors. In PET, ^{11}C-labelled ligands with high affinity to neuroreceptors are administered intravenously and the accumulation of the radioactive ligand in sections of the living human brain can be measured. The positron camera records the gamma-radiation produced upon the disintegration of ^{11}C-labelled atoms. This is a highly sensitive technique which, because of the short half-life of the ^{11}C-atom (20.3 min), results in an acceptable dose of radiation absorbed in experiments with human subjects. By the use of selective ligands for various neuroreceptor systems and mathematical models describing the ligand receptor binding, data concerning the relative distribution of receptors in different brain areas, as well as their characteristics with regard to density and affinity, can be determined (WAGNER et al. 1983; FARDE et al. 1985; WONG ET AL. 1986; SEDVALL et al. 1986). This report will describe some recent developments in this field and their significance for the further development of clinical psychopharmacology.

2 Selective Ligands for PET Analysis of Dopamine Receptor Subtypes

SCH 23390 and raclopride are selective ligands for D_1 and D_2 dopamine receptor subtypes respectively. These compounds were labelled with ^{11}C and administered to healthy human subjects. As illustrated in Fig. 1, both of these ligands accumulated markedly in the dopamine receptor-rich basal ganglia of healthy human subjects (FARDE et al. 1987a). Using the biologically inactive enantiomers of the ligands it could be demonstrated that the binding of the (−)enantiomers was stereoselective (FARDE et al. 1987d; L. FARDE, C. HALLDIN, and G. SEDVALL, unpublished data). Binding of [^{11}C]-SCH 23390 differed from that of raclopride with regard to accumulation of radioactivity in the neocortex; [^{11}C]-SCH 23390 accumulated significantly more there than in the rest of the cortices. Subsequent biochemical studies using the ^3H-labelled ligands and post-mortem brain tissue indicated that the cortical binding of SCH 23390 is due both to D_1 and 5-HT_2 receptor binding (HALL et al. 1987). Thus, a significant amount of the total binding of [^3H]-SCH 23390 could be blocked by low ketanserine concentrations. These results demonstrate the high densities of D_1 as well as D_2 receptors in the human basal ganglia. They also demonstrated the lower but significant density of D_1 receptors in the human neocortex. [^3H]-raclopride binding indicated that the density of D_2 receptors in the human neocortex is very low or nonexistent.

3 Demonstration of D_2 Receptor Occupancy in Schizophrenic Patients Treated with Antipsychotic Drugs

When [^{11}C]-SCH 23390 and [^{11}C]-raclopride were injected in tracer doses into schizophrenic patients who had been treated with conventional doses of chemically different types of antipsychotic drugs, interesting results were obtained. Thus, antipsychotic drugs such as sulpiride and flupentixol did not interfere significantly with [^{11}C]-SCH 23390 binding. After flupentixol treatment there was possibly a small diminution of the binding in the basal ganglia of the D_1 receptor ligand. However, all chemically different classes of antipsychotic drugs, including conventional as well as unconventional antipsychotics, produced a substantial (65%–84%) blockade of [^{11}C]-raclopride binding (FARDE et al. 1987c). Calculation of the reduction of receptor binding in relation to the binding obtained in untreated schizophrenic patients indicated that such a marked blockade occupancy of D_2 receptors is induced by all the antipsychotic drugs. This is in contrast to the antidepressant nortriptyline which did not significantly interfere with [^{11}C]-raclopride binding (Table 1). These results demonstrate, for the first time, a significant effect of clinical doses of psychotherapeutic agents on specific biochemical systems in the living human brain. This methodology will be useful for a further analysis of the detailed relationships between D_2 receptor occupancy and various psychological effects of antipsychotic drugs in human subjects.

Table 1. D_2 receptor occupancy in patients treated with psychoactive drugs

	Dose (mg)	Receptor occupancy (%)
Phenothiazines		
chlorpromazine	100 b. i. d.	80
thioridazine	100 t. i. d.	75
perphenazine	4 b. i. d.	79
Thioxanthenes		
flupentixol	5 b. i. d.	74
Butyrophenones		
haloperidol	4 b. i. d.	84
Diphenylbutyls		
pimozide	4 b. i. d.	77
Debenzodiazepines		
clozapine	300 b. i. d.	65
Substituted benzamides		
sulpiride	400 b. i. d.	82
Tricyclic antidepressants		
nortriptyline	25 b. i. d.	− 3

Receptor occupany was defined as the percentage reduction of specific [^{11}C]-raclopride binding in relation to the expected binding in the absence of drug treatment.

4 Determination of D_2 Receptor Characteristics in Drug-Naive Schizophrenic Patients

Using a saturation procedure, D_2 receptor characteristics such as the B_{max} and K_d values could be determined in healthy human subjects and drug-naive schizophrenic patients using [^{11}C]-raclopride (FARDE et al. 1986, 1987b). The studies demonstrated similar densities and affinities of D_2 receptors in the major basal ganglia of the drug-naive schizophrenic patients and in the healthy controls. These results do not support the concept of a general alteration of D_2 receptor characteristics in the pathophysiology of schizophrenia. Patients previously treated with high doses of antipsychotic drugs were shown to have relatively high receptor densities immediately after withdrawal of the treatment (L. FARDE, G. SEDVALL, and F.-A. WIESEL, unpublished data). These high densities may be the result of receptor induction after long-term antipsychotic drug treatment as has previously been demonstrated in animals.

5 Determination of Benzodiazepine Receptor Characteristics in Healthy Human Subjects

Using the selective benzodiazepine antagonist Ro 15-1788 labelled with ^{11}C the distribution of benzodiazepine receptor binding in vivo could be determined in the brain of healthy human volunteers (PERSSON et al. 1985). After intravenous injection of [^{11}C]-Ro 15-1788, a marked accumulation of radioactivity was observed in all the major cortices. About 90% of this binding could be blocked to by prior injection of high doses of unlabelled Ro 15-1788, indicating the specificity of the binding to benzodiazepine receptors. Using a saturation assay, in vivo B_{max} and K_d values of benzodiazepine receptors could also be determined in the major cortices in living human subjects (A. PERSSON, S. PAULI, C. HALLDIN, and G. SEDVALL, unpublished data).

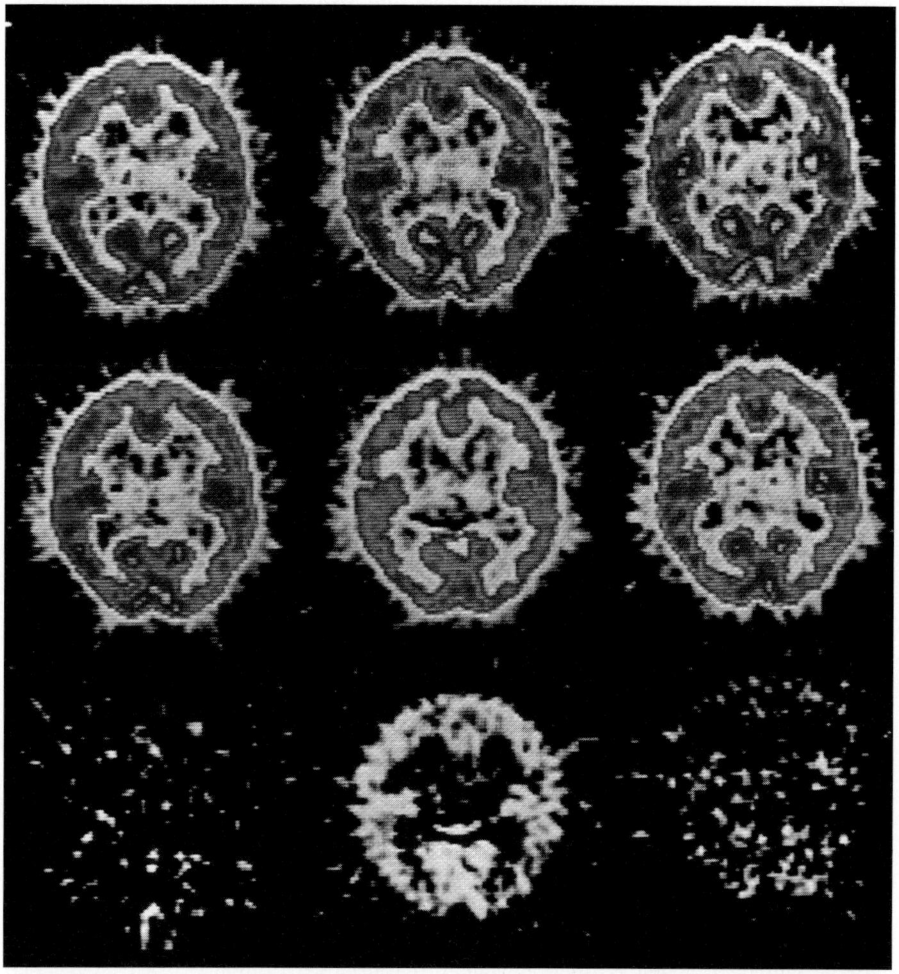

Fig. 2. PET images showing the distribution of radioactivity in a section through the brain of a healthy man after repeated intravenous injections of a tracer dose of the benzodiazepine antagonist [^{11}C]-Ro 15-788. *Upper panel* shows distribution of radioactivity before, and 2 h and 24 h after administration of a placebo tablet. *Middle panel* shows distribution of radioactivity before, and 2 h and 24 h after oral administration of 30 mg diazepam. *Lower panel* shows benzodiazepine receptor occupancy (radioactivity in middle panel subtracted from radioactivity in upper panel), before, and 2 and 24 h after oral administration of 30 mg diazepam. The results demonstrate that 2 h after diazepam administration benzodiazepine receptors are about 50% occupied. Only a faint trace of receptor occupancy remains 24 h after the benzodiazepine administration

6 Determination of Central Benzodiazepine Receptor Occupancy in Benzodiazepine-Treated Healthy Volunteers

In order to determine the degree of benzodiazepine receptor occupancy during conventional benzodiazepine treatment, healthy human volunteers were injected with [^{11}C]-Ro 15-1788 before, and at various time points after, oral administration of diazepam. As shown in Fig. 2 there was a marked blockade of [^{11}C]-Ro 5-1788 binding in the brain during the first few hours after oral administration of 30 mg diazepam. Twenty-four hours after the diazepam administration, when concentrations of diazepam and its major metabolite, desmethyl diazepam, were still high, there was just a minimal indication of remaining effects on the cerebral benzodiazepine receptors (S. PAULI, A. PERSSON, and G. SEDVALL, unpublished data). This first demonstration of an effect of conventional benzodiazepine treatment on biochemical receptor functions in the living human brain will allow a further analysis of the relationships between benzodiazepine receptor interaction and the various psychological effects of diazepam in living human subjects.

7 Conclusions

The data briefly reviewed in this report demonstrate the possibility of studying specifically and quantitatively some aspects of neuroreceptor function in the brain of living human subjects. For dopamine and benzodiazepine receptor systems, data can be obtained allowing the quantitative characterization of receptor functions of patients with neuropsychiatric disorders. The methods also allow a quantitative analysis of the effects of drugs on such receptor systems in the brain of living human subjects. PET will accordingly be useful for a detailed analysis of the relationships between in vivo receptor occupancy and neuropsychological effects induced by new and previously available psychopharmacological agents.

Acknowledgments. This study was supported by grants from the Swedish Medical Research Council (03560), the Bank of Sweden Tercentenary Fund and the National Institute of Mental Health (MH 41205-1).

References

Farde L, Ehrin E, Eriksson L, Greitz T, Hall H, Hedström C-G, Litton J-E, Sedvall G (1985) Substituted benzamides as ligands for visualization of dopamine receptor binding in the human brain by positron emission tomography. Proc Natl Acad Sci USA 82:3863–3867

Farde L, Hall H, Ehrin E, Sedvall G (1986) Quantitative analysis of D2 dopamine receptor binding in the living human brain by PET. Science 231:258–261

Farde L, Halldin C, Stone-Elander S, Sedvall G (1987a) PET analysis of human dopamine receptor subtypes using ^{11}C-SCH 23390 and ^{11}C-raclopride. Psychopharmacology (in press)

Farde L, Wiesel F-A, Hall H, Halldin C, Stone-Elander S, Sedvall G (1987b) PET determination of striatal D2-dopamine receptors in drug-naive schizophrenic patients. Arch Gen Psychiatry 192:278–284, 1987

Farde L, Wiesel F-A, Hall H, Halldin C, Sedvall G (1987c) Central D2-dopamine receptor occupancy in schizophrenic patients treated with antipsychotic drugs. Arch Gen Psychiatry 145:71–76, 1988

Farde L, Pauli S, Hall H, Stone-Elander S, Eriksson L, Halldin C, Högberg T, Nilsson L, Sjögren I (1987d) Stereoselective binding of ^{11}C-FLB 472 – a search for extrastriatal central D2-dopamine receptors by PET. Psychopharmacology (in press 1988)

Hall H, Farde L, Sedvall G (1987) Human dopamine receptor subtypes – in vitro binding analysis using ^{3}H-SCH 23390 and ^{3}H-raclopride. J Neural Transm (in press)

Persson A, Ehrin E, Eriksson L, Farde L, Hedström C-G, Litton J-E, Mindus P, Sedvall G (1985) Imaging of ^{11}C-labelled Ro 15-1788 binding to benzodiazepine receptors in the human brain by positron emission tomography. J Psychiatr Res 19:609–622

Sedvall G, Farde L, Persson A, Wiesel F-A (1986) Imaging of neurotransmitter receptors in the living human brain. Arch Gen Psychiatry 43:995–1005

Wagner HN, Burn HD, Dannals RF, Wong DF, Långström B, Duelfer T, Frost JJ, Ravert HT, Links JM, Rosenbloom SV, Lukas SE, Kramer AV, Kuhar MJ (1983) Imaging dopamine receptors in the human brain by positron tomography. Science 221:1261–1266

Wong DF, Gjedde A, Wagner HN (1986) Quantification of neuroreceptors in the living human brain. I. Irreversible binding of ligands. J Cereb Blood Flow Metab 6:147–153

Pharmacokinetics of Neuroleptic Drugs and the Utility of Plasma Level Monitoring

S. G. DAHL

Abstract

Variability in response to antipsychotic drug treatment may be caused by variable patient compliance, interactions with other drugs, pharmacokinetic variations and variations in concentration–response relationships at the receptor level. Pharmacokinetic variations may in some cases be compensated by individual dosage adjustments based on plasma drug level measurements. The interpatient variability in response to a certain time-course of drug concentrations at the receptor site could hitherto only be assessed by clinical judgement. New methods for in vivo assessment of receptor occupancy hold promise for possible measurement of parameters accounting for at least part of the interindividual variation in drug response at the receptor level.

Monitoring of fluphenazine, perphenazine, thiothixene and sulpiride plasma levels by specific chemical assay methods seems to offer some guidance to individualization of drug doses. Definite therapeutic plasma level ranges have not been established for chlorpromazine and haloperidol. However, monitoring plasma levels of chlorpromazine or haloperidol might be of value when drug-induced toxicity is suspected, and as a means of controlling patient compliance.

1 Pharmacokinetics of Neuroleptic Drugs in Man

Many pharmacokinetic studies of neuroleptics have demonstrated substantial patient-to-patient variation in the ratio of steady-state plasma level to daily dose, as illustrated in Fig. 1. The reason for such variation, which generally is largest after oral administration, resides in the pharmacokinetics of the drugs which will be briefly reviewed in this article. References not given here may be found in previous reviews by DAHL (1981, 1986) and by JØRGENSEN (1986).

As indicated in Table 1, the dibenzoxazepine loxapine and the butyrophenones, phenothiazines and thioxanthenes have similar pharmacokinetic properties, which are distinctively different from those of the benzamides and diphenylbutyl-piperidines.

1.1 Butyrophenones, Dibenzoxazepines, Phenothiazines and Thioxanthenes

In most cases the plasma concentrations of drugs from these classes reach a peak 2–3 h after oral administration and 0.5–1 h after conventional intramuscular administration. The rate of absorption from intramuscular depot preparations is slower, and may depend on the ester form.

Department of Pharmacology, Institute of Medical Biology, University of Tromsø, P.O. Box 977, N-9001 Tromsø, Norway.

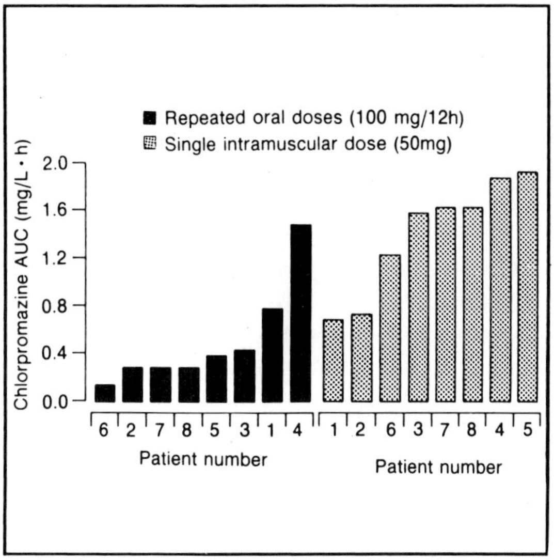

Fig. 1. Interpatient variation in area under the curve (*AUC*) of plasma concentration of chlorpromazine versus time after oral and intramuscular administration in the same patients. (From DAHL and STRANDJORD 1977)

Table 1. Pharmacokinetic parameters of neuroleptic drugs; normal ranges of observed values are given

Drug class	Butyrophenones, dibenzoxazepines[a] phenothiazines, thioxanthenes	Benzamides	Diphenylbutyl-piperidines
Systemic availability of oral doses (%)	10–70	80–100[b]	
Apparent volume of distribution (l/kg)	10–40	1–5	
Main pathway of elimination	Hepatic metabolism, renal excretion of metabolites	Renal excretion of unchanged drug	Hepatic metabolism, renal excretion of metabolites
Biological half-life (h)	10–30 h	3–10 h	50–200[c]
Time to reach steady-state plasma levels after oral doses	2–5 days	12–40 h	1–4 weeks

From DAHL (1981, 1986) and JØRGENSEN (1986).
[a] Data for loxapine only.
[b] Bioavailability of sulpiride may be more variable and depending on tablet formulation.
[c] Half-life of 3 weeks has been reported for intramuscular fluspirilene.

Plasma fluphenazine concentration peaks of up to 4 ng/ml, in some cases coinciding with extrapyramidal or autonomic side effects, have been observed during the first 24 h after intramuscular injections of fluphenazine decanoate (CHANG et al. 1985). In the same study the plasma levels then remained stable at around 1 ng/ml for the next 14 days. The enanthate seems to produce a more constant rate of release of fluphenazine than does the decanoate, and peak plasma levels of fluphenazine have been observed 2–7 days after intramuscular injection of fluphenazine enanthate (ALTAMURA et al. 1985; CHANG et al. 1985).

On the other hand, perphenazine decanoate has been demonstrated to produce smaller fluctuations in plasma drug levels than perphenazine enanthate (BOLVIG HANSEN and LARSEN 1983). Another study demonstrated that intramuscular injections of zuclopenthixol acetate in Viscoleo produced peak plasma drug levels 24–36 h later (AMDISEN et al. 1986).

Most drugs belonging to these four classes have apparent volumes of distribution in the range 10–40 l/kg, and the plasma levels after therapeutic doses are in the nanomolar range. It appears that distribution equilibrium between plasma and the rest of the body is not attained until 8–12 h after administration of single doses of chlorpromazine (MAXWELL et al. 1972; DAHL and STRANDJORD 1977; LOO et al. 1980), levomepromazine (DAHL 1976) and trifluoperazine (MIDHA et al. 1983). Haloperidol seems to be distributed in the body faster than the phenothiazines, reaching a distribution equilibrium 4–6 h after administration (CRESSMAN et al. 1974; FORSMAN and ÖHMAN 1976; HOLLEY et al. 1983; CHENG et al. 1987).

Hepatic metabolism and renal excretion of metabolites is the main pathway of elimination of these neuroleptics, and in many cases up to 20–30 different metabolites are formed. The elimination half-lives of the drugs are usually between 10 and 30 h, and steady-state plasma concentrations are reached after 2–5 days of treatment. These values represent the usual range of variation, and elimination half-lives as long as 80 h have been observed in single individuals (DAHL et al. 1977).

It is well known that clinical effects of neuroleptics may persist for weeks and months after termination of drug therapy, and it has been suggested, based on clinical observations and measurements of plasma haloperidol levels in one individual, using a new and extremely sensitive assay technique for plasma haloperidol, that the usual elimination phase with a half-life of 10–30 h may be followed by a slower elimination phase with ultra-low plasma drug concentrations (HUBBARD et al. 1987).

Steady-state plasma levels of neuroleptics may be reached more rapidly by giving larger loading doses initially, a practice which, according to COFFMAN et al. (1987), has gained acceptance among psychiatrists. Clinical studies have shown, however, that the loading dose strategy does not induce a faster reduction of psychotic symptoms, and offers little more than an increase in the frequency and severity of side effects (CLARK et al. 1970; ERICKSEN et al. 1976; COFFMAN et al. 1987).

1.2 Diphenylbutyl-piperidines

The pharmacokinetic properties of the diphenylbutyl-piperidines are mainly determined by their high lipid solubilities compared to those of other neuroleptics. Absorption after oral administration is slow and peak drug concentrations in plasma occur after about 6 h. These drugs are extensively distributed to the tissues, and a slow release from deep tissue compartments delays their elimination, which occurs mainly via hepatic metabolism and excretion of metabolites. The elimination half-lives in man are in the range 50–200 h.

1.3 Benzamides

The benzamides (sulpiride, sultopride, tiapride) are relatively hydrophilic compounds that are mainly excreted unchanged in the urine, with elimination half-lives usually in the range 3–10 h. Half-lives as long as 14–15 h have been observed for sulpiride in single patients showing normal renal function (BRESSOLLE et al. 1984).

The low lipid solubilities of the benzamides compared to those of the classical neuroleptics are reflected in their relatively small apparent volumes of distribution, which are in the range 1–5 l/kg as shown in Table 1 (WIESEL et al. 1980; BRESSOLLE et al. 1984). In spite of their relatively small apparent volumes of distribution, the average steady-state plasma concentrations of benzamides are only slightly higher than those of the phenothiazines, when both are given in similar daily doses. The reason for this small difference in plasma levels is the shorter elimination half-lives of the benzamides.

2 Pharmacodynamic and Pharmacokinetic Variance in Neuroleptic Drug Treatment

A major problem in antipsychotic drug treatment is variation in therapeutic response between different patients. This may be due to erratic patient compliance, interactions with other drugs, pharmacokinetic variations and variations in concentration–response relationships at the receptor level. Interpatient variability both in the pharmacokinetics and in the concentration–response relationships of a drug may be caused by disease, diet, physical exercise and advanced age, and may depend on genetic factors.

Up to now, inherent variations in concentration–response relationships at the receptor level could only be compensated for by dosage adjustment after clinical evaluation. New methods for in vivo assessment of receptor occupancy using positron emission tomography and other techniques hold promise for measurement of parameters describing part of the interindividual variations in drug effects at the receptor level (SEDVALL et al. 1986).

Substantial interpatient variations in the ratio of plasma level to daily dose have been observed for loxapine, in many but not all studies reported for haloperidol, and for the phenothiazines. Significantly smaller interindividual variations in plasma level: dose ratios have been observed after intramuscular than after oral administration of chlorpromazine, haloperidol, levomepromazine and perphenazine, which indicates that variation in presystemic metabolism may be important after oral intake (Dahl 1986).

It is possible that the observed variation in plasma levels of neuroleptics in many cases has been partly due to variability in the assay method. On the other hand, Van Putten et al. (1985) suggested that the lack of correlation between daily doses and plasma levels of haloperidol reported by others was due mainly to erratic patient compliance.

Compared to the variation between patients, the steady-state plasma levels of neuroleptics usually remain fairly stable in each individual as long as the daily dose of neuroleptic and of any concomitant drugs remain unchanged. As discussed earlier (Dahl 1986), this has been reported from many pharmacokinetic studies. A similar pattern of variation was recently found in a group of hospitalized patients who received a fixed intramuscular dose of zuclopentixol decanoate for 6 months or longer (Szukalski et al. 1986).

A relatively high correlation between plasma level and dose has been reported after oral administration of penfluridol (Cooper et al. 1975). It appears that oral administration of diphenylbutyl-piperidines may produce less interindividual variation in plasma drug levels relative to daily dose than has been observed with all other neuroleptics except the benzamides (Jørgensen 1986).

Fairly high correlations between steady-state plasma levels and daily doses have been reported for benzamides (Bressolle et al. 1984; Roos et al. 1986; Wiesel et al. 1980). In one study, the steady-state serum levels of sulpiride varied 4-fold in 25 patients treated with sulpiride 800 mg/day, while the steady-state serum levels of chlorpromazine varied 20-fold in 25 other patients receiving chlorpromazine 400 mg/day (Alfredsson et al. 1984).

3 Plasma Drug Level Monitoring

One of the main prerequisites for meaningful plasma drug level monitoring is that sufficiently well defined therapeutic and toxic plasma level ranges be established in clinical studies with appropriate experimental design and methodology. In such studies with neuroleptics there should be:

- Well-defined patient group
- Washout period 1 week or longer
- Fixed drug doses – randomly allocated
- Observation period of 2 weeks or longer
- Reliable rating method
- No concomitant neuroleptics
- Blood sampling before drug intake
- Specific and accurate assay method
- Data on single patients reported

As discussed recently by VAN PUTTEN and MARDER (1986), studies of plasma levels and therapeutic response to neuroleptic drugs are of limited value if the drug doses are determined individually by clinical judgement. However, most studies of plasma level–response relationships with neuroleptics reported in the literature have not applied a fixed-dose schedule. Measuring plasma levels of a neuroleptic for which no therapeutic or toxic plasma level range has been established on a firm scientific basis is likely to produce more harm than benefit.

3.1 Therapeutic and Toxic Plasma Level Ranges

As discussed in previous reviews (DAHL 1986; DAHL and HALS 1987), studies of plasma concentration–therapeutic effect relationships have been reported for chlorpromazine, fluphenazine, haloperidol, perphenazine, sulpiride, thioridazine and thiothixene. These studies used specific chemical assay methods, randomly allocated, fixed drug doses, and no co-administration of other neuroleptics. The following conclusions, summarized in Table 2, were drawn from these studies:

- Responders and non-responders to treatment with chlorpromazine have plasma drug levels within the same ranges after 4 weeks of treatment. However, most patients who respond well to chlorpromazine treatment have plasma drug levels of 30–100 ng/ml, and there seems to be no advantage in obtaining plasma chlorpromazine levels above 100 ng/ml.
- A therapeutic plasma level "window" for fluphenazine between 0.5 and 2.5 ng/ml has been proposed.
- No definite therapeutic and toxic plasma level ranges have been established for haloperidol. However, plasma haloperidol levels above 20–30 ng/ml seem to offer no therapeutic advantage, and are probably related to an increased risk of drug toxicity.
- Optimal therapeutic response to perphenazine treatment, and a low risk of extrapyramidal side effects, may be obtained by maintaining plasma perphenazine levels between 0.8 and 2.4 ng/ml.

Table 2. Suggested therapeutic and toxic plasma levels of neuroleptics. (From DAHL and HALS 1987)

Compound	Suggested range (ng/ml)[a]	
	Therapeutic	Toxic
Chlorpromazine	30–100[b]	>100–150
Fluphenazine	0.2–2.0	> 2.0
Haloperidol	5–20[b]	> 20–30
Perphenazine	> 0.8	> 2.4
Thiothixene	2–15	> 15
Sulpiride	<500	

[a] Measured 8–12 h after oral dose.
[b] Some studies found no plasma level-effect relationship.

- Response of "negative" symptoms in schizophrenia to treatment with sulpiride seems to be associated with plasma drug levels below 500 ng/ml.
- A therapeutic plasma level window between 2 and 15 ng/ml has been suggested for thiothixene.
- No therapeutic plasma level range has been established for thioridazine.

Several studies which have reported statistically significant relationships between haloperidol plasma levels and therapeutic response have been criticized, and there has been a lively debate in the literature concerning the clinical relevance of such findings (VAN PUTTEN et al. 1985; SMITH 1985; KIRCH et al. 1985; VAN PUTTEN and MARDER 1986; MILLER and HERSHEY 1986).

From the individual data presented in the original studies with haloperidol it seems obvious that statistical significance in fitting experimental data to some mathematical equation does not in itself demonstrate a clinically relevant relationship between drug concentration and response. From all the data that have been published it must still be concluded that a therapeutic window for haloperidol has not been so well defined that it may provide a general basis for a plasma drug level monitoring programme. Similar conclusions were reached in a flexible-dose study where haloperidol plasma levels were measured with the neuroleptic radioreceptor assay in 22 patients (ZOHAR et al. 1986), and in a recent review by VOLAVKA AND COOPER (1987). After having adjusted haloperidol doses to a lower threshold level for therapeutic response in 33 acutely psychotic patients, MCEVOY et al. (1986) found that individual plasma haloperidol levels ranged from 1.0 to 12.2 ng/ml, with a mean of 4.9 ng/ml.

A flexible-dose study with 28 patients who received five consecutive intramuscular depot injections of fluphenazine at 2-week intervals, reported significantly higher plasma fluphenazine levels in responders to the treatment than in non-responders (RIMÓN et al. 1986). In this study the blood samples were collected 12 h after administration of the neuroleptic, and the responders had plasma fluphenazine levels in the range 2–4 ng/ml, while the non-responders had plasma levels in the range 0.8–1.8 ng/ml. These ranges are slightly higher than the ranges observed in previous studies with oral fluphenazine (Table 2), which may be due to differences in experimental design (flexible- versus fixed-dose schedules), and the fact that the blood samples were collected when blood levels were increasing, 12 h after the injections, in the study by RIMÓN et al. (1986).

3.1.1 Additional Requirements for Monitoring of Neuroleptic Plasma Levels

In addition to the existence of sufficiently well defined therapeutic and toxic plasma drug level ranges, other criteria must be fulfilled for meaningful monitoring of neuroleptic plasma levels. The low therapeutic plasma concentrations of most neuroleptics require extremely sensitive assays, and a specific and reproducible assay method is a prerequisite.

A certain concentration–response relationship of a neuroleptic in an individual will be changed if other neuroleptics are given at the same time. In addition to pharmacodynamic interactions affecting concentration–response relationships at the receptor level, the concentrations of neuroleptic drugs may also be affected by pharmacokinetic drug interactions. Plasma levels of neuroleptics may be influenced by other drugs, among them certain anticholinergics (ALTAMURA et al. 1986), beta-blockers (SILVER et al. 1986) and antiepileptics (JANN et al. 1985; KIDRON et al. 1985; ERESHEFSKY et al. 1986).

It is obvious, therefore, that plasma concentrations of a neuroleptic, measured by gas-liquid chromatography (GLC), high-performance liquid chromatography (HPLC) or other chemical methods, cannot provide any meaningful guidelines for individualizing drug doses in patients who are treated with more than one neuroleptic. Interpretation of plasma levels of neuroleptics may be extremely difficult if other drugs are given at the same time, and in both cases it is doubtful whether monitoring of neuroleptic plasma levels offers any real benefit.

Plasma concentrations of neuroleptics may fluctuate substantially during the dose interval, and specimens for therapeutic monitoring should be collected prior to administration of the next dose, when the plasma drug levels are most stable. Meaningful results cannot be obtained if the blood samples are taken at random during the day.

3.1.2 Active Metabolites and the Radioreceptor Assay

Some of the neuroleptic drug metabolites which have been found in plasma from psychiatric patients also have antidopaminergic activity in vivo (MOREL et al. 1987). Although some neuroleptics have many different metabolites, only a small number of these may be expected to be clinically active (DAHL 1982). Nevertheless, it may be expected that the contribution from metabolites to the effects of neuroleptics may be different from patient to patient, due to pharmacokinetic variations (DAHL 1982; HITZEMANN et al. 1986; LEWIS 1986).

The neuroleptic radioreceptor assay, which is based on binding to dopamine D_2 receptors and measures the total activity of drugs and metabolites in the sample, has been used in a number of studies of the relationship between neuroleptic serum level and therapeutic response. A recent survey of such studies which had been reported in the literature up to 1985, concluded that the radioreceptor assay seems to offer little advantage over chemical assay methods in therapeutic plasma level monitoring (DAHL and HALS 1987). The reason for this may be that the dopamine receptor-blocking activity in plasma is not directly correlated with the neuroleptic drug-induced dopamine receptor-blocking activity in the brain, since different neuroleptics and neuroleptic drugs metabolites may have different plasma–brain distribution properties.

SZUKALSKI et al. (1986) reported that 15 chronic schizophrenic patients who responded favourably to intramuscular injections of 200 mg zuclopentixol decanoate every third week, had significantly higher pre-injection neuroleptic serum levels than 11 non-responding patients. HITZEMANN et al. (1986) measured plasma neuroleptic activity by radioreceptor assay and plasma fluphenazine levels by GLC in a fixed-dose study where 15 schizophrenic patients were treated witih oral fluphenazine for 2 weeks. On average, only about half of the neuroleptic activity in plasma could be accounted for by the fluphenazine levels measured by GLC, and some patients had up to 5 times higher neuroleptic serum activity than could be accounted for by fluphenazine alone.

3.2 Concentration-Dependent Effect on Negative Symptoms

The schizophrenic syndrome has been divided into two subgroups of symptoms, classified as negative and positive (ANDREASEN 1982; ANDREASEN and GROVE 1986), and it has been proposed that schizophrenia where negative symptoms are present may be characterized by a stronger genetic component than schizophrenia with predominantly positive symptoms (DWORKIN and LENZENWEGER 1984). A recent study indicated that sleep EEG patterns may provide a possible marker for negative symptoms (GANGULI et al. 1987), and others have pointed out that negative symptoms in schizophrenia may be difficult to distinguish from drug-induced parkinsonism (PROSSER et al. 1987).

Many neuroleptics are not as effective in treating anhedonia, affective flattening and other negative symptoms as in treating hallucinations, delusions and other positive symptoms, and only a few neuroleptics have been demonstrated to have a therapeutic effect on negative symptoms (LECRUBIER 1986; MELTZER 1987). These drugs, which also have effects on positive symptoms, include sulpiride, clozapine, pipothiazine and some diphenylbutyl-piperidines.

ALFREDSSON et al. (1984, 1985) found a relationship between serum levels of sulpiride and recovery from autistic and depressive schizophrenic symptoms, and a favourable treatment response associated with drug levels below 500 ng/ml. GERLACH et al. (1985) reported from a cross-over study that sulpiride had an antipsychotic effect and a therapeutic profile not significantly different from that of haloperidol. It is possible that the apparent similarity of the clinical profiles of haloperidol and sulpiride observed in the latter study was related to the relatively high sulpiride doses that were given, since 12 out of 13 patients had plasma sulpiride concentrations above 500 ng/ml after 9–12 weeks of treatment. Other studies have indicated that negative symptoms of schizophrenia respond favourably to doses of neuroleptics 4–5 times lower than those required for treating positive symptoms (LECRUBIER 1986).

Pharmacokinetic variations resulting in different plasma drug levels after similar doses might easily disguise a possible concentration-dependent relationship such as the effect of a neuroleptic upon negative and positive symptoms. The 3- to 5-fold range of interpatient variation in plasma levels relative to daily dose which has been observed for benzamides and diphenylbutyl-piperidines may seem less important than the range of variation observed with phenothiazines and other "classical" neuroleptics. Nevertheless, the sulpiride data discussed above indicate that it would be an advantage to include plasma level measurements in studies of the effects of neuroleptics – and benzamides – upon negative symptoms in schizophrenia, in order to control the variation of pharmacokinetic factors.

4 Future Trends in Psychopharmacology – Towards "Molecular Pharmacokinetics"?

Recent years have brought a rapid development to, and an increased interest in the field of molecular biology. Basic studies of the molecular structures of biological macromolecules and of small molecules which may act as drugs, neurotransmitters or hormones have provided new understanding of the molecular mechanisms of macromolecule-ligand interactions resulting in biological effects.

Molecular modelling using semi-empirical calculations ("molecular mechanics") and modern computer graphics have provided new powerful tools for studies of molecular structures of drugs and biological macromolecules, and mechanisms of drug–receptor interactions at the molecular level (WEBER et al. 1986). Such calculations are usually based on solid-state molecular structures determined by X-ray crystallography and require a powerful computer.

Many studies of structure–activity relationships have been done in the search for an active conformation or "pharmacophore pattern" common on the neuroleptic drugs. However, the molecular conformational requirements for the therapeutic action of neuroleptics are still not completely known. Molecular modelling studies (S. G. DAHL, P. A. KOLLMAN, S. N. RAO and U. C. SINGH, unpublished results) confirmed our hypothesis, derived from crystal structures, that psychoactive phenothiazines have molecular conformations different from those of their inactive metabolites (DAHL et al. 1986).

These studies have revealed new aspects of drug–receptor interactions which are clearly fundamental for understanding the basic processes involved at the molecular level. It is possible that the insight gained by these new methods may help to explain the mode of action of neuroleptics at the molecular level, and to design new drugs with more specific effects upon the schizophrenic syndrome. Up to now, neuroleptics have usually been classified by their chemical group, clinical profile, pharmacokinetic properties, and profile in animal behavioural tests and in receptor binding assays. It is possible that in the future new insights into their mode of action at the molecular level will make it feasible to classify neuroleptics according to their molecular structure and dynamics.

So far, almost all studies of molecular structures of neuroleptics have focused mainly upon drug–receptor interactions. However, the first three-dimensional structure of a cytochrome P-450, crystallized in a camphor complex, has recently been determined by X-ray crystallography (POULOS et al. 1985). This may represent a starting point for future studies of molecular mechanisms of drug metabolism and genetic polymorphism, as well as of other processes involved in drug disposition in the body, and perhaps signals the development of "molecular pharmacokinetics" as a new subdiscipline.

References

Alfredsson G, Härnryd C, Wiesel F-A (1984) Effects of sulpiride and chlorpromazine on depressive symptoms in schizophrenic patients – relationship to drug concentrations. Psychopharmacology 84:237–241

Alfredsson G, Härnryd C, Wiesel F-A (1985) Effects of sulpiride and chlorpromazine on autistic and positive psychotic symptoms in schizophrenic patients – relationship to drug concentrations. Psychopharmacology 85:8–13

Altamura AC, Curry SH, Montgomery S, Wiles D (1985) Early unwanted effects of fluphenazine esters related to plasma fluphenazine concentrations in schizophrenic patients. Psychopharmacology 87:30–33

Altamura AC, Buccio M, Colombo G, Terzi A, Cazzullo CL (1986) Combination therapy with haloperidol and orphenadrine in schizophrenia. L'Encéphale 12:31–36
Amdisen A, Aaes-Jørgensen T, Thomsen NJ, Madsen VT, Nielsen MS (1986) Serum concentrations and clinical effect of zuclopenthixol in acutely disturbed, psychotic patients treated with zuclopenthixol acetate in Viscoleo. Psychopharmacology 90:412–416
Andreasen NC (1982) Negative symptoms in schizophrenia. Definition and reliability. Arch Gen Psychiatry 39:784–788
Andreasen NC, Grove WM (1986) Evaluation of positive and negative symptoms in schizophrenia. Psychiatrie Psychobiol 1:108–121
Bolvig Hansen L, Larsen N-E (1983) Plasma levels of perphenazine related to clinical effect and extrapyramidal side-effects. In: Gram LF, Usdin E, Dahl SG, Kragh-Sørensen P, Sjöqvist F, Morselli PL (eds) Clinical pharmacology in psychiatry. Bridging the experimental-therapeutic gap. Macmillan, London, pp 175–181
Bressolle F, Bres J, Blanchin MD, Gomeni R (1984) Sulpiride pharmacokinetics in humans after intramuscular administration at three dose levels. J Pharm Sci 73:1128–1136
Chang S, Javaid JI, Dysken MW, Casper RC, Janicak PG, Davis JM (1985) Plasma levels of fluphenazine decanoate treatment in schizophrenia. Psychopharmacology 87:55–58
Cheng YF, Paalzow LK, Bondesson U, Ekblom B, Ericksson K, Ericksson SO, Lindberg A, Lindström L (1987) Pharmacokinetics of haloperidol in psychotic patients. Psychopharmacology 91:410–414
Clark ML, Ramsey HR, Ragland RE, Rahhal DG, Serafetinides EA, Costiloe JP (1970) Chlorpromazine in chronic schizophrenia: behavioral dose-response relationships. Psychopharmacologia 18:260–270
Coffman JA, Nasrallah HA, Lyskowski J, McCalley-Whitters M, Dunner FJ (1987) Clinical effectiveness of oral and parenteral rapid neuroleptization. J Clin Psychiatry 48:2024
Cooper SF, Dugal R, Albert J-M, Bertrand M (1975) Penfluridol steady-state kinetics in psychiatric patients. Clin Pharmacol Ther 18:325–329
Cressman WA, Bianchine JR, Slotnick VB, Johnson PC, Plostnieks J (1974) Plasma level profile of haloperidol in man following intramuscular administration. Eur J Clin Pharmacol 7:99–103
Dahl SG (1976) Pharmacokinetics of methotrimeprazine after single and multiple doses. Clin Pharmacol Ther 19:435–442
Dahl SG (1981) Pharmacokinetic aspects of new antipsychotic drugs. Neuropharmacology 20:1299–1302
Dahl SG (1982) Active metabolites of neuroleptic drugs: possible contribution to therapeutic and toxic effects. Ther Drug Monit 4:33–40
Dahl SG (1986) Plasma level monitoring of antipsychotic drugs – clinical utility. Clin Pharmacokin 11:36–61
Dahl SG, Hals P-A (1987) Pharmacokinetic and pharmacodynamic factors causing variability in response to neuroleptic drugs. In: Dahl SG, Gram LF, Paul SM, Potter WZ (eds) Clinical pharmacology in psychiatry. Selectivity in psychotropic drug action – promises or problems? Springer, Berlin Heidelberg New York, pp 266–274 (Psychopharmacology series, vol 3)
Dahl SG, Strandjord RE (1977) Pharmacokinetics of chlorpromazine after single and chronic dosage. Clin Pharmacol Ther 21:437–448
Dahl SG, Strandjord RE, Sigfusson S (1977) Pharmacokinetics and relative bioavailability of levomepromazine after repeated administration of tablets and syrup. Eur J Clin Pharmacol 11:305–310
Dahl SG, Hough E, Hals P-A (1986) Phenothiazine drugs and metabolites: molecular conformation and dopaminergic, alpha adrenergic and muscarinic cholinergic receptor binding. Biochem Pharmacol 35:1263–1269
Dworkin RH, Lenzenweger MA (1984) Symptoms and genetics of schizophrenia: implications for diagnosis. Am J Psychiatry 141:1541–1546
Ereshefsky L, Jann MW, Saklad SR, Davis CM (1986) Bioavailability of psychotropic drugs: historical perspective and pharmacokinetic overview. J Clin Psychiatry 47 [Suppl]:6–15
Ericksen SH, Hurt SW, Davis JM (1976) Dosage of antipsychotic drugs. N Engl J Med 294:1296–1297
Forsman A, Öhman R (1976) Pharmacokinetic studies of haloperidol in man. Curr Ther Res 20:319–336

Ganguli R, Reynolds CF III, Kupfer D (1987) Electroencephalographic sleep in young, never-medicated schizophrenics. Arch Gen Psychiatry 44:36–44

Gerlach J, Behnke K, Heltberg J, Munk-Andersen E, Nielsen H (1985) Sulpiride and haloperidol in schizophrenia: a double-blind cross-over study of therapeutic effect, side effects and plasma concentrations. Br J Psychiatry 147:283–288

Hitzemann RJ, Garver DL, Mavroidis M, Hirschowitz J, Zemlan F (1986) Fluphenazine activity and antipsychotic response. Psychopharmacology 90:270–273

Holley FO, Magliozzi JR, Stanski DR, Lombrozo L, Hollister LE (1983) Haloperidol kinetics after oral and intravenous doses. Clin Pharmacol Ther 33:477–484

Hubbard JW, Ganes D, Midha KK (1987) Prolonged pharmacological activity of neuroleptic drugs. Arch Gen Psychiatry 44:99–100

Jann MW, Ereshefsky L, Saklad SR, Seidel DR, Davis CM, Burch NR, Bowden CL (1985) Effects of carbamazepine on plasma haloperidol levels. J Clin Psychopharmacol 5:106–109

Jørgensen A (1986) Metabolism and pharmacokinetics of antipsychotic drugs. In: Bridges JF, Chasseaud LF (eds) Progress in drug metabolism, vol 9. Taylor and Francis, London, pp 111–174

Kidron R, Averbuch I, Klein E, Belmaker RH (1985) Carbamazepine-induced reduction of blood levels of haloperidol in chronic schizophrenia. Biol Psychiatry 20:219–222

Kirch DG, Bigelow LB, Wyatt RJ (1985) The interpretation of haloperidol plasma levels. Arch Gen Psychiatry 42:838–839

Lecrubier Y (1986) Schizophrénie: La prescription des neuroleptiques antiproductifs et antidéficitaires en France. Psychiatrie Psychobiol 1:139–147

Lewis MH, Steer RA, Favell J, McGimsey J, Clontz L, Trivette C, Jodry W, Shroeder SR, Kanoy RC, Mailman RB (1986) Thioridazine metabolism and effects on stereotyped behaviour in mentally retarded patients. Psychopharmacol Bull 22:1040–1044

Loo JCK, Midha KK, McGilveray IJ (1980) Pharmacokinetics of chlorpromazine in normal volunteers. Communic Psychopharmacol 4:121–129

Maxwell JD, Carella M, Parkes JD, Williams R, Mould GP, Curry SH (1972) Plasma disappearance and cerebral effects of chlorpromazine in cirrhosis. Clin Sci 43:143–151

McEvoy JP, Stiller RL, Farr R (1986) Plasma haloperidol levels drawn at neuroleptic threshold doses: a pilot study. J Clin Psychopharmacol 6:133–138

Meltzer HY (1987) Effect of neuroleptics on the schizophrenic syndrome. In: Dahl SG, Gram LF, Paul SM, Potter WZ (eds) Clinical pharmacology in psychiatry. Selectivity in psychotropic drug action – promises or problems? Springer, Berlin Heidelberg New York, pp 244–265 (Psychopharmacology series, vol 3)

Midha KK, Korchinski ED, Verbeek RK, Roscoe RMH, Hawes EM, Cooper JK, McKay G (1983) Kinetics of oral trifluoperazine disposition in man. Br J Clin Pharmacol 15:380–382

Miller DD, Hershey LA (1986) A "therapeutic window" for haloperidol? J Clin Psychopharmacol 6:250–251

Morel E, Lloyd KG, Dahl SG (1987) Anti-apomorphine effects of phenothiazine drug metabolites. Psychopharmacology 92:68–72

Poulos TL, Finzel BC, Gunsalus IC, Wagner GC, Kraut J (1985) The 2.6-Å crystal structure of *Pseudomonas putida* cytochrome P-450. J Biol Chem 260:16122–16130

Prosser ES, Csernansky JG, Kaplan J, Thiemann S, Becker TJ, Hollister LE (1987) Depression, parkinsonian symptoms, and negative symptoms in schizophrenia treated with neuroleptics. J Nerv Ment Dis 175:100–105

Rimón R, Kampman R, Laru-Sompa R, Wiles DH (1986) Serum and cerebrospinal fluid levels of fluphenazine – Relationship to treatment response in schizophrenic patients. Human Psychopharmacol 1:23–27

Roos RAC, Van der Velde EA, Buruma OJS, De Wolff FA (1986) Assessment of the therapeutic range of tiapride in patients with tardive dyskinesia. J Neurol Neurosurg Psychiatry 49:1055–1058

Sedvall G, Farde L, Persson A, Wiesel F-A (1986) Imaging of neurotransmitter receptors in the living human brain. Arch Gen Psychiatry 43:995–1005

Silver JM, Yudofsky SC, Kogan M, Katz BL (1986) Elevation of thioridazine plasma levels by propranolol. Am J Psychiatry 143:1290–1292

Smith RC (1985) Replies. Arch Gen Psychiatry 42:835–838, 839–840

Szukalski B, Lipska B, Welbel L, Nurowska K (1986) Serum levels and clinical response in long-term pharmacotherapy with zuclopenthixol decanoate. Psychopharmacology 89:428–431
Van Putten T, Marder SR (1986) Variable dose studies provide misleading therapeutic windows. J Clin Psychopharmacol 6:55–56
Van Putten T, Marder SR, Mintz J (1985) Plasma haloperidol levels: clinical response and fancy mathematics. Arch Gen Psychiatry 42:835
Volavka J, Cooper TB (1987) Review of haloperidol blood level and clinical response: looking through the window. J Clin Psychopharmacol 7:25–30
Weber HP, Lybrand T, Singh U, Kollman P (1986) Analysis of the pharmacological properties of clozapine analogues using molecular electrostatic potential surfaces. J Mol Graphics 4:56–60
Wiesel F-A, Alfredsson G, Ehrnebo M, Sedvall G (1980) The pharmacokinetics of intravenous and oral sulpiride in healthy human subjects. Eur J Clin Pharmacol 17:385–391
Zohar J, Shemesh Z, Belmaker RH (1986) Utility of neuroleptic blood levels in the treatment of acute psychosis. J Clin Psychiatry 47:600–603

Neuroleptic Drugs in the Treatment of Acute Psychosis: How Much Do We Really Know?

B. M. COHEN

Abstract

The efficacy of neuroleptic antipsychotic drugs has been well demonstrated and neuroleptics are the standard treatment of acute psychosis. However, important aspects of neuroleptic treatment, including course of response, optimal doses, and mechanism of action, remain poorly studied or controversial. Placebo-controlled studies of the onset of the response of acute psychosis to neuroleptics are few and yield conflicting results. Studies of the relationship of doses and blood levels to the therapeutic effects of neuroleptics suggest that the optimal range of doses and levels is narrow and that commonly used doses are too high. Finally, studies of the mechanism of action of neuroleptics suggest that the dopamine hypothesis is based on unsupported assumptions concerning drug effects, drug distribution, and effective doses of drug. Alternative hypotheses, that the antipsychotic effects of the neuroleptics are mediated, at least in part, through α_1-adrenergic or serotonin 5-HT_2 receptor antagonism, are reviewed. The evidence regarding these issues and controversies is discussed, and specific approaches to increase our understanding and enhance our use of the neuroleptics are suggested.

1 Introduction

Neuroleptic antipsychotic drugs have been in widespread use for over 30 years. While alternative treatments are available, including standard treatments such as electroconvulsive therapy (ECT) and lithium, and less proven treatments such as carbamazepine and valproate, most patients presenting with acute psychosis are still treated with neuroleptics. Such treatment is justifiable, as the antipsychotic efficacy of the neuroleptics is well documented. In fact, the efficacy of the neuroleptics may be greatest in patients with acute psychosis, as patients with chronic psychosis often show only partial or minimal response (BALDESSARINI 1985).

Despite their long and frequent use and intensive study, there are numerous issues concerning the neuroleptic drugs which have never been thoroughly addressed. Among these issues, the course of response to neuroleptics, the optimal doses of neuroleptic drugs, and the mechanisms by which the neuroleptic drugs produce their therapeutic effects are all matters of current controversy. A brief review of these controversies and the implications of recent studies which address these issues are presented below.

Clinical Pharmacology, Laboratory, Mailman Research Center, McLean Hospital, Belmont, MA 02178, USA.

2 Course of Response of Acute Psychosis to Neuroleptic Drugs

2.1 Onset of Antipsychotic Effects

Some studies suggest that response of psychosis to neuroleptic treatment occurs, and can even be complete, within hours. Others suggest that response, especially complete response, requires weeks of treatment (BALDESSARINI et al. 1988 a). Most studies are open in design, making the results hard to interpret since spontaneous remissions and responses to environmental change, especially hospitalization, may be frequent and marked in psychotic patients (GOTTSCHALK 1979).

There have been very few placebo-controlled studies of the course of response of acute psychosis to neuroleptics. In addition, like the open studies, the controlled studies yield contradictory results as to when the beneficial effects of neuroleptics are first seen and how rapidly they progress. RESHKE (1974) reported 30% greater symptom reduction with haloperidol than placebo in the first 2 h after dosing. GOTTSCHALK et al. (1975) reported 50% symptom reduction at 1 day following a single dose of thioridazine. However, LERNER et al. (1979) saw no advantages of haloperidol over diazepam in 1 day of treatment. Patients receiving each treatment improved approximately 70%. Similarly, while ABSE et al. (1960) reported 30% symptom reduction at 1 week of chlorpromazine treatment, JOHNSTONE et al. (1978), studying flupentixol, and SCHOOLER et al. (1976), studying chlorpromazine, both reported that 3–4 weeks of treatment were needed to achieve that degree of improvement. CASEY et al. (1960), studying chlorpromazine, noted that complete remission of symptoms required months of treatment even in acute psychosis.

Patient populations, drugs, doses, and rating scales varied between studies and may explain the differences in the rate of response reported. However, to a striking degree, the rate of improvement observed seems to follow the predesignated length of each study. Clearly more and larger studies with standardized techniques and active and inactive placebos, but also with ratings blinded as to time (e.g., performed from videotapes) would be useful to establish the time course of antipsychotic drug effects in acute psychosis. Currently, the course of such effects is unknown.

2.2 Length of Treatment with Neuroleptic Drugs

While the course of onset of neuroleptic drug effects in acute psychosis is unclear despite study, the optimal length of treatment is both unclear and little studied. For acute psychosis, the length of drug treatment tends to be determined on the basis of evaluations of residual symptoms, the perceived risks to the patient should relapse occur when the drug is withdrawn, and knowledge of the average length of acute episodes of psychosis. However, it is not known if neuroleptic treatment itself changes the length of episodes of illness, as has been claimed for antidepressant drugs (PRIEN and KUPFER 1986). In addition, neuroleptic-induced side effects, especially akathisia, can mimic psychotic symptoms. Misidentified as a symptom of psychosis rather than as a drug-induced side effect, akathisia can lead to unnecessary prolongations of treatment and inappropriate increases in doses of drug (COHEN and LIPINSKI 1986a). As with other psychotropic medications used in the treatment of episodic illness, studies to determine the most appropriate length of treatment of acute psychosis with neuroleptic drugs are sorely needed.

2.3 Offset of Neuroleptic Effects

2.3.1 Persistence of the Behavioral Effects of Neuroleptics

There is a growing body of evidence which suggests that the effects of neuroleptic drugs may persist long after the termination of treatment. Side effects, including the life-threatening symptoms of the neuroleptic malignant syndrome (ITOH et al. 1977), have been reported to last for days to weeks after medication is discontinued (HUBBARD et al. 1987; CURRY et al. 1970; MIDHA et al. 1980), and clinical relapse, even in chronic patients who seem unable to remain symptom-free without the administration of neuroleptics, may not occur for weeks or months after the drug is stopped (BALDESSARINI 1985). We have observed what may be a parallel phenomenon in animals. Rats given single, moderate doses of haloperidol exhibited signs of central dopaminergic blockade (apomorphine antagonism) for at least 30 days after treatment (CAMPBELL and BALDESSARINI 1985; CAMPBELL et al. 1985). It is not known whether these extended effects of neuroleptics are due to continued presence of the drug in tissue long after dosing or long-lasting physiological changes which develop after even brief exposure to medication.

2.3.2 Persistence of Drug in Tissue

Plasma elimination half-lives for neuroleptics in man and rat are usually reported as being approximately 24 h (BALDESSARINI 1985), which would argue against the likelihood that drug effects lasting for weeks are due to drug remaining in tissue. However, most studies of the pharmacokinetics of neuroleptics follow drug concentrations for less than 48 h even though distribution phases may occur for days after dosing (OHMAN et al. 1977; DAHL and STRANDJORD 1977). In addition, there may be enterohepatic recirculation of neuroleptics (SUNDARESAN and RIVERA-CALIMLIN 1975; FORSMAN and OHMAN 1977). Therefore, true *terminal elimination* half-lives are almost certainly not measured in studies lasting less than several days.

Longer-term studies suggest that neuroleptics may remain at substantial concentrations in tissue long after administration has stopped. Thus, older studies of phenothiazines given to volunteers and patients show excretion of metabolites in urine for days to weeks after a single dose (LUTZ 1965; JOHNSON et al. 1967) and for months after the discontinuation of extended treatment (CAFFEY et al. 1963; FORREST and FORREST 1963; KURLAND et al. 1965; COWEN and MARTIN 1968; SVED et al. 1971; SAKALIS et al. 1972). Similarly, in a study which addressed our report of persistent effects of single doses of haloperidol given to rats, HUBBARD et al. (1987) gave a single, moderate (5 mg), oral dose of haloperidol to several volunteers. Each of the subjects reported side effects for a week after dosing. In addition, for one subject, blood was drawn periodically for 270 h (11 days) after dosing, and haloperidol in plasma was determined by a sensitive HPLC assay. While half-lives calculated from early data points were similar to those typically reported in the literature (13–37 h), apparent elimination half-life increased with the time of follow-up and a terminal value of 508 h (21 days!) was reached at the end of the period monitored. Similarly, ERESHEFSKY et al. (1986) studied haloperidol concentrations in plasma by RIA in three human subjects for up to 336 h (14 days) after a single dose. As in the experiment by HUBBARD et al., apparent half-life of the drug increased with the time of measurement, and an overall plasma half-life of 91 h (4 days) was estimated by log-linear regression on all data obtained between 12–336 h.

These results in human subjects are provocative, although the studies are few and the number of patients followed is small. In rats, SOUDIJN et al. (1967) and BRAUN et al. (1967), using tritiated haloperidol, reported that up to 13% of the drug was still present in tissue 96 h after an acute s.c. dose and that concentrations of the drug in brain became relatively unchanging (elimination was unmeasurably slow) by 72 h. OHMAN et al. (1977) measured haloperidol concentrations in serum by gas chromatography (GC) in rats up to 216 h (9 days) after dosing. They estimated an apparent terminal elimination half-life of 4 days at the furthest time points measured. Interestingly, they also noted that beyond 4 days after dosing, haloperidol concentrations in brain were at virtually identical levels in all cohorts, irrespective of the dose (0.05–0.75 mg/kg i.p.) of haloperidol received. The authors suggested that a slowly turning-over, but saturable pool represents most of the haloperidol in brain by several days after dosing. In similar experiments, we observed substantial concentrations of haloperidol in brain for over 2 weeks after single doses (0.3 mg/kg) of haloperidol were given i.p. to rats. The half-life of haloperidol in brain estimated by log-linear regression on data obtained 1–14 days after dosing was 13.7 days (COHEN et al. 1988 a), comparable to the half-life of 9.7 days calculated from the disappearance of the behavioral effects (apomorphine antagonism) of haloperidol at the same dose (CAMPBELL et al. 1985).

2.3.3 Clinical Significance of the Persistence of Neuroleptic Drugs

The importance of establishing whether drug levels and effects persist at extended times after dosing are clear. The information gained would be crucial for delineating drug distribution and metabolism and, thus, is essential for understanding drug mechanisms of action, making decisions about drug dosing, timing, and withdrawal in clinical care, and designing research protocols. Persistent drug in tissue may explain the extended therapeutic as well as the extended adverse effects sometimes seen after treatment with neuroleptics is discontinued. Better data on persistent effects might help to guide treatment with neuroleptics, supporting reduced or intermittent dosing, and possibly sparing patients unnecessary side effects.

Knowledge of a persistent pool of drug in brain is also relevant to the design of studies of presumably drug-free patients. The current common use of patients off drugs for only a few days or weeks as equivalent to patients in a drug-naive state might well be reconsidered in the light of evidence that there is drug in active sites in brain for months after treatment.

In a more speculative vein, the persistence of drug at an important site of action after a single dose of medication might produce extended therapeutic as well as side effects. That is, *time* after dosing might be more important than repeated dosing in achieving an antipsychotic effect. Currently, the effects of time and repeated dosing are confounded, and it is not clear which is crucial to drug effect (ANTELMAN et al. 1983). Interestingly, antidepressant effects have been reported to develop with time after single doses of tricyclic antidepressants (POLLOCK et al. 1985), which are chemically similar to the phenothiazine antipsychotic agents. Whether antipsychotic effects would increase with time after a single dose of neuroleptics has never been tested.

3 Optimal Doses of Neuroleptic Drugs

3.1 Standard Dosing Customs

Like choice of drug, which may largely be determined by familiarity, dose of neuroleptic may largely be determined not by evidence on dose-response relationships, but, rather, by common, and often local, customs of practice. Thus, one can find recommendations for low dose, moderate dose, and high dose therapies (BALDESSARINI et al. 1988a). It is interesting to note in this regard, that a study of dosing comparing practices in a hospital in the Federal Republic of Germany and a hospital in Manhattan serving a population of largely European origin observed five-fold greater doses of neuroleptics being given for the same conditions in the United States (DENBAR et al. 1962). These higher doses are most easily understood as representing differences in custom, not differences of drug metabolism or illness in Europe and the United States.

3.2 Blood Levels of Neuroleptic Drugs and Clinical Response

As with other investigators, our own interest in dose-response relationships led us to attempt to define correlations between blood levels and clinical effects of neuroleptic drugs. For blind studies in which fixed doses of drug were given for 2 weeks, we picked what we believed were low doses of neuroleptics, 200 mg/day thioridazine and 6 mg/day haloperidol, hoping to observe the upswing of a drug level-to-response curve. Interestingly, the curve which fitted the data best was a so-called inverted U; that is, patients with the highest as well as the lowest levels of medication showed the poorest response, on average (COHEN 1983; COHEN et al. 1988b). This was surprising since at the doses chosen we expected to avoid excessive levels of drug in all but the rarest of our patients (COHEN 1983).

Our experience has been a common one. Of 15 fixed dose, randomized, blind studies of neuroleptic treatment of acute psychosis, 11 (73%) have reported observing similar inverted U relationships between drug level and drug effects (COHEN and BALDESSARINI 1985; BALDESSARINI et al. 1988b, for review). Among these 11 studies, despite the choice of neuroleptic doses typically used in clinical practice [mean dose = 604 mg equivalents of chlorpromazine (CPZ-eq) per day], fully 25% of the patients treated had levels of drug which appeared to be excessive (COHEN and BALDESSARINI 1985). These findings imply that the optimal range of levels may be narrow and may occur at relatively low doses of neuroleptics.

3.3 Dose of Neuroleptic Drugs and Clinical Effects

3.3.1 Dose of Neuroleptic Drugs and Therapeutic Response

Blind, randomized, *dose*-response studies of neuroleptics are few, but their results show a remarkable concordance with the results of blood level-response studies. Combining the data from three studies which compared more than one dose of haloperidol in the acute treatment of psychosis, an inverted U relationship appeared between response at 2–4 h and dose of drug (BALDESSARINI et al. 1988 b). Optimal improvement occurred between doses of 10–15 mg. Both higher and lower doses were associated with a poorer response. The ED_{50} for drug effect was around 6 mg. Similarly, combining data from six studies comparing the efficacy of more than one dose of fluphenazine decanoate in the maintenance treatment of chronic or recurrent psychosis, optimal effects were achieved at doses of 10–30 mg drug received every other week (BALDESSARINI et al. 1988 b). High doses led to a markedly worse effect. The ED_{50} for beneficial effects was approximately 5 mg of drug received per 2 weeks, implying that even this relatively low dose would be adequate for many patients. Finally, of greatest relevance to the current argument, we combined the results of nine studies comparing multiple doses of neuroleptics in the subacute treatment of psychosis (BALDESSARINI et al. 1988 b). In these studies, acutely psychotic patients were treated for 1–6 weeks. Doses were converted to CPZ-eq to allow an analysis of the combined data from the individual studies. There was no evidence that higher doses led to greater improvement. In fact, for doses over 800 mg CPZ-eq/day, improvement on average was less than that observed with lower doses.

3.3.2 Dose of Neuroleptic Drugs and Side Effects

Side effects as well as therapeutic effects may correlate with dose and blood level of medication (HANSEN et al. 1982; KEEPERS et al. 1983). For this reason, it has been speculated that the decrease of beneficial effects observed for moderate to high doses of drug are due to increased side effects (COHEN and BALDESSARINI 1985). There is evidence suggesting that therapeutic effects may occur at doses below those which lead to significant side effects in most patients (BISHOP et al. 1965). Thus, in a fixed dose study of perphenazine, HANSEN et al. (1982) observed that the drug level-response curve lay to the left of the drug level-side effects curve. Similarly, in countries where lower doses of neuroleptics (200–400 mg CPZ-eq per day) are typically employed, therapeutic benefits remain striking, but side effects, including tardive dyskinesia, seem to be less prevalent and less severe (GARDOS et al. 1980; DOONGAJI et al. 1982).

3.4 Clinical Observations on the Use and Efficacy of Low–Moderate Doses of Neuroleptics

Our own experience supports the interpretation that therapeutic benefits can be maintained and side effects reduced at lower doses of drug than are commonly recommended in textbooks and commonly employed in the United States (COHEN and LIPINSKI 1986a). We performed a survey of dosing practices and patient response comparing patients admitted to the Clinical Research Center of the Mclean Hospital 11 years ago before we began using lower doses of neuroleptics, and 1 year ago after our drug level studies were completed but the use of lower doses of neuroleptics had become routine (VUCKOVIC and COHEN 1987). Patients were not on fixed dose protocols in either period of study and were receiving physicians choice of medications and dose. Despite patient populations which were equivalent in age and illness, mean daily doses for the treatment of psychosis went from approximately 600 mg CPZ-eq in 1976 to 250 mg CPZ-eq in 1985. Length of stay and condition on discharge were equivalent in both years, and side effects were less frequent and less severe in 1985 when patients received lower doses of medication.

These dose changes were not achieved without other changes in treatment. We recognize that high doses of neuroleptics may be so commonly prescribed for acutely psychotic patients not because they produce greater or more rapid antipsychotic effects, but because they produce needed sedative effects in patients who are often agitated, hyperactive, and insomniac (COHEN and LIPINSKI 1986a). To compensate for the loss of sedative side effects when using lower doses of neuroleptics, we prescribe benzodiazepine sedative tranquilizers, mostly lorazepam at doses of 1–4 mg/day, when agitation, psychomotor hyperactivity, or insomnia require treatment. Such drugs are often helpful during the first week or two of treatment of acute psychosis, after which they appear unnecessary and are tapered and discontinued. This practice of using low doses of neuroleptics supplemented by sedative tranquilizers is becoming increasingly more common in the United States and is currently receiving formal study in several centers as an alternative to higher dose treatment with neuroleptics (MODELL et al. 1985; COHEN and LIPINSKI 1986b; ARANA et al. 1986; SALZMAN et al. 1986).

4 Mechanisms of Therapeutic Action of Neuroleptic Drugs

4.1 Critique of the Hypothesis that Dopamine Antagonism Explains the Antipsychotic Effects of Neuroleptic Drugs

4.1.1 Problems Arising from Drug and Dose Selection

All neuroleptics are dopamine antagonists (CARLSSON 1978; PEROUTKA and SNYDER 1980), and dopamine antagonism is frequently postulated as necessary and sufficient to explain the beneficial effects of the neuroleptic drugs (BALDESSARINI 1985). However, following the success of chlorpromazine as an antipsychotic drug, all of the neuroleptics chosen for clinical trials were picked precisely because they produced signs of dopamine antagonism, like chlorpromazine, in test systems (BALDESSARINI 1985). Therefore, it is hardly surprising that the neuroleptics are all dopamine-blocking drugs but it is unconvincing to argue from this shared but predetermined potency that dopamine antagonism is necessary for the therapeutic effects of neuroleptics (COHEN and LIPINSKI 1986 b).

In fact, the neuroleptics share a number of pharmacological effects including antagonism of α_1-adrenergic, serotonin 5-HT_2, and histamine H_1 receptors in addition to antagonism of dopamine D_2 receptors (COHEN et al. 1979; PEROUTKA and SNYDER 1980). Of these multiple effects, the potency of neuroleptics as dopamine antagonists in test systems correlates most highly with the doses of neuroleptics commonly recommended for clinical use (PEROUTKA and SNYDER 1980; SEEMAN 1980). This correlation is offered as the strongest available evidence that dopamine antagonism explains the antipsychotic effect of neuroleptic drugs. However, drawing conclusions from such correlations requires the acceptance of the assumption that both the potency of neuroleptics as neurotransmitter antagonists and the optimal clinical doses of neuroleptics are accurately known. The potency of neuroleptics in preclinical tests of dopamine antagonism *can* be accurately measured. The potency of neuroleptics in the clinic, as discussed above, is largely a matter of speculation. Doses of drugs recommended for clinical use are not based on adequate dose-response studies. In fact, they are based largely on data from preclinical experiments, most notably experiments testing dopamine blockade (BALDESSARINI 1985; COHEN and LIPINSKI 1986 b). For this reason, it is hardly surprising, and not informative, that recommended clinical doses correlate highly with the known dopamine antagonist potency of neuroleptics.

Furthermore, in clinical use, doses of neuroleptics are probably chosen as producing adequate (not optimal) therapeutic effects and tolerable side effects. In practice, and especially with slow-acting drugs like the neuroleptics, the temptation is great to increase doses beyond those necessary to produce antipsychotic effects (COHEN 1983; COHEN and LIPINSKI 1986 a). Thus, doses may be determined not by clinical need, but by the limitations imposed by side effects (COHEN and LIPINSIKI 1986 a; BALDESSARINI et al. 1988 b). Since for the neuroleptics, such side effects will often be extrapyramidal (dopamine antagonist) effects, standard clinical doses will correlate highly with the potency of neuroleptics as dopamine antagonists, but this correlation may imply little regarding the therapeutic mechanisms of these drugs.

4.1.2 Problems of Inferring Mechanisms of Action from In Vitro Studies

In comparing the results of preclinical, particularly in vitro, experiments and clinical data, it is important to recognize that doses of drug given, as are always used in correlational analyses, may reflect poorly the amount of drug in tissue (SUNDERLAND and COHEN 1987). The strong correlation observed between dose of neuroleptics used clinically and dopamine antagonist potency of neuroleptics measured in vitro has been interpreted as evidence that dopamine antagonism determines the antipsychotic potency of neuroleptics. However, accepting this interpretation requires the acceptance of the assumption that there is no systematic difference between drugs studied in bioavailability or blood-to-brain distribution (COHEN and LIPINSKI 1981). Experiments comparing the blood-to-brain distribution of a variety of neuroleptic agents indicate that high-potency drugs such as haloperidol and fluphenazine concentrate in brain 20–40-fold over their levels in serum or plasma (COHEN et al. 1980; SUNDERLAND and COHEN 1987), while low-potency agents, such as chlorpromazine and thioridazine, do not concentrate in brain, being at similar levels in both sites (SUNDERLAND and COHEN 1987). In clinical surveys, the difference in the dose prescribed between high- and low-potency drugs is only 15–30-fold (BALDESSARINI et al. 1984). Thus, differences in distribution could account for the entire difference in clinical dosing between drugs. That is, in clinical use, while antipsychotic drugs may be given at very different doses and attain different concentrations in blood, they may all be at very similar concentrations in the brain (COHEN and LIPINSKI 1986b; SUNDERLAND and COHEN 1987).

If true, this argues against dopamine blockade as the determining factor in therapeutic effect, since potencies of various neuroleptic drugs at dopamine receptors are quite different (COHEN et al. 1979; PEROUTKA and SNYDER 1980; SEEMAN 1980). By comparison, the neuroleptics all have very similar potencies as α_1-adrenergic antagonists and, for most neuroleptics, as serotonin 5-HT_2 antagonists. Drug distribution studies would argue that these sites might well be involved in mediating the therapeutic effects of the neuroleptic drugs.

4.2 Alternative Hypotheses of Neuroleptic Drug Action are Supported by In Vivo Studies

If distribution varies widely and explains the differences in dosing between neuroleptic drugs, then neuroleptics which are equipotent as alpha adrenergic antagonists in the test tube might differ greatly in potency when given to animal or human subjects. In particular, the order of potency of the neuroleptic drugs as α_1-adrenergic antagonists in vivo might parallel their order of potency in clinical use. There are two small in vivo studies in animals which support this possibility: the order of potency of the neuroleptics haloperidol, clopenthixol, thioridazine, and clozapine in increasing the turnover of norepinephrine, presumably in consequence of alpha adrenergic antagonism (CARLSSON 1978), and the order of potency of fluphenazine, haloperidol, and chlorpromazine in blocking the adrenergic inhibition of cerebellar pyramidal cells (MARWAHA et al. 1981) were in each study precisely concordant with the order of clinical potency of the same drugs.

These studies, and those of an experiment discussed below, yield results not predicted by in vitro experiments and argue that α_1-adrenergic antagonism might contribute to the therapeutic effects, not just the side effects, of the neuroleptic drugs.

4.3 The Importance of the Adrenergic Effects of Neuroleptic Drugs

4.3.1 Side Effects as a Clue to the Mechanisms of Therapeutic Effects

Observations of the side effects of neuroleptics were initially responsible for our interest in the effects of the neuroleptic drugs on neurotransmitter systems other than dopamine (COHEN and LIPINSKI 1986a). Specifically, even though our patients were treated with relatively low doses of neuroleptics, we saw a high prevalence of akathisia. Concordant with results in order centers (VAN PUTTEN et al. 1974, 1984), neuroleptic-induced akathisia was present in moderate-to-marked degree in two-thirds of 100 patients consecutively treated with neuroleptics in our in-patient units. Patients received antimuscarinic, antiparkinsonian agents and benzodiazepine anxiolytics as needed, but neither of these treatments was strikingly and consistently effective in ameliorating akathisia.

On the basis of a report by STRANG (1967) on the efficacy of propranolol in the treatment of idiopathic restless leg syndrome, a syndrome with a clinical presentation very similar to akathisia, we treated several patients with neuroleptic-induced akathisia with propranolol. The effects of such treatment were striking (LIPINSKI et al. 1983; ZUBENKO et al. 1984; COHEN and LIPINSKI 1986a). Clinical improvement occurred in most cases. Doses required for effective treatment were low (30–90 mg/day propranolol), and response was rapid, appearing within hours. The efficacy of this treatment has since been confirmed in several double-blind, placebo-controlled studies (ADLER et al. 1985, 1986; LIPINSKI and COHEN, to be published).

Akathisia is not common in idiopathic Parkinson's disease and does not respond well to and may even worsen during treatment with antiparkinsonian agents (ADLER et al. 1986). Thus, it seemed unlikely that akathisia was caused by dopamine antagonism alone. The response of akathisia to propranolol suggested that the syndrome might be related to the α-adrenergic antagonism produced by the neuroleptics, perhaps reflecting increased norepinephrine turnover in the face of α-adrenergic blockade. Since akathisia is commonly observed with all neuroleptics (VAN PUTTEN et al. 1975, 1984), the findings implied further that all neuroleptics, at doses used in clinical practice, might produce physiologically significant adrenergic antagonism. This suggested, in turn, that such antagonism might be related to the therapeutic effects of the drugs, not just the side effects of some neuroleptic drugs.

4.3.2 A Test of the Contribution of Noradrenergic and Dopaminergic Antagonism to the Effects of Neuroleptics

The possibility that all neuroleptics produce physiologically significant α-adrenergic blockade at doses typically used was tested in an animal paradigm (COHEN and LIPINSKI 1986b). Reductions of signal transmission through dopaminergic and adrenergic receptors, whether caused by receptor blockade, neurotransmitter depletion, or chemical or surgical lesions of monoamine tracts, lead to compensatory increases in postsynaptic dopamine or adrenergic receptors (CREESE and SIBLEY 1981; BYLUND and U'PRICHARD 1983; COHEN and LIPINSKI 1986b). These receptor increases are a reliable consequence of receptor blockade and can be used to test the effects of drugs on dopamine and adrenergic receptors in vivo.

Rats were treated with standard doses of typical and atypical neuroleptics, including haloperidol, fluphenazine, chlorpromazine, thioridazine, and clozapine, all known to be effective antipsychotic agents. After 4 weeks of treatment, the characteristics of dopamine D_2 and α_1-adrenergic receptors were determined in brain (COHEN and LIPINSKI 1986b). Significant increases of dopamine receptors were observed in rats after treatment with haloperidol and fluphenazine; modest increases in dopamine receptors, which did not reach statistical significance, were observed in rats treated with chlorpromazine and thioridazine; and no apparent change in dopamine receptors was observed in rats treated with clozapine. By comparison, maximal, statistically significant increases in α_1-adrenergic receptors were observed after treatment with each and every one of the neuroleptics studied.

For the dopamine receptor, these results are consistent with those of past experiments. Haloperidol treatment consistently leads to antagonism of dopamine receptors, as measured by receptor upregulation. Clozapine treatment rarely leads to such upregulation (BURT et al. 1977; MULLER and SEEMAN 1978; SEVERSON et al. 1984). Increases in dopamine receptor density have been observed in only one (ALLIKMETS et al. 1981) of seven experiments (KOBAYASHI et al. 1978; ALLIKMETS et al. 1981; SEEGER et al. 1982; LEE and TANG 1984; RUPNIAK et al. 1984; SEVERSON et al. 1984; COHEN and LIPINSKI 1986b) with clozapine. Similarly, neither molindone (MELLER 1982; SEVERSEN et al. 1984) nor sulpiride (LEE and TANG 1984; RUPNIAK et al. 1984) appear to cause significant dopamine blockade in animals, as measured by receptor upregulation.

Only one other investigator has studied α_1-adrenergic receptor upregulation following neuroleptic treatment. As seen in our experiment, MULLER and SEEMAN (1977) observed significant increases in both dopamine D_2 and α_1-adrenergic receptors in rats after chronic treatment with haloperidol. Thus, upregulation of α_1-adrenergic receptors, and by implication, α-adrenergic antagonism appears to be a consistent property of the neuroleptic drugs, while physiologically significant dopamine antagonism may not be.

4.4 Multiple Neurotransmitters and the Antipsychotic Effects of Neuroleptic Drugs

These findings do not disprove the dopamine hypothesis of antipsychotic drug action. Neither do they prove an adrenergic hypothesis of neuroleptic action. Rather, they suggest that the adrenergic effects of neuroleptic drugs may contribute to their therapeutic effects and suggest that such effects require more study. As a corollary, the serotonin antagonist effects of the neuroleptic drugs, which are nearly equal to their adrenergic effects, also deserve increased study.

The long preoccupation of the drug companies in producing dopamine antagonist drugs and of investigators in studying the dopamine antagonist effects of the neuroleptics is being tempered by more attention to drugs with other actions and more attention to the other actions of current drugs. Thus, it may soon be possible to study relatively pure dopamine, α_1-adrenergic, and serotonin antagonists in patients. Only with such drugs, can the contribution of different neurotransmitter-specific actions to the overall therapeutic effect of the antipsychotic drugs be determined. It may be that blockade of a single receptor (e.g., the dopamine D_2 receptor) is necessary and sufficient to produce antipsychotic effects. However, it may be that the blockade of other receptors is also sufficient. Finally, it may not only be a reflection of the similarity of monoamine receptors that all of the well-proven antipsychotic drugs are nonspecific antagonists. The simultaneous blockade of multiple neurotransmitter receptors may be necessary to induce lasting therapeutic effects.

5 General Conclusions

While the neuroleptics are in constant use, what we know regarding issues as critical as optimal dosing, course of response, and mechanisms of action is quite limited and largely based on custom or experimental results which are incomplete or contradictory. Neuroleptics are likely to remain the mainstay of treatment of psychoses for the immediate future. More knowledge of their effects will yield better treatment. In addition, neuroleptics are the best-proven antipsychotic agents, and as such still represent one of our best source of clues to the underlying pathophysiology of the psychoses. While the development of new antipsychotic drugs is indisputably worthwile, the continued study of the older, neuroleptic antipsychotic drugs is also important.

References

Abse DW, Dahlstrom WG, Tolley AG (1960) Evaluation of tranquilizing drugs in the management of acute mental disturbance. Am J Psychiatry 116:973–980

Adler L, Angrist B, Peselow E et al. (1985) Efficacy of propranolol in neuroleptic-induced akathisia. J Clin Psychopharmacol 5:164–166

Adler LA, Reiter S, Corwin V, Hemdal P, Angrist B (1986) Differential effects of propranolol and benztropine in neuroleptic-induced akathisia (abs). American College of Neuropsychopharmacology annual meeting, p 210

Allikmets LH, Zarkovsky AM, Nurk AM (1981) Changes in catalepsy and receptor sensitivity following chronic neuroleptic treatment. Eur J Pharmacol 75:145–147

Antelman SM, Kocan D, Edwards DJ et al. (1983) Haloperidol catalepsy shows sensitization which depends on passage of time rather than repeated treatment. Neurosci Soc Abs 9:566

Arana GW, Ornsteen ML, Kanter F, Friedman HL, Greenblatt DJ, Shader RI (1986) The use of benzodiazepines for psychotic disorders: a literature review and preliminary clinical findings. Psychopharmacol Bull 22:77–87

Baldessarini RJ (1985) Drugs and the treatment of psychiatric disorders. In: Gilman AG et al. (eds) Goodman and Gilman's pharmacologic basis of therapeutics, 7th edn. MacMillan, New York, pp 387–445

Baldessarini RJ, Katz B, Cotton P (1984) Dissimilar dosing with high-potency and low-potency neuroleptics. Am J Psychiatry 141:748–752

Baldessarini RJ, Cohen BM, Teicher MH (1988a) Pharmacologic treatment of psychoses with neuroleptic agents. In: Treatment of acute psychosis: current concepts and controversies. Aaronson, New York (in press)

Baldessarini RJ, Cohen BM, Teicher MH (1988b) Significance of neuroleptic dose and plasma level in the pharmacologic treatment of psychoses. Arch Gen Psychiatry 45:79–91

Bishop MP, Gallant DM, Sykes RF (1965) Extrapyramidal side effects and therapeutic response. Arch Gen Psychiatry 13:155–162

Braun GA, Poos GI, Soudihn W (1967) Distribution, excretion and metabolism of neuroleptics of the butyrophenone type. Part II. Distribution, excretion and metabolism of haloperidol in Sprague-Dawley rats. Eur J Pharmacol 1:58–62

Burt DR, Creese I, Snyder SH (1977) Antischizophrenic drugs: chronic treatment elevates dopamine receptor binding in brain. Science 196:326–328

Bylund DB, U'Prichard DC (1983) Characterization of α1- and α2-adrenergic receptors. Int Rev Neurobiol 24:343–431

Caffey EM, Forrest IS, Frank TV, Klett CJ (1963) Phenothiazine excretion in chronic schizophrenics. Am J Psychiatry 120:578

Campbell A, Baldessarini RJ (1985) Prolonged pharmacologic activity of neuroleptics. Arch Gen Psychiatry 42:637

Campbell A, Baldessarini RJ, Kula NS (1985) Prolonged antidopamine actions of single doses of butyrophenones in the rat. Psychopharmacology (Berlin) 87:161–166

Carlsson A (1978) Antipsychotic drugs, neurotransmitters, and schizophrenia. Am J Psychiatry 135:164–173

Casey JF, Lasky JJ, Klett CJ, Hollister LE (1960) Treatment of schizophrenic reactions with phenothiazine derivatives. Am J Psychiatry 117:97–105

Cohen BM (1983) The clinical utility of plasma neuroleptic levels. In: Stancer HC (ed) Guidelines for the use of psychotropic drugs. Spectrum, Jamaica, pp 246–260

Cohen BM, Baldessarini RJ (1985) Blood neuroleptic levels as a guide to clinical treatment. Directions Psychiatry 4(37):1–7

Cohen BM, Lipinski JF (1981) Radioreceptor assays and blood levels of neuroleptics. In: Usdin E, Bunney WE, Davis JM (eds) Neuroreceptors: Basic and clinical aspects. Wiley, New York, pp 199–214

Cohen BM, Lipinski JF (1986a) The treatment of acute psychosis with non-neuroleptic agents. Psychosomatics S27:7–16

Cohen BM, Lipinski JF (1986b) In vivo potencies of antipsychotic drugs in blocking alpha 1 and dopamine D2 receptors: implications for drug mechanisms of action. Life Sci 39:2571–2580

Cohen BM, Herschel M, Aoba A (1979) Neuroleptic, antimuscarinic, and anti-adrenergic activity of chlorpromazine, thioridazine, and their metabolites. Psychiatry Res 1:199–208

Cohen BM, Herschel M, Miller EM et al. (1980) Radioreceptor assay of haloperidol tissue levels in the rat. Neuropharmacology 19:663–668

Cohen BM, Campbell A, Baldessarini RJ (1988a) Persistent brain levels and behavioral effects of haloperidol after single doses. Arch Gen Psychiatry (in press)

Cohen BM, Lipinski JF, Waternaux C (1988b) Plasma levels of thioridazine and its metabolites by HPLC and RRA and clinical effects. J Clin Psychopharmacol (in press)

Cowen MA, Martin WC (1968) Long-term chlorpromazine retention and its modification by steroids. Am J Psychiatry 125:139–141

Creese I, Sibley DR (1981) Receptor adaptation to centrally acting drugs. Annu Rev Pharmacol Toxicol 21:357–391

Curry SH, Marshall JHL, Davis JM, Janowsky DS (1970) Chlorpromazine plasma levels and effects. Arch Gen Psychiatry 22:189–196

Dahl SG, Strandjord RE (1977) Pharmacokinetics of chlorpromazine after single and chronic dosage. Clin Pharmacol Ther 21:437–448

Denber HCB, Bente D, Rajotte P (1962) Comparative analysis of the action of butyrylperazine at Manhattan State Hospital and the University Psychiatric Clinic at Erlangen. Am J Psychiatry 119:203–206

Doongaji DR, Jeste DV, Jope NM et al. (1982) Tardive dyskinesia in India. J Clin Psychopharmacol 2:341–344

Ereshefsky L, Jann MW, Saklad SR, Davis CM (1986) Bioavailability of psychotropic drugs: historical perspective and pharmacokinetic overview. J Clin Psychiatry 47 [Suppl]:6–15
Forrest IS, Forrest FM (1963) On the metabolism and action mechanism of the phenothiazine drugs. Exp Med Surg 21:231–240
Forsman A, Ohman R (1977) Applied pharmacokinetics of haloperidol in man. Curr Ther Res 21:396–411
Gardos G, Samu I, Kallos M et al. (1980) Absence of severe tardive dyskinesia in Hungarian schizophrenic outpatients. Psychopharmacology (Berlin) 71:29–34
Gottschalk LA (1979) A preliminary approach to the problems of relating the pharmacokinetics of phenothiazine to clinical response with schizophrenic patients. In: Gottschalk LA (ed) Pharmacokinetics of psychoactive drugs: further studies. Spectrum, New York, pp 63–81
Gottschalk LA, Biener R, Noble EP, Birch H, Wilbert DE, Heiser JF (1975) Thioridazine plasma levels and clinical response. Compr Psychiatry 16:323–337
Hansen CB, Larsen N-E, Gulmann N (1982) Dose-response relationship of perphenazine in the treatment of acute psychoses. Psychopharmacology (Berlin) 27:112–115
Hubbard JW, Ganes D, Midha KK (1987) Prolonged pharmacologic activity of neuroleptic drugs. Arch Gen Psychiatry 44:99–100
Itoh H, Ohtsuka N, Ogita K et al. (1977) Malignant neuroleptic syndrome: its present status in Japan and clinical problems. Folia Psychiatr Neurol Jpn 31:565–576
Johnson PC, Charalampous KD, Braun GA (1967) Absorption and excretion and tritiated haloperidol in man (a preliminary report). Int J Neuropsychiatry 3 [Suppl 1):524–525
Johnstone EC, Crow TJ, Frith CD, Carney MWP, Price JS (1978) Mechanism of the antipsychotic effect in the treatment of acute schizophrenia. Lancet I:848–851
Keepers GA, Clappison VJ, Casey DE (1983) Initial anticholinergic prophylaxis for neuroleptic-induced extrapyramidal syndromes. Arch Gen Psychiatry 40:1113–1117
Kobayashi RM, Fields JZ, Hruska RE et al. (1978) Brain neurotransmitter receptors and chronic antipsychotic drug treatment: a model for tardive dyskinesia. In: Usdin E (ed) Animal models in psychiatry. Pergamon, New York, pp 405–409
Kurland AA, Huang CL, Hallam KJ, Hanlon TE (1965) Further studies of chlorpromazine metabolism and relapse rate. J Psychiatr Res 3:27–35
Lee T, Tang SW (1984) Loxapine and clozapine decrease serotonin (S_2) but do not elevate dopamine (D_2) receptor numbers in the rat brain. Psychiatry Res 12:277–285
Lerner Y, Lwow EI, Levitin A, Belmaker RH (1979) Acute high-dose parenteral haloperidol treatment of psychosis. Am J Psychiatry 136:1061–1064
Lipinski JF, Zubenko GS, Cohen BM et al. (1983) Propranolol in the treatment of neuroleptic-induced akathisia. Lancet I:685–686
Lutz EG (1965) Dissipation of phenothiazine effect and recurrence of schizophrenic psychosis. Dis Nerv Sys 26:355–357
Marwaha J, Hoffer BJ, Geller HM, Freedman R (1981) Electrophysiologic interations of antipsychotic drugs with central noradrenergic pathways. Psychopharmacology (Berlin) 73:126–133
Meller E (1982) Chronic molindone treatment: relative inability to elicit dopaminereceptor supersensitivity in rats. Psychopharmacology (Berlin) 76:222–227
Midha KK, Cooper JK, Hubbard JW (1980) Radioimmunoassay for fluphenazine in human plasma. Commun Psychopharmacology 4:107–114
Modell JG, Lenox RH, Weiner S (1985) Inpatient clinical trial of lorazepam for the management of manic agitation. J Clin Psychopharmacol 5:109–113
Muller P, Seeman P (1977) Brain neurotransmitter receptors after long-term haloperidol: dopamine, acetycholine, serotonin, α-noradrenergic and naloxone receptors. Life Sci 21:1751–1758
Muller P, Seeman P (1978) Dopaminergic supersensitivity after neuroleptics: time-course and specificity. Psychopharmacology (Berlin) 60:1–11
Ohman R, Larsson M, Nilsson IM et al. (1977) Neurometabolic and behavioural effects of haloperidol in relation to drug level in serum and brain. Nauny Schmiedebergs Arch Pharmacol 299:105–114
Peroutka SJ, Snyder SH (1980) Relationship of neuroleptic drug effects at brain dopamine, serotonin, α-adrenergic, and histamine receptors to clinical potency. Am J Psychiatry 137:1518–1522

Pollock BG, Perel JM, Shostok M (1985) Rapid achievement of antidepressant effect with intravenous chlorimipramine. New Engl J Med 312:1130
Prien RJ, Kupfer DJ (1986) Continuation drug therapy for major depressive episodes: how long should it be maintained? Am J Psychiatry 143:18–23
Reschke RW (1974) Parenteral haloperidol for rapid control of severe, disruptive symptoms of acute schizophrenia. Dis Nerv Syst 35:112–115
Rupniak NMJ, Kilpatrick G, Hall MD et al. (1984) Differential alterations in striatal dopamine receptor sensitivity induced by repeated administration of clinically equivalent doses of haloperidol, sulpiride or clozapine in rats. Psychopharmacology (Berlin) 84:512–519
Sakalis G, Curry SH, Mould GP, Lader MH (1972) Physiologic and clinical effects of chlorpromazine and their relationship to plasma level. Clin Pharmacol Ther 13:931–946
Salzman C, Green AI, Rodriguez-Villa F, Jaskiw GI (1986) Benzodiazepines combined with neuroleptics for management of severe disruptive behavior. Psychosomatics 27:17–22
Schooler NR, Sakalis G, Chan TL, Gershon S, Goldberg SC, Collins P (1976) Chlorpromazine metabolism and clinical response in acute schizophrenia: a preliminary report. In: Gottschalk LA, Merlis S (eds) Pharmacokinetics, psychoactive drug blood levels and clinical response. Spectrum, New York, pp 199–219
Seeger TF, Thal L, Gardner EL (1982) Behavioral and biochemical aspects of neuroleptic-induced dopaminergic supersensitivity: studies with chronic clozapine and haloperidol. Psychopharmacology (Berlin) 76:182–187
Seeman P (1980) Brain dopamine receptors. Pharmacol Rev 32:229–313
Severson JA, Robinson HE, Simpson GM (1984) Neuroleptic-induced striatal dopamine receptor supersensitivity in mice: relationship to dose and drug. Psychopharmacology (Berlin) 84:115–119
Soudijn W, van Wijngaarden I, Allewijn F (1967) Distribution, excretion and metabolism of neuroleptics of the butyrophenone type. Part I. Excretion and metabolism of haloperidol and nine related butyrophenone-derivatives in the wistar rat. Eur J Pharmacol 1:47–57
Strang RR (1967) The symptoms of restless legs. Med J Aust 24:1211–1213
Sundaresan PR, Rivera-Calimlim L (1975) Distribution of chlorpromazine in the gastrointestinal tract of the rat and its effect on absorptive function. J Pharmacol Exp Ther 194:593–602
Sunderland T, Cohen BM (1987) Blood and brain concentrations of neuroleptic in the rat. Psychiatry Res 20:299–305
Sved S, Perales A, Palaic D (1971) Chlorpromazine metabolism in chronic schizophrenics. Br J Psychiatry 119:589–596
Van Putten T (1975) The many faces of akathisia. Compr Psychiatry 16:43–47
Van Putten T, Mutalipessi CR, Malkin MD (1974) Phenothiazine-induced decompensation. Arch Gen Psychiatry 30:102–105
Van Putten T, May PRA, Marder SR (1984) Akathisia with haloperidol and thiothixene. Arch Gen Psychiatry 41:1036–1039
Vuckovic A, Cohen BM (1987) A comparison of low and moderate doses of antipsychotic medication. Am J Psychiatry (in press)
Zubenko GS, Lipinski JF, Cohen BM, Barreira P (1984) Comparison of metoprolol and propranolol in the treatment of akathisia. Psychiatry Res 11:143–149

Observations on the Use of Depot Neuroleptics in Schizophrenia

D. A. W. JOHNSON

Abstract

This paper reviews some of the advantages and disadvantages of long-term maintenance therapy with neuroleptics in schizophrenia. The need to separate first-illness schizophrenia from chronic schizophrenia is illustrated. The reduction in the risk of a further acute relapse with continued medication and the likely duration of maintenance therapy are discussed. The true meaning of a further relapse to the patient in terms of reduced social and work function is also discussed. The advantages of using long-acting depot injections for drug administration are stressed. The complex issue of the correct dosage for maintenance is reviewed, with no proven advantage for either very high doses or very low doses. The frequency of depressive symptoms in schizophrenia is reviewed and the possible aetiologies discussed.
The decision to use short- or long-term drug therapy, and whether to use a particular method of drug administration (oral or long-acting depot injections) should be separate issues. Depot injections may, on occasions, be the appropriate method of drug administration for short-term therapies, just as oral drugs have a place in the longer-duration maintenance treatments.

1 Advantages of Depot Administration

The advantages of depot administration are now widely accepted. It overcomes many of the problems of oral administration, giving a more predictable and constant plasma level, both in different individuals and in the same individual on different occasions. Parenterally administered drugs bypass the initial biotransformation process of the gut and liver, so that for a given dose a higher concentration of unaltered free drug is presented selectively to the brain. Probably the most important clinical advantage is the control it gives to the therapist over medication compliance. It has been repeatedly demonstrated that non-compliance with oral medication is high (37%–65% in day patients and outpatients). Urinalyses have demonstrated both the absence of prescribed drugs in 6%–8% of inpatients, suggesting long periods of constant defaulting, and the presence of drugs never prescribed for the patient in 10% of cases (BALLINGER et al. 1974, 1975).

The problems of compliance are complex and depend on many factors involving not only the patient but also the patient's family and its attitude towards mental illness and its treatment by drugs: the family's attitude towards the particular patient's mental state; the success of doctor–patient communication; and the

University Hospital of South Manchester, Manchester M20 8LR, UK.

qualities of the staff administering treatment. The complexity of the problem makes anticipation or prevention very difficult. We are not discussing a situation where patients either take their drugs correctly or not at all; the nature of compliance may vary. To make a sensible decision concerning future medication, whether for the treatment of the patient or modification of side-effects, the prescribing psychiatrist must have a knowledge of the exact dose and type of drug actually received by the patient, not just the prescription offered. This precise knowledge can be achieved only by the use of depot injections. An additional advantage is that the use of depot injections reduces the risk of overdose or abuse. This is potentially an important consideration, not only for the patient but also for the family. In the United Kingdom, the most common source of drugs used in an overdose is medication prescribed for the patient; the next most common source is medication prescribed for another member of the family.

2 Use of Oral Drugs in Maintainance Therapy

The principal potential advantage of oral medication is the flexibility of prescription provided by the short duration of action. However, we must remember that neuroleptic drugs can be stored in the body lipids. After a relatively short period of regular treatment with oral drugs, these drugs cease to be truly short acting since they, or their metabolites, can remain active for weeks or even months after discontinuation of treatment. As a consequence, the maintenance use of oral drugs introduces the same limitation as depot injections, a delay in response to dose reduction or discontinuation of treatment.

A number of studies have demonstrated that under research conditions schizophrenic patients can be equally well maintained on oral or depot medication. Since it is the same free drug molecule that is available to the brain whatever the route of drug administration, it is to be expected that under favourable conditions the outcome, both in terms of therapeutic gain and side-effects, will be more similar than different, despite pharmacokinetic differences. Unfortunately, research conditions and normal clinical practice are likely to be dissimilar in many respects; in particular, research substantially increases the number of staff–patient contacts.

3 Maintenance Neuroleptics in Schizophrenia

The efficacy of maintenance neuroleptic treatment in the prevention of psychotic relapse and rehospitalization in chronic schizophrenia, under different cultural and clinical conditions, has been well established and recently reviewed by a number of authors (Glazer 1984; Hogarty 1984; Johnson 1984; Kane 1984; Leff 1984). However, it is clear that not all patients benefit equally, and a few patients apparently receive no benefit (Fig. 1). These non-responsive patients have

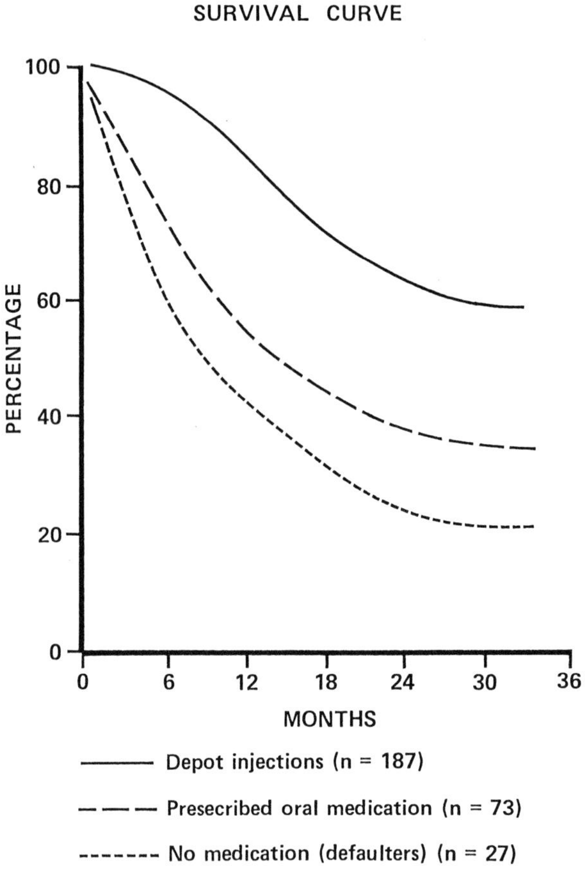

Fig. 1. Survival curves for chronic schizophrenic patients treated with oral neuroleptics ($n=73$, ---) or depot neuroleptics ($n=187$, —), or drug free (defaulters; $n=27$, ----). Survival is defined as no acute relapse of the schizophrenic symptoms in the defined period

not received as much systematic study as they might have done, but certainly in some cases the antipsychotic effect is absent in the presence of blood levels of neuroleptics within what is considered to be the therapeutic range, and in the presence of evidence of dopaminergic blockade as indicated by elevated prolactin levels. The reasons for poor or non-response, the problem of whether patients always remain non-responders and the final outcome of this small group of patients needs urgent research.

An epidemiologically based patient sample suggested that the relapse rate for patients with chronic schizophrenia maintained on depot medication over 2 years is likely to be 28%–37% despite an adequate dose (JOHNSON 1976a). Three different prospective studies also suggest that medication should be continued for an unknown period in excess of 5 years with continuing benefit for these patients (JOHNSON 1976b, 1981b, 1983).

3.1 First-Illness Schizophrenia

The issue as to whether long-term maintenance therapy should be prescribed for first-illness schizophrenia is less clear. Only one double-blind placebo-controlled trial of maintenance drug therapy has been published (KANE et al. 1982). In the patients with a final diagnosis of schizophrenia the drug effect over one year was significant ($p < 0.01$), with no relapses in the drug-treated group compared to a relapse rate of 41% in the placebo group. A drug discontinuation study by JOHNSON (1979) found that patients with a first-illness schizophrenia had a better prognosis over the 2 years following recovery if they received medication for at least 12 months. MAY et al. (1981) reported that neuroleptic treatment during the patient's first hospital admission was associated with a better outcome, and the lack of neuroleptic treatment with a worse outcome, over the following 3 years. However, neither group was controlled for ongoing treatment. CROW et al. (1986) showed that the outcome in terms of relapse for patients who had been ill for 1 year before the prescription of neuroleptics was very much worse than for those who started drug treatment within 1 year of onset. This effect appeared stronger than the expected prophylactic effect of maintenance neuroleptics. The results of these studies collectively suggest a need for early drug treatment for a first illness with continuing maintenance therapy for a period of not less than 1 year.

3.2 Study of Relapse

If long-term medication is required it is reasonable that the use of drug holidays should be explored. Unfortunately, all studies investigating this strategy have strongly suggested that the patient will be highly disadvantaged, with a significantly increased risk of relapse after an interval without medication of 3 months after the first missed injection (JOHNSON 1976b, 1981b, 1983; DENCKER and ELGEN 1980; WISTEDT 1981). In addition, it has been suggested that intermittent medication may increase the risk of tardive dyskinesia (FRIEDHOFF and ALPORT 1978).

So far, the presence or absence of relapse has been reported without any attempt to explain its real meaning. If we are to understand the full consequences of schizophrenia and the full significance of drug therapy to patients, and to become capable of fully evaluating the true risk–benefit ratio, then we must know the full implications of a relapse. What are the changes in patients' symptoms and level of function, and for what period of time? What does it mean in terms of treatments received by the patient? Is there a difference in the nature of a relapse taking place with the partial protection of drugs and a relapse without medication? Does a relapse have an effect on the long-term outcome of schizophrenia and, in particular, does it increase the risk of negative symptoms? So far, most research has concentrated on the acute positive symptoms with little attention being paid to the other aspects of relapse.

HOGARTY et al. (1975) demonstrated that it took 12 months before the benefits of rehabilitation became general to the patient group as a whole, and improvements were continuing after 18 months. JOHNSON (1981b) found that even 12 months after the resolution of acute symptoms only 40% of patients had resumed their prerelapse level of function, and only 50% were reported by their families to have resumed their prerelapse level of social function, even though their prerelapse level of function may have been well below their premorbid function. Some 3%–5% of patients still remained inpatients. These results were confirmed in a further study (JOHNSON et al. 1983) which found that, 6–18 months after recovery from an acute episode of illness, less than 50% of patients had resumed their prerelapse level of work or social function. More recent research (D. A. W. JOHNSON, unpublished data) suggests that in many patients a change of work and social function actually takes place some months before the development of acute symptoms, and this again confirms that most patients are significantly disadvantaged in their level of function 18 months after the event. This study also suggests that there are important differences in the ways patients and their families perceive these changes. Patients see themselves as being more occupied but with a lower level of satisfaction than their families. Collectively, these studies strongly suggest that the period of illness activity is much longer and more disruptive than a consideration of the acute positive symptoms alone would suggest.

The consequences of a relapse in terms of the additional treatment prescribed are also important. JOHNSON et al. (1983) found that at the time of a relapse patients were likely to receive up to three times their normal maintenance dose. After an interval of 18 months following recovery they had received 20% more neuroleptics than controls who had remained stable, and their prescriptions at that time were on average approximately one-third higher than those of the controls, suggesting the excess of drugs for relapsed patients was likely to increase over the next few months. A more recent analysis (D. A. W. JOHNSON, unpublished data) of treatments prescribed to relapsed patients, compared to controls who remained relapse-free, confirmed the substantial increase in exposure to neuroleptic drugs both at the time of relapse and over the next 18 months, and also the increased use of anticholinergic drugs (50%), benzodiazepines (25%–50%) and antidepressants (4%–9%). There was also an increased exposure to electroconvulsive therapy (ECT). The higher dose and number of drugs prescribed must increase the risks to patients in many ways, not least in the increased risk of tardive dyskinesia.

The question of whether patients who relapse without the partial protection of drugs have a different type and severity of relapse from those remaining on drugs has only been investigated in the setting of drug-discontinuation studies, when the discontinuation itself is likely to be a relevant cause of relapse. JOHNSON et al. (1983) strongly suggested that the nature of a relapse following drug discontinuation was both more acute and more severe. There was an increased risk both to the patient ($p < 0.05$) and society ($p < 0.01$) as measured by the increased presence of attempted self-injury and antisocial behaviour. The management strategies adopted at the time also reflected this difference. More patients in the drug-discontinued group who relapsed required inpatient treatment ($p < 0.001$) and were admitted under compulsory powers of the Mental Health Act ($p < 0.01$). In normal clinical practice the issue is likely to be more complex, since patients who relapse on medication may have a higher level of environmental stress than patients who relapse without maintenance medication.

It has been suggested (STEVENS 1982) that recurring acute attacks with partial remission may cause an accumulative deficit with an increased risk of negative symptoms. So far, there is no direct research to confirm this hypothesis, but the findings already reported that social and work deficits continue to be present for long periods after the resolution of acute symptoms emphasise the need for further research.

3.3 Correct Maintenance Dosage

The issue of the correct dose for maintenance is complex and unclear. Perhaps this is not surprising, since the illness itself is subject to many influences, and prescribed drugs are only one factor influencing progress.

The relationship between plasma levels, drug dose and clinical response gives no clear guidelines for clinical practice. It has been suggested that there is a therapeutic window for treatment response, with a lower critical dose below which there is no therapeutic response, and a higher dose above which the therapeutic response diminishes. Two recent studies (JOHNSTONE et al. 1983; SMITH et al. 1984) demonstrated a paradoxical response, with an increase beyond a critical dose reversing the therapeutic gain of a lower dose. Previous papers have also reported exacerbations of psychotic symptoms on high doses of neuroleptics which improve on reduction of medication (CURRY et al. 1970; VAN PUTTEN et al. 1974; SIMPSON et al. 1976).

The possibility that very high doses may increase the therapeutic effect, particularly amongst patients resistant to standard neuroleptic doses, has been investigated by a number of authors. The consensus is that very high doses have failed to prove beneficial either in improving the overall level of response (both in maintenance therapy and in the treatment of the acute attack) or in the speed of symptom resolution in acute psychosis. MCCREADIE et al. (1979) suggested that high doses may be useful if used only for patients who fail to achieve reasonable plasma levels on standard doses, but so far this hypothesis has not been fully explored.

The need to study the minimum dose that will maintain the majority of patients is, perhaps, the most important issue concerning dosage at the present time. BALDESSARINI and DAVIS (1980) reviewed the controlled studies that permitted estimates of the equivalent dose of chlorpromazine to be plotted against reduction of relapse. They found no significant differences between the effects of doses between 100 and 2000 mg/day, and no mean difference in outcome between doses above and below 310 mg. KANE (1984) suggested that these findings may indicate that patients can generally be maintained on doses lower than 300 mg chlorpromazine or equivalent per day.

In a trial of 10% of the existing dose prescription of fluphenazine decanoate, KANE et al. (1983) compared a low-dose group (1.25–5.0 mg every 2 weeks) with a standard dose (12.5–50.0 mg every 2 weeks) over 12 months, in outpatients. The relapse rates were significantly higher in the low-dose group (56% versus 7%). KANE (1984) subsequently studied a group of patients on 20% of the standard dose and reported a reduced relapse rate of 20% over 12 months. MARDER et al.

(1984) reported a double-blind comparison of a low-dose group recieving 20% of the previous dose with a standard group (5 mg versus 25 mg fluphenazine decanoate every 2 weeks) in outpatients. At the end of 12 months the two doses appeared to be having an equal effect. During the second year the low-dose group became significantly disadvantaged with a wide separation of the survival curves after 15 months. The standard-dose group had a negligible relapse rate in the second year whilst the low-dose group had a fairly constant relapse rate throughout both years (31% versus 64% at 24 months). The apparent equal outcome at 12 months may be an artefact of the entry procedure into the treatment since most of the relapses in the standard-dose group occurred within the first 3 months. It is likely that some early relapses occurred before stabilisation on the standard-dose therapy had been established.

These low-dose studies indicate that if relapse is the sole criterion of assessment than standard-dose therapy is superior. However, the authors suggest that the risk of side-effects may be less, and the comfort and function of the patient improved, by the use of low doses. It has also been suggested that any relapse as a consequence of a reduced dose may have a less dramatic onset than relapse following complete withdrawal of medication, so remedial therapy may be offered. A more recent double-blind controlled trial of a 50% dose reduction in maintenance treatment in stable outpatients with minimum residual symptoms and good social function (JOHNSON et al. 1987) showed a significantly higher relapse rate in the low-dose group at 12 months (10% versus 32%). After an interval of 24–36 months from dose reduction 56%–76% had experienced a relapse and 76%–79% had resumed their former dosage. No clear advantage was shown for the lower dose in either reduction of side-effects or improved social function, but a reduced prevalence or lower rate of symptom emergence for tardive dyskinesia was suggested. However, it was recognised that individual patients may be able to survive on very small doses for long intervals. The issue of the correct maintenance dose requires further research.

4 Depression in Schizophrenia

The importance of depression in schizophrenia has only recently been researched (Table 1). A survey of stable patients maintained in the community reported that affective symptoms were those most frequently complained of by the patients (CHEADLE et al. 1978). One study found that patients on maintenance therapy were more than twice as likely to experience depression as an acute schizophrenic relapse (JOHNSON 1981 a), and another study found that depression gave an equal risk of hospital admission as an acute psychotic relapse (FALLOON et al. 1978). Other studies have suggested a particularly high risk in the post-psychotic period (MCGLASHAN and CARPENTER 1976; KNIGHTS and HIRSCH 1981). A careful consideration of depression is important for many reasons, not least that, although the exact relationship between suicide and clinical depression in schizophrenia is uncertain, reviews of the literature clearly suggest an important association with a particular correlation between post-psychotic depression and suicide.

Table 1. Frequency of depression in schizophrenia

Year	Authors	%
1967	HELMCHEN and HIPPIUS	50
1973	HIRSCH et al.	15
1976	MCGLASHAN and CARPENTER (review)	25 (P.P.D.)
1976	MCGLASHAN and CARPENTER	50 (P.P.D.)
1978	CHEADLE et al. (Salford Register)	57
1978	FALLOON et al.	40
	Admissions: Depression 16%	
	Schizophrenia 13%	
1981	KNIGHTS and HIRSCH	54
1981 a	JOHNSON	
	1st Illness: No drugs	
	Prodrome	29
	Acute phase	19
	Chronic illness at relapse	
	No drugs	30
	On drugs	38
	Remission on drugs	
	Antidepressants prescribed	15
	Psychiatrist's assessment	25
	Nurse + self-assessment	26

P.P.D., Post-psychotic depression.

The problem of depression in schizophrenia is complex and it is clear that at present the aetiology and significance are not completely understood. It is suggested that the subject should be analysed under a number of headings.

4.1 Personality

Since the illness occurs in the presence of a wide spectrum of premorbid states the personality of the patient cannot be ignored. It has been suggested that depressed schizophrenic patients were more likely to be living alone, have suffered an early parental loss, have been treated for a previous depression, have had previous attempts at self-harm, have had some undesirable life-events in the previous six months and have had more hospital admissions (ROY et al. 1983).

4.2 Genetic Predisposition

A number of authors have suggested that depressed schizophrenic patients have more relatives who suffer from depressive illnesses, but no satisfactory controlled trials have evaluated this hypothesis. An alternative genetic theory suggests that it is the depressive response to neuroleptic drugs that is determined by inheritance (GALDI et al. 1981). This depression may represent an extrapyramidal component of a dopaminergic-related disorder. A strong argument against this hypothesis as a frequent cause of depression is that many depressions improve with continuing neuroleptic treatment.

4.3 Post-psychotic Depression

It is generally accepted that the 6–12 months after recovery is a time of particular risk both for depression and other forms of relapse. The theories of aetiology fall into two principal categories – the theory of psychological development and the suggestion that depression occurring at this time is only an apparent phenomenon due to the differential response of symptoms.

The arguments for psychological development have not been supported by research studies and the clinical syndromes described have no consistent features. At present these theories are based only on clinical impressions or anecdotal reports. In contrast, the "revealed" depression theory has been subjected to prospective analysis and it is likely that this must explain at least some of the depression reported in this period. It is important to note that both theories suggest that the appearance of depression at this time is an index of progress. The issues have been debated extensively (McGlashan and Carpenter 1976; Galdi 1986; Hirsch 1986).

4.4 Depression as a Symptom of Schizophrenia

The frequency of depression, its presence in all phases of the illness (whether or not therapy is being given), the presence of the revealed depressive syndrome, and the observation that it responds to continuing neuroleptic treatment, all suggest that at least some depression is secondary to the primary schizophrenic illness. The argument would be even stronger if a relationship with prognosis or outcome were found. Recent research suggests that depression in schizophrenia should not be regarded as a single entity; post-psychotic depression and non-post-psychotic depression are likely to have different aetiologies and, therefore, relationships to outcome. Patients who experience an episode of depression more than 12 months after recovery from an acute episode of schizophrenia are more likely to have an illness with a relapsing course, and to relapse within 3 years of their previous illness. The risks of relapse with post-psychotic depression are no different from those in patients who do not experience significant mood changes (Johnson 1987).

4.5 Relationship with Neuroleptic Drugs

It is possible for drugs to be associated with depressive symptoms in two ways:

1. Neuroleptic drugs may produce a true pharmacogenic depression.

2. Neuroleptic drugs may produce a neurological or psychological syndrome which is similar to depression so that either the patient or therapist can confuse the syndrome with true depression. It is suggested that such an extrapyramidal syndrome (akinesia or akinetic depression) can be produced.

There are many reasons for believing that, even if neuroleptic drugs can cause depression on occasions, this must be a minority cause. Historically, depression was recorded before the use of drugs. Depression has been identified as a prodrome to first-illness schizophrenia, before the patient has been introduced to drugs. In double-blind placebo trials the placebo group has experienced an excess of depression. Post-psychotic depression resolves on continuing neuroleptic medication.

HIRSCH (1984) reports that over 30 papers have been published supporting the argument for pharmacogenic depression, but the evidence from structured research is sparse. Nevertheless, a number of observations have been reported that are relevant. An increased incidence of extrapyramidal side-effects has been noted amongst depressed patients. A relationship with high-dose regimens has also been reported. Several studies have suggested that different neuroleptic drugs have different effects on mood, with flupentdixol likely to cause less depression. The issue is complex and no final conclusion can be made at this time. However, one important conclusion has been generally agreed upon and that is that depot medication is no more likely to cause depression than oral medication.

It is agreed that akinesia can be confused with depression even if the syndrome is not one of true depression. The syndrome responds very rapidly to a challenge test with anticholinergic drugs. JOHNSON (1981 a) estimated that 10%–15% of depressions might be due to this cause, and also suggested that symptoms of muscle weakness or muscle stiffness are invariably present even in the absence of overt extrapyramidal symptoms.

4.6 Schizo-Affective Psychosis

A number of psychiatrists have suggested the existence of a separate category of illness – schizo-affective psychosis. The subject has been reviewed by a number of authors (BROCKINGTON et al. 1978, 1979). At the present time there is no consensus on the definition, natural history or prognosis of this condition. It remains a useful research hypothesis, but at the present time is of unproven clinical value.

References

Baldessarini RJ, Davis JM (1980) What is the best maintenance dose of neuroleptics in schizophrenia? Psychiatr Res 3:115–122

Ballinger BR, Simpson E, Stewart MJ (1974) An evaluation of drug administration in a psychiatric hospital. Br J Psychiatry 125:202–207

Ballinger BR, Ramsay AC, Stewart MJ (1975) Methods of assessment of drug administration in a psychiatric hospital. Br J Psychiatry 127:494–498

Brockington IF, Kendell RE, Kellett JM, Curry SH, Wainwright S (1978) Trials of lithium, chlorpromazine and amitriptyline in schizo-affective patients. Br J Psychiatry 133:162–168
Brockington IF, Kendell RE, Leff JP (1979) Prognostic implications of six alternative definitions of schizophrenia. Arch Gen Psychiatry 36:25–31
Cheadle AJ, Freeman HL, Korrer J (1978) Chronic schizophrenic patients in the community. Br J Psychiatry 132:211–227
Crow TJ, Macmillan JF, Johnson AL, Johnstone EC (1986) The Northwich Park Study of first episodes of schizophrenia. Br J Psychiatry 148:120–127
Curry SH, Marshall JHL, Davis JM, Janowsky DS (1970) Chlorpromazine levels and effects. Arch Gen Psychiatry 22:289–295
Dencker SJ, Elgen K (1980) Depot neuroleptic treatment in schizophrenia. Acta Psychiatr Scand [Suppl] 279:61, 5–103
Falloon I, Watt DC, Shepherd M (1978) A comparative trial of pimozide and fluphenazine decanoate in the continuation therapy of schizophrenia. Psychol Med 8:59–70
Friedhoff AJ, Alport M (1978) Receptor sensitivity modification as a patient treatment. In: Lipton MA, DiMascio M, Killam K (eds) Psychopharmacology: a generation of progress. Raven, New York
Galdi J (1986) Depression "revealed" in schizophrenia. In: Kerr A, Snaith P (eds) Contemporary issues in schizophrenia. Gaskell, London, pp 462–467
Galdi J, Rieder RD, Silber D, Bonata RR (1981) Genetic factors in the response to neuroleptics in schizophrenia: a psychopharmacogenetic study. Psychol Med 11:713–728
Glazer AC (1984) Depot fluphenazine: risk/benefit ratio. J Clin Psychiatry 45:28–35
Helmchen H, Hippius H (1967) Depressive syndrome im Verlauf neuroleptischer Therapie. Nervenarzt 38:455–458
Hirsch SR (1984) Depression in schizophrenia. In: Hirsch SR (ed) Seminar schizophrenia. Update, London, pp 27–30
Hirsch SR (1986) Depression "revealed" in schizophrenia. In: Kerr A, Snaith P (eds) Contemporary issues in schizophrenia. Gaskell, London, pp 467–469
Hirsch SR, Gaind R, Rohde RD, Stevens BC, Wing JK (1973) Outpatient maintainance of chronic schizophrenic patients with long-acting fluphanozine: double blind placebo trial. Br Med J 1:633–637
Hogarty GE (1984) Depot neuroleptics: the relevance of psychosocial factors – a United States perspective. J Clin Psychiatry 45:36–42
Hogarty GE, Goldberg SC, Schooler NR (1975) Drug and sociotherapy in the aftercare of schizophrenic patients. In: Greenblatt M (ed) Drugs in combination with other therapies. Grune and Stratton, New York
Johnson DAW (1976a) The expectations of outcome for maintenance therapy in chronic schizophrenia. Br J Psychiatry 128:246–250
Johnson DAW (1976b) The duration of maintenance therapy in chronic schizophrenia. Acta Psychiatr Scand 53:298–301
Johnson DAW (1979) Further observations on the duration of depot neuroleptic maintenance therapy in schizophrenia. Br J Psychiatry 135:524–530
Johnson DAW (1981a) Studies of depressive symptoms in schizophrenia. Br J Psychiatry 139:89–101
Johnson DAW (1981b) Long-term maintenance treatment in chronic schizophrenia. Some observations on outcome and duration. Acta Psychiatr Belg 8:161–172
Johnson DAW (1983) Chronic schizophrenia: is additional medication necessary? World Congress of Psychiatry, Vienna
Johnson DAW (1984) Observations on the use of long-acting depot neuroleptic injections in the maintenance treatment of schizophrenia. J Clin Psychiatry 45:13–21
Johnson DAW (1987) The significance of depression in the prediction of relapse in chronic schizophrenia. Br J Psychiatry (in press)
Johnson DAW, Pasterksi G, Ludlow JM, Street K, Taylor RDW (1983) The discontinuance of maintenance neuroleptic therapy in chronic schizophrenic patients: drug and social consequences. Acta Psychiatr Scand 67:339–352
Johnson DAW, Pasterski G, Ludlow JM, Street K, Taylor RDW (1987) Double-blind comparison of half dose and standard dose flupenthixol decanoate in the maintenance treatment of stabilised outpatients with schizophrenia. Br J Psychiatry (in press)

Johnstone EC, Crow TJ, Ferrier IN, Frith CD, Owens DGC, Bourne RC, Gamble SJ (1983) Adverse effects of anticholinergic medication on positive schizophrenic symptoms. Psychol Med 13:513–527
Kane JM (1984) The use of depot neuroleptics: Clinical experience in the United States. J Clin Psychiatry 45:5–12
Kane JM, Rifkin A, Quitkin F, Nayak D, Ramos-Lorenzi J (1982) Fluphenazine vs. placebo in patients with remitted acute first episode schizophrenia. Arch Gen Psychiatry 39:70–73
Kane JM, Rifkin A, Woerner M (1983) Low-dose neuroleptic treatment of outpatient schizophrenics. Arch Gen Psychiatry 40:893–896
Knights A, Hirsch SR (1981) Revealed depression and drug treatment for schizophrenia. Arch Gen Psychiatry 38:806–811
Leff J (1984) Psychosocial relevance and benefit of neuroleptic maintenance: experience in the United Kingdom. J Clin Psychiatry 45:43–49
Marder SR, van Putten T, Mintz J, McKenzie J, Lebell M, Faltico G, May PR (1984) Cost benefits of two doses of fluphenazine. Arch Psychiatry 41:1025–1029
May PRA, Tuma AH, Dixon WJ (1981) Schizophrenia: a follow-up study of the results of five forms of treatment. Arch Gen Psychiatry 125:12–19
McCreadie RG, Flanagan WL, McNight J, Jorgensen A (1979) High dose flupenthixol decanoate in chronic schizophrenia. Br J Psychiatry 135:75–79
McGlashan TH, Carpenter WT (1976) Postpsychotic depression in schizophrenia. Arch Gen Psychiatry 33:231–239
Roy A, Thompson R, Kennedy S (1983) Depression in schizophrenia. Br J Psychiatry 142:456–470
Simpson GM, Varga E, Haher GJ (1976) Psychotic exacerbations produced by neuroleptics. Dis Nervous Syst 37:367–369
Smith RC, Baumgartner R, Misra CH (1984) Haloperidol: Plasma levels and prolactin response as predictors of clinical improvement in schizophrenia: chemical v. radioreceptor plasma level assays. Arch Gen Psychiatry 41:1044–1049
Stevens JR (1982) Neurology and neuropathology of schizophrenia. In: Henn FA, Nasrallah HA (eds) Schizophrenia as a brain disease. Oxford University Press, New York
Van Putten T (1974) Why do schizophrenic patients refuse to take their drugs? Arch Gen Psychiatry 31:67–72
Wistedt B (1981) A depot withdrawal study. A controlled study of the clinical effects of withdrawal of depot fluphenazine decanoate and depot flupenthixol decanoate in chronic schizophrenic patients. Acta Psychiatr Scand 65:65–84

Neuroleptic Side Effects: Acute Extrapyramidal Syndromes and Tardive Dyskinesia

D. E. Casey [1] and G. A. Keepers [2]

Abstract

The neuroleptic-induced motor system side effects of acute extrapyramidal syndromes (EPS) and tardive dyskinesia (TD) are the major limitations of these drugs. Effective strategies for managing these problems are based on the clinical presentations, pathophysiological processes, and a complex interaction of patient and treatment variables. New concepts about the causes and long-term outcome of acute EPS and TD are emerging to challenge some of the commonly held views about these syndromes. The primary method of preventing undue side effects is to use the lowest effective dose of both neuroleptic and anti-EPS drugs. The pressing need is for novel compounds which treat schizophrenia and are free of the undesirable motor system effects (a nonneuroleptic neuroleptic).

1 Introduction

Since the beginning of their use in the 1950s, antipsychotic drugs have been labeled "neuroleptics" because of their ability to produce neurological syndromes of motor dysfunction. The movement disorders commonly seen with neuroleptic drugs include the acute extrapyramidal syndromes (EPS) which occur with the initiation of treatment, and tardive dyskinesia (TD) which occurs during or at the cessation of extended neuroleptic therapy. Though the acute EPS were once thought to indicate the lower threshold of antipsychotic efficacy, they are now regarded as detrimental side effects which compromise therapeutic benefits and are unrelated to the antipsychotic effects. TD, which was recognized in the late 1950s (Schönecker 1957; Sigwald et al. 1959; Uhrbrand and Faurbye 1960) and was officially labeled as such in 1964 (Faurbye et al. 1964), has led to a careful reconsideration of the proper indications for neuroleptic use.

While acute EPS are thought of as troublesome but acceptable, TD is considered the most serious side effect of neuroleptic drugs. This perspective deserves reevaluation. Acute EPS are highly prevalent – occurring in up to 90% of patients – and are a major cause of physical and mental impairment, which adds to the existing disabilities of psychotic patients. In contrast, TD occurs in a minority of patients (approximately 15%–20%), it is usually mild in severity, and causes little or no impairment to patients except in severe cases.

[1] Psychiatry Service, VA Medical Center; Departments of Psychiatry and Neurology, Oregon Health Sciences University, Portland, OR, USA, and Department of Animal Behavior, Oregon Regional Primate Research Center, Beaverton, OR, USA.

[2] Psychiatry Service, VA Medical Center; Department of Psychiatry, Oregon Health Sciences University, Portland, OR, USA.

The goals of this chapter are to review our current knowledge about the acute and late-onset dyskinesias. The relative contributions of patient and treatment variables will be summarized and algorithms outlining strategies for managing acute EPS and TD will be provided.

2 Acute Extrapyramidal Syndromes

2.1 Clinical Manifestations

Dystonia is an involuntary muscular spasm producing a briefly sustained or fixed abnormal posture, such as torticollis, trismus, oculogyric crisis, laryngeal-pharyngeal constriction, tongue protrusion, or bizarre positions of the limbs and trunk. It is sometimes misdiagnosed as hysterical conversion reactions, malingering, seizures, or catatonia (Table 1). However, the vast majority of these and other unusual symptoms that appear within the first 96 h of starting neuroleptic therapy should be considered as acute dystonic reactions and managed accordingly (KEEPERS and CASEY 1986).

Neuroleptic-induced parkinsonism, which is clinically similar to idiopathic parkinsonism, is characterized by tremor, rigidity, and bradykinesia (sometimes called akinesia). The tremor is rhythmical, with a to-and-fro motion and is usually greater at rest. Cogwheel rigidity is most easily examined in the arms. Bradykinesia is recognized by a paucity of spontaneous activity, decreased associated arm movements during walking, and a mask-like facial expression. Bradykinesia is often not recognized or is misdiagnosed because it mimics withdrawal, negative symptoms of schizophrenia, or depression.

Akathisia is a subjective feeling of restlessness, sometimes described as "anxiety" or "jitters." This may be expressed through the motor activities of pacing, rocking back and forth, lifting the feet as if marching in place, or other repetitive purposeless actions. Patients can have considerable difficulty articulating their feeling of akathisia. Frequently they appear to be agitated or experiencing a psychotic decompensation (VAN PUTTEN et al. 1974) when expressing their discomfort in their thought-disordered, unique use of language.

The rabbit syndrome is an uncommon side effect characterized by rhythmical tremors in the lips and perioral area (VILLENEUVE 1972). It may occur at any time during neuroleptic therapy and appears to be a variant of drug-induced parkinsonism because it improves with antiparkinsonian medications.

Paradoxical dyskinesia refers to a seldom-reported and incompletely understood syndrome that clinically resembles TD, but pharmacologically responds like acute EPS. The symptoms may be difficult to distinguish from TD because they can involve the mouth, face, limbs, and trunk, but they are usually more repetitive and stereotyped than TD. Paradoxical dyskinesia rapidly improves or resolves with antiparkinsonian drugs or when neuroleptics are discontinued, which is the opposite of traditional TD responses (GERLACH et al. 1974; CASEY and DENNEY 1977).

Table 1. Acute extrapyramidal syndromes and tardive dyskinesia

Dyskinesia	Symptoms	Distinguish from psychiatric symptoms	Period of maximum risk (days)	Treatment
Acute dystonia	Muscle spasm of tongue, face, neck, back, oculogyric crisis	Manipulation, hysteria, seizures, catatonia	1–5	Anticholinergics/antihistaminics are diagnostic and curative (i.m. or i.v., then p.o.)
Parkinsonism	Tremor, rigidity, bradykinesia (akinesia), mask face, decreased arm swing	Depression, negative symptoms of psychosis	5–30	Reduce neuroleptic dose; antiparkinsonian agents
Akathisia	Subjective complaints or motor restlessness, pacing, rocking, shifting foot to foot	Severe agitation; psychotic decompensation	1–30	Reduce neuroleptic dose; propranolol; β-adrenergic blockers anti-EPS agents
Rabbit syndrome	Perioral tremor (parkinsonian variant?)		Variable	Anti-EPS agents
Paradoxical dyskinesia	Orofacial-lingual dyskinesias, choreoathetosis in limbs and trunk; movements are more stereotyped than TD	Stereotypy or mannerisms of psychosis	Variable	Reduce neuroleptic dose; anti-EPS agents
Tardive dyskinesia	Orofacial-lingual dyskinesia, choreoathetosis in limbs and trunk	Stereotypy or mannerisms of psychosis	Months to years (unmasked on neuroleptic withdrawal)	Prevention best; treatment unsatisfactory; lower neuroleptic dose

2.2 Pathophysiology

Despite more than 30 years of neuroleptic research, little is known about the specific pathophysiologies underlying these acute EPS. It is tempting to parsimoniously correlate all the acute EPS with the onset of dopamine receptor blockade which occurs within a few hours of starting neuroleptics. However, there is a major temporal problem with this proposal since some acute EPS may not develop for several days to weeks.

The preponderance of data suggests that dystonia is due to a hypodopaminergic state secondary to dopamine receptor blockade, but there is also an argument for a hyperdopaminergic state (RUPNIAK et al. 1986). A critical, as yet undetermined balance between multiple neurotransmitters may be involved, as dystonia usually occurs on the day after single dosing, when blood levels are falling (GARVER et al. 1976) or on the 2nd day of continuous treatment when blood levels are rising (KEEPERS et al. 1983).

Neuroleptic-induced parkinsonism takes several days or weeks to develop, which is a considerable time after receptor blockade has been established. The partial or complete tolerance to parkinsonism that evolves over several months is also unexplained. This time course is consistent with the evolution of dopamine hypersensitivity and may be a better fit of the model than its application to TD (CASEY 1987a, b).

Akathisia is the least-understood EPS. There is not a good neuroanatomical localization of this syndrome and it is poorly responsive to antiparkinsonian drugs (KEEPERS and CASEY 1986). The recently identified effectiveness of propranolol, a nonselective β-adrenergic blocker, in akathisia (LIPINSKI et al. 1984) implicates a nondopamine role. Very little is known about the presence of β-adrenergic receptors in the extrapyramidal system or the effect of neuroleptics on these receptors. Perhaps akathisia is not an acute EPS but occurs from dysfunction outside the neuroanatomical region known as the "extrapyramidal system."

2.3 Epidemiology

EPS prevalence rates vary widely across studies, ranging from 2% to 90% (SOVNER and DIMASCIO 1978). This variability is influenced by patient, drug, and treatment phase parameters. Over the past few decades there has been a trend toward an increasing prevalence of acute EPS, as it has become more common to use higher drug dosages and more aggressive therapy with low-milligram, high-potency neuroleptics. For example, the acute dystonia rate has steadily risen from 2.3% (AYD 1961) to as much as 39% (KEEPERS et al. 1983) and was over 90% in a study evaluating high-risk young male patients (BOYER et al. 1987).

2.4 Patient Variables

Age, sex, race, and history of previous EPS strongly influence whether a patient will develop these symptoms. Young patients, particularly males, are more susceptible to dystonia, whereas the prevalence of parkinsonism is higher in older age groups. Indeed, the virtual absence of acute dystonia in elderly patients as compared to its widespread occurrence in young adults and children undoubtedly reflects important, but relatively unexplored, age-related aspects of central nervous system dopaminergic systems. Akathisia is most often seen in middle-aged females (AYD 1961; KEEPERS et al. 1983). A patient's history of previous EPS is a very strong predictor of vulnerability to future symptoms if similar treatment is reinitiated. In one study comparing two hospitalizations for 63 patients, EPS rates in the second treatment course could be predicted with 85% accuracy based on the presence or absence of EPS in the first hospitalization. This prior EPS history was more effective in predicting future EPS than a multifactorial discriminant function which included patient, drug, and time variables (KEEPERS et al. 1986).

2.5 Drug Factors

Neuroleptic characteristics also influence EPS rates. The relative balance of dopamine receptor blocking and anticholinergic properties intrinsic to each neuroleptic drug correlates with its propensity to produce EPS (SNYDER et al. 1974), though other actions of neuroleptics may also influence EPS rates (SAYERS et al. 1976). Low-milligram, high-potency drugs with minimal anticholinergic activity produce more EPS than high-milligram, low-potency drugs which have more anticholinergic aspects. Intermediate-potency drugs produce moderate rates of EPS. However, EPS rates should not be the sole consideration in neuroleptic drug choice because (a) EPS can usually be well managed with anti-EPS medications; and (b) other undesirable drug effects (e.g., hypotension, anticholinergic side effects, photosensitivity, leukopenia, etc.) should also be weighed in selecting a neuroleptic.

Although lower doses produce fewer EPS than moderate to high doses, there is no direct linear relationship. Megadoses produce the same or fewer EPS than moderate-to-high doses (KEEPERS et al. 1986). Data evaluating the correlation between neuroleptic dose and EPS have produced conflicting results which vary between no relation (TUNE and COYLE 1981) to a significant positive correlation (HANSEN et al. 1981). While it seems intuitive that there should be a correlation between drug dose and therapeutic as well as side effect rates, such associations are not easily identified. For example, if a high side effect rate plateaus with low to moderate dosages, any further increase in drug dose will show no further correlation with the already high, plateaued EPS rates. If the EPS dosage association is nonlinear, such as an inverted U-shaped curve function seen in dystonia, linear statistical analyses will show no correlation between dose level and symptoms. Only a complex mathematical analysis will identify the true inverted U-shaped function. The core problem in characterizing the dose–effect relationship (which applies to both desirable and undesirable effects) may lie in the increasing tendency to use high doses of neuroleptics which are substantially above the inflection points in sigmoid or other dose–response curves. Only by studying fixed dosages along the complete range of the dose–response curve can the relationships between parameters of drug treatment and side effects be delineated.

2.6 Treatment Phase

There are separate time courses for the different acute EPS. The large majority of dystonic reactions occur within the first 96 h after starting or rapidly increasing neuroleptic drug dosage (Keepers et al. 1983; Sramek et al. 1986). Parkinsonism and akathisia occur most commonly at the end of the 1st or 2nd week of treatment, though these symptoms may develop within the first few days of drug therapy. These two syndromes gradually resolve over several weeks to months in some patients, but persist indefinitely in others if not treated.

2.7 Therapeutic Strategies

Three distinct strategies have developed for managing drug-induced acute EPS. These are initial prophylaxis, treating existing EPS, and extended prophylaxis. Initial prophylaxis utilizes anti-EPS agents at the beginning of neuroleptic treatment to prevent EPS. Considerable controversy surrounds this approach. Proponents of prophylaxis argue that dystonic episodes can be dangerous, subtle forms of bradykinesia and akathisia are often unrecognized, and acute EPS occur at high rates in predisposed vulnerable patients. Opponents of prophylaxis argue that the anti-EPS drugs have their own drawbacks of autonomic nervous system dysfunction, memory impairment, and the risk of delirium. Interestingly, both sides of the discussion contend that their approach seeks the maximum benefit with the minimum side effects, thereby fostering a therapeutic alliance with the patient and maintaining treatment compliance.

Treatment of acute EPS with anti-EPS medicines aims to control symptoms which have emerged during neuroleptic therapy. This is standard practice. Extended prophylaxis is arbitrarily defined as continued use of anti-EPS drugs for longer than 3 months to suppress EPS. This can result from extending initial prophylaxis or from continuing anti-EPS drug treatment after symptoms emerge.

2.8 Managing Clinical Syndromes

The accompanying algorithm (Fig. 1) charts critical decision points for the effective management of the common acute EPS. It follows the logical course of clinical choices ranging from initiating neuroleptic therapy to maintaining long-term drug treatment of psychotic symptoms.

The history and evaluation are essential elements for fully estimating the EPS risk factors and the need for initial prophylaxis. Documenting the psychiatric and neurological status of patients prior to initiating drug therapy is important as this serves as a valuable baseline and reference point for interpreting symptom evolution or change.

Initial prophylaxis is recommended when there is (a) high risk of EPS; (b) predisposition to EPS; and (c) detrimental sequelae of EPS (Keepers and Casey 1986). An informed judgment about the high EPS risk is made by considering the patient characteristics (age, sex), drug properties (mg potency, dosage, anticholin-

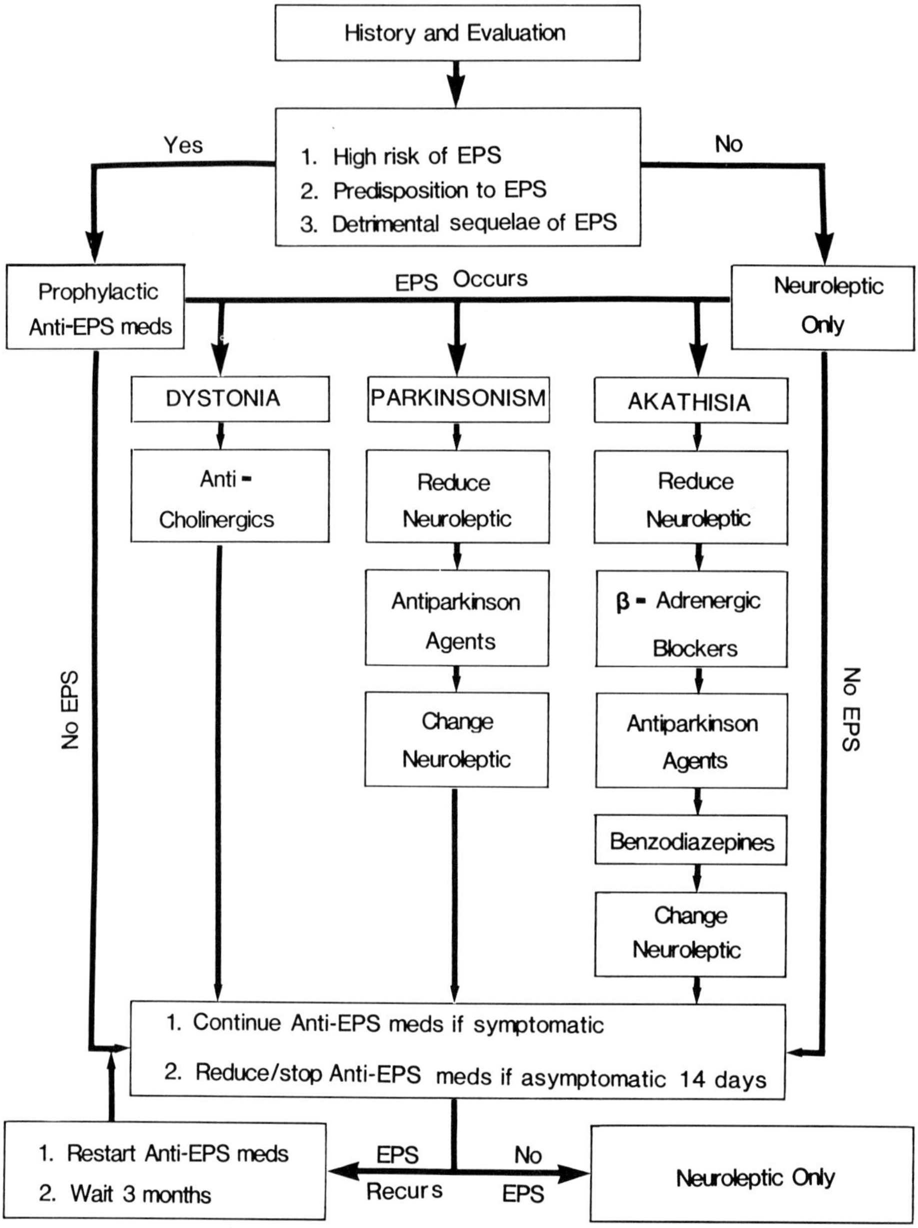

Fig. 1. An algorithm for managing neuroleptic-induced acute extrapyramidal syndromes (EPS)

ergic components), and the temporal aspects of EPS (KEEPERS et al. 1983). Previous EPS indicate that the patient is highly vulnerable to a recurrence of these symptoms if the neuroleptic drug and dose are similar to past treatments. Finally, situations where EPS would have detrimental sequelae must be considered. For example, acute dystonia in the paranoid patient may irrevocably disrupt the formative phases of the therapeutic alliance. If the balance of these considerations favors preventing EPS, initial prophylaxis with anti-EPS drugs is indicated, since it is clearly effective (Casey et al. 1980; Keepers et al. 1983). Indeed, all five studies (two prospective with 241 patients and three retrospective with 336 patients) published since 1980, evaluating the role of initial prophylaxis, found a statistically significant benefit (Moleman et al. 1982; Keepers et al. 1983; Sramek et al. 1986; Winslow et al. 1986; Boyer et al. 1987). However, if there is a low likelihood of EPS, treatment with only a neuroleptic drug is preferred because anti-EPS agents can produce their own undesirable side effects.

Treating EPS is less controversial. Dystonia is treated with parenteral anticholinergic or antihistaminic agents. These drugs are so uniformly effective in reversing dystonic reactions that a failure to improve after one to three repeated doses over a few hours should stimulate the search for other uncommon causes of dystonia associated with underlying medical illnesses.

In parkinsonism, the first strategy is to reduce the neuroleptic dose. Much of the controversy regarding anti-EPS drugs would not be relevant if lower neuroleptic doses were used more commonly. This would reduce the EPS rate and often make anti-EPS treatment unnecessary. Many patients, however, have a psychotic exacerbation when neuroleptic doses are reduced, so using antiparkinsonian medicines is the next alternative. The widely accepted anticholinergic and antihistaminic agents are equally efficacious. Amantadine, a weak dopamine agonist, has fewer side effects and is also an effective antiparkinsonian drug (Keepers and Casey 1986). Changing to another neuroleptic with a different side effect profile of fewer EPS is a further option, though this is seldom necessary.

Akathisia is one of the most difficult syndromes to treat. As in parkinsonism, neuroleptic dose reduction is the first choice. If this is not possible or is unsuccessful, β-adrenergic blockers that penetrate the blood-brain barrier should be considered. Propranolol, 30–120 mg/day in divided doses, is effective in the majority of patients (Lipinski et al. 1984). The benefit of β-adrenergic blockers in akathisia raises important theoretical questions about the role of neuroleptic drugs on these receptors. It also raises the further possibility that akathisia may not be an EPS, and may have a neuroanatomical explanation that does not include the extrapyramidal system.

In some ways it is not surprising that the underlying pathophysiology and treatment of akathisia may, at least in part, be separate from drug-induced parkinsonism. These two syndromes often coexist to produce the simultaneously distressing and occasionally bizarre presentation of a rigid, shuffling, bradykinetic (parkinsonism – too little movement) patient, constantly pacing with uncontrollable restlessness (akathisia – too much movement).

Other anti-EPS agents, including the anticholinergics, are less likely to be effective in akathisia. Benzodiazepines may offer another avenue for treating akathisia, though this class of drugs poses potential problems of dependence and abuse. Finally, changing to another neuroleptic is a viable strategy.

Extended prophylaxis with anti-EPS medications is indicated in many patients. When EPS are not present for 14 days or more, anti-EPS agents should be gradually reduced with an aim toward drug discontinuation. If EPS recur, then the previous regimen can be reinstituted. A review of five double-blind placebo-controlled extended prophylaxis studies with 166 patients published since 1980 showed that prophylaxis was effective in some aspects of all these studies. The rate of benefit ranged from 35%–90% of the patients (JELLINEK et al. 1981; MANOS et al. 1981; BAKER et al. 1983; MCINNIS and PETURSSON 1985; MANOS et al. 1986). Many patients gradually develop tolerance to EPS and can eventually do without anti-EPS drugs. Others, however, will indefinitely need extended prophylaxis with anti-EPS medications to control symptoms. While it was commonly stated in the 1970s that up to 90% of patients with EPS have it resolve within 3 months (ORLOV et al. 1971), the more recent evaluations show that 35%–90% of patients in the 1980s require indefinite prophylaxis to control neuroleptic-induced acute EPS.

Several studies with monkeys demonstrate that prior neuroleptic-induced dystonia and parkinsonism predispose or sensitize the animals toward more severe EPS during subsequent neuroleptic exposure. This issue is generally unexplored in the clinic, but has direct relevance to questions about anti-EPS treatment (CASEY 1987b).

The concern about anticholinergic drugs lowering neuroleptic blood levels is often raised. While this drug interaction occurs with some but not all neuroleptics, the most clinically relevant point is that this has not consistently produced a change in the patient's mental status (MCEVOY 1983; BAMRAH et al. 1986).

The algorithm for managing acute EPS prescribes a process for achieving the greatest benefit with the fewest risks. Adopting a single approach for all patients will not adequately address the complex interaction of patient, drug, and treatment phase variables. Failing to control EPS can lead to poor medication compliance and psychotic exacerbation. Similarly, overtreatment or unnecessary prescription of anti-EPS drugs may compound unacceptable side effects and produce the same poor compliance and relapse. With a logical stepwise strategy for managing acute EPS, these often frustrating side effects can be controlled to allow the neuroleptic drugs to exert their maximum therapeutic benefit. In the meantime, the search continues for an effective antipsychotic drug which is free of acute EPS (a nonneuroleptic neuroleptic).

3 Tardive Dyskinesia

3.1 Clinical Description

TD is characterized by the late onset of involuntary repetitive purposeless movements in predisposed patients. The original descriptions emphasized orofacial signs of chewing, tongue protrusion, lip smacking, puckering, and pursing. TD can also affect the lower and upper limbs with choreoathetosis and may produce bizarre movements in the head, neck, or hips. Rarely, dyskinesias involve irregular breathing or swallowing to cause grunting noises (CASEY 1981).

Though atypical forms of TD have been recognized for many years, recent interest has focused on the less characteristic presentations. Tardive dystonia occurs more often in younger patients (as does acute dystonia) and is predominated by sustained abnormal postures with torticollis, blepharospasm, grimacing, and truncal torsion (Burke et al. 1982). Tardive akathisia is persisting restlessness (Barnes and Braude 1985). It is unclear if these different symptoms represent distinct pathophysiological mechanisms or are better explained as symptom clusters which reflect the breadth of the TD syndrome that evolves from a common underlying pathophysiology (Casey 1987a).

3.2 Differential Diagnosis

The controversy surrounding the role of abnormal movements in psychosis dates back to at least the debates between Kraepelin and Bleuler about the existence and meaning of choreiform dyskinesias.

Kraepelin (1907) believed that abnormal movements were an integral part of the biological basis of schizophrenia:

> Some of these movements correspond exactly to the movements of expression: wrinkling of the eyebrow, distortion of the mouth, rolling the eyes, and those other facial movements which are characterized as grimacing. These movements remind one of choreic movements and are quite independent of ideas and feelings. There may be associated with them smacking of the lips, clucking the tongue, sudden grunting, sniffing, and coughing. Furthermore, in the lips we observe very rapid rhythmical movements. More often there exists a peculiar choreiform movement of the mouth which may be described as athetoid ataxia.

Kraepelin may have grouped together heterogeneous disorders of idiopathic, postinfectious, traumatic, or hereditary neurodegenerative origin by overly including some of these seemingly unrelated symptoms. Bleuler (1950) took an opposing view about the meaning of chorea in schizophrenia:

> The expressive gestures are also modified. Grimaces of all kinds, peculiar ways of shrugging the shoulders, extraordinary movements of the tongue and lips, finger play, sudden involuntary gestures – all of these peculiarities are the reasons why some authors have spoken of choreic or tetanic movements and catatonia, quite mistakenly, though.
>
> Choreal, athetotic, and tetanic phenomena are entirely different from the motor symptoms which accompany schizophrenia. The confinement of the movements to specific groups of muscles can be much better explained on a psychic than on an anatomic basis ...

The most parsimonious explanation to bring together these apparently polar viewpoints centers around issues of definition of terms and theoretical framework. Both these observant clinicians saw similar signs of "grimacing" and "irregular movements of the tongue and lips," but adopted opposite positions when interpreting these phenomena. These positions can be brought more closely together by postulating that Kraepelin combined diverse and unrelated signs within a biological framework, whereas Bleuler offered an overly strict psychological explanation for abnormal movements.

Stereotypies and mannerisms of psychosis, as well as other idiopathic dyskinesias, are included in the differential diagnosis of TD. Other disorders include blepharospasm-oromandibular dystonia (Meige syndrome), other focal and segmental dystonias, Tourette's syndrome, and simple persisting tics. Even dental problems may be associated with orofacial dyskinesias. The neuroleptic-induced acute EPS must also be distinguished from TD. These syndromes are usually easily recognized, though paradoxical dyskinesias may be difficult to identify.

Other drug-induced dyskinesias are uncommonly seen with extended use of anticholinergics or antihistaminics. Chorea as well as stereotyped behavior and psychosis can occur with chronic amphetamine abuse. Several anticonvulsants, oral contraceptives, chloroquine and other antimalarial drugs can also evoke reversible orofacial and limb dyskinesias.

Hereditary and systemic illnesses such as Huntington's and Wilson's diseases may initially resemble TD and/or psychosis, but are usually distinguishable by clinical signs, laboratory tests, and family history. Endocrinopathies of hyperthyroidism and hypoparathyroidism, as well as systemic lupus erythematosis, and encephalitis can also be associated with dyskinesias (CASEY 1981).

3.3 Epidemiology

The prevalence of TD varies greatly from 0.5%–100% (CASEY 1987a). This wide range undoubtedly reflects many different variables, including the populations at risk, characteristics of past and present treatment, and criteria for diagnosis. Conservative estimates of average TD prevalence rates are 15%–20%, but may exceed 70% in high-risk populations such as the elderly. Spontaneous dyskinesia (SD) rates average 5%. Though most prevalence studies show TD is higher than SD, a few do not. This has led some to question whether TD exists as a discrete drug-related side effect. A study that initially reported no significant difference between prevalence of TD (67%) and SD (53%) in chronically psychotic schizophrenics (OWENS et al. 1982) did show a significant drug effect when the data were reanalyzed with age-matched groups (CROW et al. 1982).

Though TD prevalence rates have increased approximately 20% over the past two decades, SD rates have increased similarly (HANSEN et al. 1986). The difference between the TD and SD rates has remained relatively stable at approximately 15% when similar patient groups are compared. When TD rates were low, SD rates were also low, as in the 1960s, and when TD rates were high, SD rates were high, as in the 1980s. Perhaps greater awareness and vigilance account for increases in both TD and SD, since it is unlikely that nondrug factors would produce SD increases that match the purported TD drug-induced increases. Both TD and SD were probably underdiagnosed 20 years ago, and may be overdiagnosed currently.

Also, perhaps TD and SD are associated. Symptoms can be phenomenologically similar and share risk factors of increasing age and female sex (CASEY and HANSEN 1984). Perhaps a preexisting vulnerability interacts with additional elements, such as central nervous system disease (schizophrenia, dementia), drugs (neuroleptics), and environment (toxins), to convert a covert predisposition to dyskinesias to clinically overt symptoms (CASEY 1985b). This proposal could account for both the findings of a naturally occurring 5% SD base rate and an uncorrected 20% TD rate to yield a corrected net neuroleptic drug contribution of 15%.

On the other hand, the incidence rate of new cases of TD is remarkably consistent at approximately 3%–4% per year in the few studies that have evaluated this question prospectively (BARNES et al. 1983; KANE et al. 1984a).

3.4 Risk Factors

3.4.1 Patient Variables

Age, Sex, and Psychiatric Diagnosis. TD frequency increases with increasing age, and usually occurs more often in females (1.7:1.0 ratio). Affective disorders as a risk factor for TD have been noted in several reports (CASEY 1984a; KANE et al. 1984b). These observations suggest that schizophrenics may be less vulnerable to TD when compared to either other psychiatric patients or the nonpsychiatrically ill population exposed to neuroleptics.

3.4.2 Treatment Variables

Neuroleptic Dose and Duration of Treatment. Identifying a relationship between TD and parameters of drug exposure (i.e., total, average, or peak dose; duration of treatment) has been a complicated problem. Most retrospective studies looking at long treatment durations failed to find an association between drug measures and TD (BALDESSARINI et al. 1980; KANE and SMITH 1982). However, the few investigations showing a positive correlation evaluated short treatment periods of 3 years or less (CRANE and SMEETS 1974; TOENNIESSEN et al. 1985). This raises the possibility of a period of increased vulnerability. A recent study with a fixed age group (average = 65 years) showed that the largest increase in TD prevalence occurred in the first 3 years of neuroleptic treatment. There was no significant difference in TD in those patients treated between 5 and 25 years (TOENNIESSEN et al. 1985). In contrast, a prospective study in younger patients (average = 28 years) showed a steady annual incidence of 3%–4%, with equal vulnerability in all of the first 5 treatment years evaluated (KANE et al. 1984a). Perhaps the varying results in these two studies are due to the large age differences. The question of whether drug blood levels and TD are positively correlated cannot yet be answered.

Neuroleptic Drug Type. Several conflicting studies on drug types do not answer the question of whether one agent or chemical class is more or less liable to produce TD. Proponents of any particular perspective in the argument can marshal inadequate data to partially support their own view.

It is also unclear if the purportedly "atypical" neuroleptics such as clozapine will be less likely to cause TD. Sulpiride is another compound claiming atypical neuroleptic status, based in part on its low EPS rate (and speculated low TD risk). Alternatively, its EPS profile may be explained by low brain drug levels secondary to poor penetration of the blood-brain barrier. One conservative viewpoint is that any drug that suppresses TD, which sulpiride does, carries the risk of producing TD.

Hypotheses about different drug types, dopamine receptors, and neuronal pathways are intriguing and important, but they are not yet well enough established to guide clinical practice. Unfortunately, prospective studies comparing typical and atypical drugs are not available. In spite of this, the proposals about unique mechanisms are so attractive that they undoubtedly will and should be exploited in future studies.

Other Drug Factors. Periodically discontinuing neuroleptic treatment has been offered as a method for decreasing TD risk. However, this increases the risk of psychotic relapse and has been associated with the increased prevalence of irreversible TD (Jeste et al. 1979). There is no consensus about the etiologic role of anticholinergics in TD. Correlational data exist both for and against such an association (Kane and Smith 1982; Casey 1987a). Anticholinergic drugs may temporarily aggravate existing TD, but symptoms generally return to baseline levels when these drugs are discontinued.

Acute EPS have also been variably associated with TD risk. Identifying the relationship between acute EPS and the later evolution of TD will be difficult, because acute EPS are influenced by patient parameters, drug characteristics, and the widely divergent treatment and prophylaxis practices with anti-EPS drugs. The retrospective associations of anticholinergic agents and TD may actually be indirect measures of EPS and TD correlations since anticholinergics are used to treat EPS.

The role of organic brain disease, such as dementia or mental retardation, may be an additional risk factor for TD. Though these associations have been difficult to define, there is face validity to the rationale that existing deficits in an organ enhance the expression of other dysfunctions in the same organ.

3.5 Etiology

There is no direct evidence of central nervous system pathology to explain TD. Attempts to address this issue with radiological (CT scans), light-microscopic, endocrinological (prolactin and growth hormone), and biochemical (comparing D_1 and D_2 receptor numbers, cerebrospinal fluid) studies have not shown consistent significant differences between TD and non-TD patients (Casey 1987a). Therefore, theories about neuroleptics and TD have derived from indirect measures.

The most widely held theory of TD is the dopamine hypersensitivity hypothesis. This proposes that the nigrostriatal dopaminergic system becomes functionally overactive as a consequence of extended neuroleptic-induced dopamine receptor blockade. Though the human postmortem data comparing dopamine receptors in schizophrenic TD and non-TD patients do not support this hypothesis, there are ample clinical pharmacologic data to support a role for dopamine. Chronic neuroleptic treatment produces TD, acute neuroleptic treatment suppresses TD, and drug discontinuation may unmask TD. Similarly, acute dopamine agonists usually increase TD. The standard interpretation of these data is that dopamine has a primary role in TD. An alternate explanation of these observations is that dopamine plays a secondary or modulatory role on the as yet unknown primary pathophysiology of TD which may involve other neurotransmitters or neuroanatomical systems (Gerlach 1985; Casey 1987a).

Animal models of TD provide data both for and against the dopamine hypersensitivity hypothesis. Rodents show increased behavioral responses to dopamine agonists following dopamine antagonist treatment of a single dose, a few days, several weeks, and 1 year (Schelkunov 1967; Klawans and Rubovits 1972; Tarsy and Baldessarini 1973; Christensen et al. 1976; Clow et al. 1979). Furthermore, the changes seen in all these treatment periods are reversible. Biochemical changes of increased D_2 receptor numbers in the treated animals correlate with behavioral changes in most but not all studies (WADDINGTON et al. 1983). Many of these observations are not compatible with the essential clinical aspects of TD: symptoms without agonist provocation, individual vulnerability, late onset, and potential irreversibility.

Spontaneous chewing in rodents, which increases with neuroleptic treatment, has also been proposed as a model of TD (WADDINGTON et al. 1983). However, this has also been proposed as a paradigm for acute EPS (RUPNIAK et al. 1983). Other models include central nervous system destruction with unilateral 6-hydroxydopamine lesions and cortical ablation (UNGERSTEDT 1971; R. GLASSMAN and H. GLASSMAN 1980).

The cebus monkey model of TD most closely fits the human syndrome as it corresponds to the critical factors of symptom similarity, individual vulnerability, chronic neuroleptic treatment, and reversible/irreversible course (GUNNE and BARANY 1976; CASEY 1984b). Data from these studies suggest that γ-aminobutyric acid (GABA) as well as dopamine may be involved, since there was decreased glutamic acid decarboxylase in the substantia nigra, medial globus pallidus, and subthalamic nucleus in TD monkeys when compared to neuroleptic-treated but non-TD monkeys (GUNNE and HÄGGSTRÖM 1985).

A noradrenergic dysfunction theory of TD has also been proposed (JESTE et al. 1986). This derives in part from data showing significantly greater dopamine β-hydroxylase activity in TD patients than those without TD. Additionally, drugs which improve or aggravate TD affect both norepinephrine and dopamine.

With the notable exception of TD in monkeys, animal models of TD are more appropriately characterized as paradigms of acute and chronic neuroleptic treatment. Though the purported rodent models of TD are almost uniformly accepted, they are limited by many findings which are not compatible with the clinical TD syndrome. Many of the data from animal models could be used to argue that the observed behavioral and biochemical changes underlie either the acute EPS side effects or the desirable therapeutic antipsychotic actions, rather than only correlate with the undesirable TD effect (CASEY 1985a).

3.6 Treatment

There is no uniformly safe and effective treatment for TD. The long list of agents used to investigate the pharmacology and possible therapeutic approaches for TD attests to their general ineffectiveness for many patients (GERLACH et al. 1986). From these studies one can conclude that there are either many treatments for TD or that there are no treatments for TD.

Reducing dopamine function is the most effective way of suppressing TD. However, this strategy, whether by presynaptic depletion (tetrabenazine, reserpine) or postsynaptic blockade (neuroleptics), is not recommended for the sole purpose of suppressing TD unless symptoms are severe and distressing. The concern is that treatment aimed only at symptom suppression may aggravate TD or limit the possibility of spontaneous recovery. However, when psychosis and TD are present, neuroleptics in the lowest effective doses are indicated in those patients who have benefited from previous neuroleptic treatment.

The conceptually attractive approach of desensitizing the hypersensitive dopamine system by treatment with dopamine agonists has mostly been unsuccessful. These results may lend further support to the proposal that dopamine hypersensitivity is not the primary pathophysiology underlying TD.

Other compounds which affect acetylcholine, GABA, serotonin, the α- and β-adrenergic receptors, neuropeptides, opiates, and other drugs, have all produced variable and inconsistent results (JESTE and WYATT 1982; CASEY 1985d; GERLACH et al. 1986).

3.7 Long-Term Outcome

It is widely believed that continued neuroleptic treatment will inevitably worsen TD. This has led to admonitions against using neuroleptic drugs in all patients with TD, but produces the unacceptable consequences of inadequately treated psychotic patients. However, the reversible course of TD, even in some patients continuing neuroleptic therapy, has been recognized since the earliest reports (UHRBRAND and FAURBYE 1960).

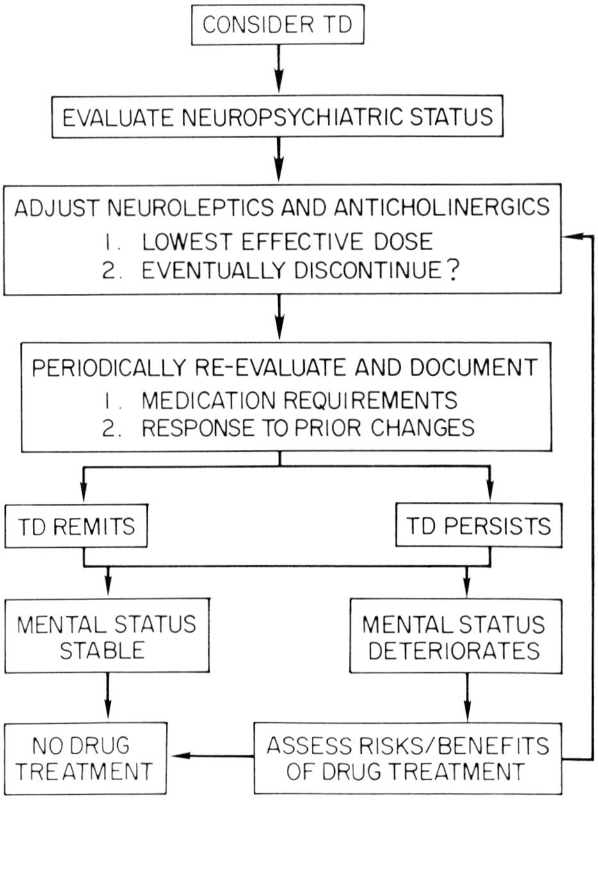

Fig. 2. An algorithm for managing tardive dyskinesia (TD). (From CASEY and GERLACH 1984, Fig. 1, p. 184)

Improvement across studies varies widely from 0%–92% (CASEY 1985c). As in the prevalence of TD onset, this range undoubtedly reflects multiple factors of patient, drug, and time variables. Younger patients are more likely to improve, whereas older patients are less likely to do so. Yet, this trend does not exclude symptom resolution in any age group, as some elderly patients have had TD improve over 5–8 years. Duration of follow-up and degree of improvement are positively associated (CASEY et al. 1986). Discontinuing neuroleptic drugs and early recognition are also directly correlated with a favorable outcome (QUITKIN et al. 1977; KANE et al. 1986).

These data offer some reason for cautious optimism in TD. Neuroleptic drugs, with an emphasis on the lowest effective dose (Fig. 2), can be used to treat psychosis and not inevitably aggravate or produce irreversible TD.

4 Summary

The motor side effects are the major limitations of neuroleptic drugs. Acute EPS of dystonia, parkinsonism, and akathisia, which occur in up to 90% of patients, are the major causes of treatment-related problems, though TD has been more the focus of attention in the past decade. Each of the acute and late-developing syndromes has its own clinical characteristics, underlying pathophysiology, risk factors, treatment strategies, and outcomes. Far more research is needed on all these syndromes before developing a cohesive, unified explanation of motor system dysfunction and antipsychotic drug effects.

New drugs which act through different mechanisms are clearly needed. One important impediment to achieving this goal is the lack of precise screening models. It is not yet clear if the models of catalepsy and reversal of stimulant-induced stereotypy are selecting for compounds which have motor effects and/or antipsychotic properties. The high correlations between these two characteristics suggest that the currently available drugs, with rare notable exceptions, have been selected primarily on the basis of motor system involvement.

Finding new drugs without good screening tools is a substantial challenge, but well worth the effort. A drug which treats schizophrenia effectively and is free of extrapyramidal side effects (a non neuroleptic neuroleptic) will be a giant step forward in knowledge and patient care.

Acknowledgments. This work was supported in part by funds from the Veterans Administration Research Program (DEC and GAK) and by NIMH grant MH36657 (DEC). M. Karr prepared the typescript.

References

Ayd FJ (1961) A survey of drug-induced extrapyramidal reactions. JAMA 175:1054–1060

Baker LA, Cheng LY, Amara IB (1983) The withdrawal of benztropine mesylate in chronic schizophrenic patients. Br J Psychiatry 143:584–590

Baldessarini RJ, Cole JO, Davis JM, Gardos G, Preskorn SH, Simpson GM, Tarsy D (1980) Tardive dyskinesia: a task force report. American Psychiatric Press, Washington DC

Bamrah JS, Kumar V, Krska J, Soni SD (1986) Interactions between procyclidine and neuroleptic drugs. Br J Psychiatry 149:726–733

Barnes TRE, Braude WM (1985) Akathisia variants and tardive dyskinesia. Arch Gen Psychiatry 42:874–878

Barnes TRE, Kidger T, Gore SM (1983) Tardive dyskinesia: a 3-year follow-up study. Psychol Med 13:71–81

Bleuler E (1950) Dementia praecox or the group of schizophrenias. International Universities Press, New York, p 191

Boyer WF, Bakalar NH, Lake CR (1987) Anticholinergic prophylaxis of acute haloperidol-induced dystonic reactions. J Clin Psychopharmacol 7:164–166

Burke RE, Fahn S, Jankovic J, Marsden CD, Lang AE, Gollomp S, Ilson J (1982) Tardive dystonia: late-onset and persistent dystonia caused by antipsychotic drugs. Neurology 32:1335–1346

Casey DE (1981) The differential diagnosis of tardive dyskinesia. Acta Psychiat Scand 63 [Suppl 291):71–87

Casey DE (1984a) Tardive dyskinesia and affective disorders. In: Gardos G, Casey DE (eds) Tardive dyskinesia and affective disorders. American Psychiatric Press, Washington DC, pp 1–20

Casey DE (1984b) Tardive dyskinesia – animal models. Psychopharmacol Bull 20:376–379

Casey DE (1985a) Behavioral effects of long-term neuroleptic treatment in cebus monkeys. In: Casey DE, Chase T, Christensen AV, Gerlach J (eds) Dyskinesia: research and treatment. Springer, Berlin Heidelberg New York, pp 211–216

Casey DE (1985b) Spontaneous and tardive dyskinesia: clinical and laboratory studies. J Clin Psychiatry 46(4):42–47

Casey DE (1985c) Tardive dyskinesia: reversible and irreversible. In: Casey DE, Chase T, Christensen AV, Gerlach J (eds) Dyskinesia: research and treatment. Springer, Berlin Heidelberg New York, pp 88–97

Casey DE (1985d) Tardive dyskinesia: nondopaminergic treatment approaches. In: Casey DE, Chase T, Christensen AV, Gerlach J (eds) Dyskinesia: research and treatment. Springer, Berlin Heidelberg New York, pp 137–144

Casey DE (1987a) Tardive dyskinesia. In: Meltzer H (ed) Psychopharmacology: The third generation of progress. Raven, New York, pp 1411–1419

Casey DE (1987b) Neuroleptic-induced parkinsonism increases with repeated treatment in monkeys. In: Dahl SG, Gram LF, Paul SM, Potter WZ (eds) Clinical pharmacology in psychiatry IV. Selectivity in psychotropic drug action – promise or problems. Springer, Berlin Heidelberg New York, pp 243–247

Casey DE, Denney D (1977) Pharmacological characterization of tardive dyskinesia. Psychopharmacology (Berlin) 54:1–8

Casey DE, Gerlach J (1984) Tardive dyskinesia. In: Stancer HC, Garfinkel PE, Rakoff VM (eds) Guidelines for the use of psychotropic drugs: a clinical handbook. Spectrum, Jamaica, NY, pp 183–203

Casey DE, Hansen TE (1984) Spontaneous dyskinesias. In: Jeste DV, Wyatt RJ (eds) Neuropsychiatric movement disorders. American Psychiatric Press, Washington DC, pp 68–95

Casey DE, Gerlach J, Christensson E (1980) Dopamine, acetylcholine, and GABA effects in acute dystonia in primates. Psychopharmacology (Berlin) 70:83–87

Casey DE, Povlsen UJ, Meidahl B, Gerlach J (1986) Neuroleptic-induced tardive dyskinesia and parkinsonism: changes during several years of continuing treatment. Psychopharmacol Bull 22:250–253

Christensen AV, Fjalland B, Moller Nielsen I (1976) On the supersensitivity of dopamine receptors induced by neuroleptics. Psychopharmacology (Berlin) 48:1–6

Clow A, Jenner P, Marsden CD (1979) Changes in dopamine-mediated behavior during one year's neuroleptic administration. Eur J Pharmacol 57:365–375

Crane GE, Smeets RA (1974) Tardive dyskinesia and drug therapy in geriatric patients. Arch Gen Psychiatry 30:341–343

Crow TJ, Cross AJ, Johnstone EC, Owen F, Owens DG, Waddington JL (1982) Abnormal involuntary movements in schizophrenia: are they related to the disease process or its treatment? Are they associated with changes in dopamine receptors? J Clin Psychopharmacol 2:336–340
Faurbye A, Rasch PJ, Bender Peterson P, Brandenborg G, Pakkenberg H (1964) Neurologic symptoms in the pharmacotherapy of psychoses. Acta Psychiatr Scand 40:10–26
Garver DL, Davis JM, Dekirmenjian H, Ericksen S, Gosengeld L, Haraszti J (1976) Dystonic reactions following neuroleptics: time course and proposed mechanisms. Psychopharmacology (Berlin) 47:199–201
Gerlach J (1985) Pathophysiological mechanisms underlying tardive dyskinesia. In: Casey DE, Chase T, Christensen AV, Gerlach J (eds) Dyskinesia: research and treatment. Springer, Berlin Heidelberg New York, pp 98–103
Gerlach J, Reisby N, Randrup A (1974) Dopaminergic hypersensitivity and cholinergic hypofunction in the pathophysiology of tardive dyskinesia. Psychopharmacologia (Berlin) 34:21–35
Gerlach J, Casey DE, Korsgaard S (1986) Tardive dyskinesia: epidemiology, pathophysiology, and pharmacology. In: Shah NS, Donald AG (eds) Movement disorders. Plenum, New York, pp 119–147
Glassman RB, Glassman HN (1980) Oral dyskinesia in brain-damaged rats withdrawn from a neuroleptic: implication for models of tardive dyskinesia. Psychopharmacology (Berlin) 69:19–25
Gunne LM, Barany S (1976) Haloperidol-induced tardive dyskinesia in monkeys. Psychopharmacology (Berlin) 50:237–240
Gunne LM, Häggström JE (1985) Pathophysiology of tardive dyskinesia. In: Casey DE, Chase T, Christensen AV, Gerlach J (eds) Dyskinesia: research and treatment. Springer, Berlin Heidelberg New York, pp 191–193
Hansen LB, Larsen NE, Vestergard P (1981) Plasma levels of perphenazine (Trilafon) related to development of extrapyramidal side effects. Psychopharmacology (Berlin) 74:306–309
Hansen TE, Casey DE, Vollmer W (1986) Is there an epidemic of tardive dyskinesia? In: Casey DE, Gardos G (eds) Tardive dyskinesia and neuroleptics: from dogma to reason. American Psychiatric Press, Washington DC, pp 2–14
Jellinek T, Gardos G, Cole JO (1981) Adverse effects of antiparkinson drug withdrawal. Am J Psychiatry 138:1567–1571
Jeste DV, Wyatt RJ (1982) Therapeutic strategies against tardive dyskinesia. Arch Gen Psychiatry 39:803–816
Jeste DV, Potkin SG, Sinha S, Feder S, Wyatt RJ (1979) Tardive dyskinesia – reversible and irreversible. Arch Gen Psychiatry 36:585–590
Jeste DV, Lohr JB, Kaufmann CA, Wyatt RJ (1986) Pathophysiology of tardive dyskinesia: evaluation of supersensitivity theory and alternative hypotheses. In: Casey DE, Gardos G (eds) Tardive dyskinesia and neuroleptics: from dogma to reason. American Psychiatric Press, Washington DC, pp 15–32
Kane JM, Smith JM (1982) Tardive dyskinesia: prevalence and risk factors, 1959 to 1979. Arch Gen Psychiatry 39:473–481
Kane JM, Woerner M, Weinhold P, Wegner J, Kinon B, Borenstein M (1984a) Incidence of tardive dyskinesia: five-year data from a prospective study. Psychopharmacol Bull 20:387–389
Kane JM, Woerner M, Weinhold P, Kinon B, Lieberman J, Borenstein M (1984b) Incidence and severity of tardive dyskinesia in affective illness. In: Gardos G, Casey DE (eds) Tardive dyskinesia and affective illness. American Psychiatric Press, Washington DC, pp 22–28
Kane JM, Woerner M, Sarantakos S, Kinon B, Lieberman J (1986) Do low-dose neuroleptics prevent or ameliorate tardive dyskinesia? In: Casey DE, Gardos G (eds) Tardive dyskinesia and neuroleptics: from dogma to reason. American Psychiatric Press, Washington DC, pp 99–108
Keepers GA, Casey DE (1986) Clinical management of acute neuroleptic-induced extrapyramidal syndromes. In: Masserman JH (ed) Current psychiatric therapies. Grune and Stratton, New York, pp 139–157
Keepers GA, Clappison VJ, Casey DE (1983) Initial anticholinergic prophylaxis for neuroleptic-induced extrapyramidal syndromes. Arch Gen Psychiatry 40:1113–1117

Keepers GA, Hansen TE, Casey DE (1986) Prospective prediction of vulnerability to neuroleptic-induced extrapyramidal syndromes. Proc Soc Biol Psychiatry 170:222

Klawans HL, Rubovits R (1972) An experimental model of tardive dyskinesia. J Neural Transm 33:235–246

Kraepelin E (1907) Clinical psychiatry. MacMillan, New York, p 229

Lipinski JF, Zubenko GS, Cohen BM, Barreira PJ (1984) Propranolol in the treatment of neuroleptic-induced akathisia. Am J Psychiatry 141:412–415

Manos N, Gkiouzepas J, Tzotzoras T, Tzanetoglou A (1981) Gradual withdrawal of antiparkinson medication in chronic schizophrenics: any better than the abrupt? J Nerv Ment Dis 169:659–661

Manos N, Lavrentiadis G, Gkiouzepas J (1986) Evaluation of the need for prophylactic antiparkinsonian medication in psychotic patients treated with neuroleptics. J Clin Psychiatry 47:114–116

McEvoy JP (1983) The clinical use of anticholinergic drugs as treatment for extrapyramidal side effects of neuroleptic disorders. J Clin Psychopharmacol 3:288–302

McInnis M, Petursson H (1985) Withdrawal of trihexyphenidyl. Acta Psychiatr Scand 71:297–303

Moleman P, Schmitz PJM, Ladee GA (1982) Extrapyramidal side effects and oral haloperidol: an analysis of explanatory patient and treatment characteristics. J Clin Psychiatry 43:492–496

Orlov P, Kasparian G, DiMascio A, Cole JO (1971) Withdrawal of antipsychotic drugs. Arch Gen Psychiatry 25:410–412

Owens DGC, Johnstone EC, Frith CD (1982) Spontaneous involuntary disorders of movement. Arch Gen Psychiatry 39:452–461

Quitkin F, Rifkin A, Gochfeld L, Klein DF (1977) Tardive dyskinesia: are first signs reversible? Am J Psychiatry 134:84–87

Rupniak NMJ, Jenner P, Marsden CD (1983) Cholinergic manipulation of perioral behavior induced by chronic neuroleptic administration to rats. Psychopharmacology (Berlin) 79:226–230

Rupniak NMJ, Jenner P, Marsden CD (1986) Acute dystonia induced by neuroleptic drugs. Psychopharmacology (Berlin) 88:403–419

Sayers AC, Burki HR, Ruch W, Asper H (1976) Anticholinergic properties of antipsychotic drugs and their relation to extrapyramidal side effects. Psychopharmacology (Berlin) 51:15–22

Schelkunov EL (1967) Adrenergic effect of chronic administration of neuroleptics. Nature 214:1210–1212

Schönecker M (1957) Ein eigentümliches Syndrom im oralen Bereich bei Megaphen-Applikation. Nervenarzt 28:35–36

Sigwald J, Bouttier D, Raymondeaud C (1959) Quatre cas de dyskinesie facio-bucco-linguo-masticatrice à l'évolution prolongée secondaire à un traitement par les neuroleptiques. Rev Neurol (Paris) 100:751–755

Snyder S, Greenberg D, Yamamura H (1974) Antischizophrenic drugs and brain cholinergic receptors. Arch Gen Psychiatry 31:58–61

Sovner R, DiMascio (1978) Extrapyramidal syndromes and other neurological side effects of psychotropic drugs. In: Lipton MA, DiMascio A, Killam DK (eds) Psychopharmacology: a generation of progress. Raven, New York, pp 1021–1032

Sramek JJ, Simpson GM, Morrison RL, Heiser JF (1986) Anticholinergic agents for prophylaxis of neuroleptic-induced dystonic reactions: a prospective study. J Clin Psychiatry 47:305–309

Tarsy D, Baldessarini RJ (1973) Pharmacologically induced behavioral supersensitivity to apomorphine. Nature 245:262–263

Toenniessen LM, Casey DE, McFarland BH (1985) Tardive dyskinesia in the aged. Arch Gen Psychiatry 42:278–284

Tune L, Coyle JT (1981) Acute extrapyramidal side effects: serum levels of neuroleptics. Psychopharmacology (Berlin) 75:9–15

Uhrbrand L, Faurbye A (1960) Reversible and irreversible dyskinesia after treatment with perphenazine, chlorpromazine, reserpine, and electroconvulsive therapy. Psychopharmacologia (Berlin) 1:408–418

Ungerstedt U (1971) Post-synaptic supersensitivity after 6-hydroxydopamine-induced degeneration of the nigrostriatal dopamine system. Acta Physiol Scand 82 [Suppl] 367:69–93
Van Putten T, Mutalipassi LR, Malkin MD (1974) Phenothiazine-induced decompensation. Arch Gen Psychiatry 30:102–105
Villeneuve A (1972) The rabbit syndrome: a peculiar extrapyramidal reaction. Can Psychiatr Assoc J 17:69–72
Waddington JL, Cross AJ, Gamble SJ, Bourne RC (1983) Spontaneous orofacial dyskinesia and dopaminergic function in rats after 6 months of neuroleptic treatment. Science 220:530–532
Winslow RS, Stillner V, Coons DJ, Robinson MW (1986) Prevention of acute dystonic reactions in patients beginning high-potency neuroleptics. Am J Psychiatry 143:706–710

Future Treatment of Schizophrenia

J. GERLACH

Abstract

In spite of 35 years of experience with antipsychotic drugs, the psychiatrists are still faced with the limitations of these drugs: no or minimal therapeutic effect in hallucinations and delusions in about 25% of schizophrenic patients; persisting anergia and emotional withdrawal in otherwise successfully treated patients; a great spectrum of side effects, some irreversible. Quo vadis? An incidental discovery of a completely new drug, a new "chlorpromazine" would be the ideal solution, but for the present, one has to continue with the small pragmatic steps, especially within the following areas: (a) the selective antidopaminergic drugs, especially the substituted benzamides, may be further developed in the direction of antipsychotic selectivity with fewer and fewer extrapyramidal side effects; (b) the atypical clozapine ought soon to have successors, hopefully without the risk of bone marrow depression and cardiovascular side effects; (c) the D_1 antagonists as well as the D_1 agonists may imply therapeutically valuable effects; (d) the dopamine autoreceptor has long been in focus, but until now, no pure agonist has been found, and the drugs available, including (−)3-PPP, appear to have many side effects; (e) serotonin antagonists may be an interesting possibility; and (f) when it may be possible to influence brain peptides more efficiently than up to now, this area will probably provide us with several psychotropic drugs. Furthermore, during the search for new antipsychotic drugs, one must not forget to improve the practical use of available neuroleptics and of nonpharmacological, psychosocial treatment modalities.

1 Introduction

The treatment of schizophrenia has changed dramatically over the past 200 years: from primitive torture-like procedures such as the "rotating bed" and the "surprising bath" at the beginning of the nineteenth century over different treatment cures with drugs [including opium (1855), barbiturates (1903), and insuline (1934)] and electroconvulsive stimulation (1938) to the discovery of chlorpromazine, the first neuroleptic drug, in 1952. The neuroleptics became a milestone in the development of treatment of schizophrenia. These drugs could suppress or totally eliminate hallucinations, delusions and psychomotor unrest and changed the hospital milieu, which gradually became calm and useful for psychosocial treatment efforts. About two-thirds of the otherwise chronically hospitalised schizophrenic patients could be discharged over the following decade and treated from an out-patient clinic.

However, in spite of the striking improvements in the treatment of schizophrenia, there are still limitations: about 25% of the schizophrenic patients do not re-

---

Sankt Hans Hospital, Department 2, DK-4000 Roskilde, Denmark.

spond to neuroleptic treatment and may still suffer from hallucinations and paranoid ideas, some of them have to spend most of their lives in institutions, and in spite of good symptom reduction, most schizophrenics remain socially isolated and inactive. Furthermore, neuroleptics may induce serious side effects which hamper their utility in both short-term and long-term treatment. So we are still far from a satisfactory treatment of schizophrenia.

What can be expected from the future treatment of schizophrenia? If we could look in a "crystal ball", we might have the best answer. Maybe we would see a completely new drug, discovered incidentally, a drug which would not only remove the hallucinations and paranoid ideas, but would also make the schizophrenics active and talking, living happily in the society. However, until this crystal ball vision comes through, we have to deal with the more pragmatic issues, the small steps forward in the research of schizophrenic treatments.

In the following I shall deal with the following areas: (a) the new dopamine (DA)-selective and the new "broad-spectrum" antipsychotic drugs; (b) potentially new antipsychotic drugs acting in the DA system in an atypical way or on other transmitter systems; (c) improvement in the use of traditional neuroleptics; and (d) improvement of the nonpharmacological therapy.

2 New "Atypical" Antipsychotic Drugs

In the past decade, traditional neuroleptics have been modified along two parameters: the development of increasingly selective antidopaminergic drugs (e.g. sulpiride), and diminution of the antidopaminergic component of neuroleptic drugs together with an increase of antiserotonergic and antinoradrenergic potency (e.g. clozapine). These two types of antipsychotic medication have been united under the term "atypical neuroleptics", but they have no common pharmacological profile. The only common feature appears to be a relatively low level of extrapyramidal side effects.

2.1 DA Receptor-Selective Neuroleptics

The DA receptor-selective antipsychotics are characterised by a traditional antipsychotic effect combined with a low level of autonomic and sedating side effects. The antidopaminergic action of these drugs provides for an antipsychotic effect, while the lack of anticholinergic and antinoradrenergic actions results in few autonomic and cardiovascular side effects. Furthermore, the putative selectivity of some of these compounds for subgroups of D_2 receptors may result in relatively few extrapyramidal side effects.

The substituted benzamides represent a group of neuroleptics characterised by DA receptor selectivity. Sulpiride is the oldest and clinically most established member of this group. It is characterised by the following pharmacological properties:

- It binds to a functional subgroup of D_2 receptors (SEDVALL 1984).

- It increases brain DA turnover in rodents and humans, similarly to other neuroleptics (SEDVALL 1984).
- At relatively low doses, it inhibits apomorphine-induced locomotion, while higher doses are needed to counteract apomorphine-induced stereotyped behaviour. Even in very high doses, the drug induces only weak or atypical catalepsy. Traditional neuroleptics like haloperidol produce all three types of behaviour at the same dose level (ÖGREN et al. 1986). Sulpiride may even aggravate amphetamine-induced stereotyped behaviour.
- With long-term treatment, it induces no increase in D_2 receptors, but a significant increase in D_1 receptors, in contrast to traditional neuroleptics like haloperidol, which elevates the D_2 but not the D_1 receptors (JENNER et al. 1985).

How do these biochemical data relate to the clinical effect of sulpiride? In double-blind studies, sulpiride (800–2400 mg/day) has been shown to have an antipsychotic effect in chronic schizophrenic patients not significantly different from that of chlorpromazine, haloperidol and trifluoperazine (SEDVALL 1984). Figure 1 illustates the effects of sulpiride and haloperidol in a double-blind cross-over study of 20 chronic schizophrenic patients (GERLACH et al. 1985). The antipsychotic effect of the two drugs is not significantly different.

The antipsychotic effect of sulpiride appears to be best in relatively young and acute schizophrenic patients, while chronic and severely disturbed patients re-

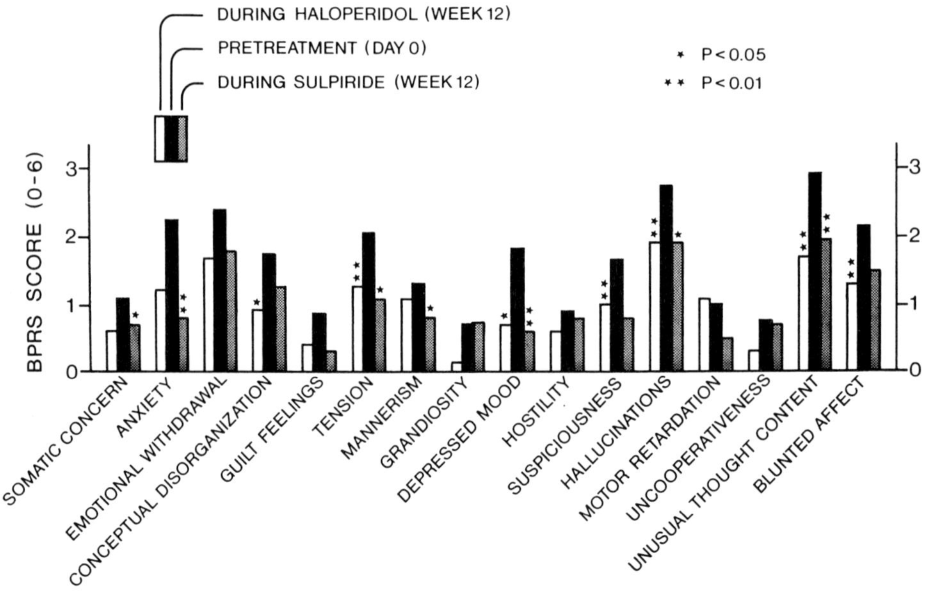

Fig. 1. Mean brief psychiatric rating scale (BPRS) scores before and following treatment with sulpiride (800–3200 mg/day) and haloperidol (6–24 mg/day) ($n = 20$). The drugs were given in randomised order in two 12-week periods, each preceded by drug-free periods (until relapse) (GERLACH et al. 1985). The significance signs above the bars indicate the difference between rating at day 0 and day 82: *$p < 0.05$; **$p < 0.01$. No significant differences were found between sulpiride and haloperidol

spond less favourably. There are few autonomic and cardiovascular side effects, corresponding to low-dose neuroleptics like haloperidol. The potential advantage of sulpiride appears to be a relatively low level of parkinsonism, although most studies only showed a trend in this direction. Another advantage may be an anti-autistic and an antidepressant effect related to sulpiride in small–moderate doses (200–600 mg) (SEDVALL 1984).

It has been claimed that sulpiride should be less liable to produce tardive dyskinesia (TD) than traditional neuroleptics. This assertion has been based on the following observations: sulpiride induces no or weak DA supersensitivity in rodents; sulpiride suppresses TD without subsequent rebound aggravation (studied in one cebus monkey with TD); uncontrolled observations worldwide indicate that only six patients have developed TD during sulpiride treatment (SEDVALL 1984). However, TD may not be related to DA supersensitivity or to rebound aggravation (GERLACH et al. 1986), and uncontrolled observations are not useful for reliable conclusions. Therefore, the relationship between sulpiride and TD has to be re-evaluated. The biochemical selectivity of sulpiride may well lead to a relatively low TD-inducing capacity.

Sulpiride is not an ideal antipsychotic drug. It has a relatively low lipophilicity and must be given in high doses in order to penetrate the blood-brain barrier in sufficient amounts. The peripheral consequences of these high doses appear to be small, but a marked prolactin secretion is a significant drawback. About a quarter of the females treated with sulpiride developed breast tension, galactorrhea, and/or amenorrhea. Another drawback of sulpiride is a low elimination half-time (7 h) which makes it necessary to give the drug relatively frequently. Maybe new substituted benzamides such as amisulpiride, remoxipride, and raclopride represent improvements in this respect. Pilot studies support this view, and controlled studies are under way.

The advantage of the D_2 DA-selective neuroleptics lies in their few side effects and their antipsychotic effect, preferentially in the so-called type I schizophrenia without neurological and intellectual deficiencies or organic defects. Maybe these drugs can contribute to separation of different subtypes of schizophrenia and of the mechanisms underlying different extrapyramidal symptoms such as parkinsonism and akathisia, and maybe they can elucidate the question about "psychotic" versus "extrapyramidal" DA receptors. That is in the future! However, the D_2-selective antagonists will hardly bring us new drugs more therapeutically effective than the existing traditional neuroleptics.

2.2 Broad-Spectrum, Nonselective Neuroleptics

The most important drug in this group is clozapine which has been the subject of a lot of animal and clinical experiments over the past 20 years. Due to the risk of agrunulocytosis, laboratories around the world have tried intensively to develop new antipsychotic drugs with clozapine-like properties, but hitherto with limited success. Therefore, clozapine appears to remain – with its advantages and its disadvantages – the principal *atypical* broad-spectrum neuroleptic with an antipsychotic effect in otherwise therapy-resistant schizophrenic patients.

Clozapine belongs to the chemical class of dibenzoazepines which also includes powerful traditional neuroleptics such as loxapine and clothiapine (BÜRKI et al. 1977). The main pharmacological characteristics of this drug are as follows:

- Clozapine binds to several types of receptors, especially serotonin (S_2), α_1-adrenergic and histaminergic (H_1) receptors (HYTTEL et al. 1985). D_1 and D_2 receptors are affected to a smaller degree, and the binding to DA receptors appears to be more loose than that for other neuroleptics (HARTVIG et al. 1986).
- In relatively low doses (up to 225 mg/day), it apparently decreases the DA turnover as shown by a decreased homovanillic acid (HVA) concentration in the cerebrospinal fluid (GERLACH et al. 1975). Higher doses of clozapine increase DA turnover like other neuroleptics (SEDVALL et al. 1978).
- Clozapine produces no catalepsy. It inhibits the locomotion, but not the stereotypies induced by apomorphine (BURKI et al. 1977). Like sulpiride, it may even potentiate amphetamine-induced stereotypy (ROBERTSON and MACDONALD 1984).
- With chronic treatment, clozapine produces no increase in D_2 receptors, but like sulpiride, it may increase D_1 receptors (JENNER et al. 1985).

Controlled clinical trials at the beginning of the 1970s demonstrated that the antipsychotic effect of clozapine was at least equal to, and often greater than,

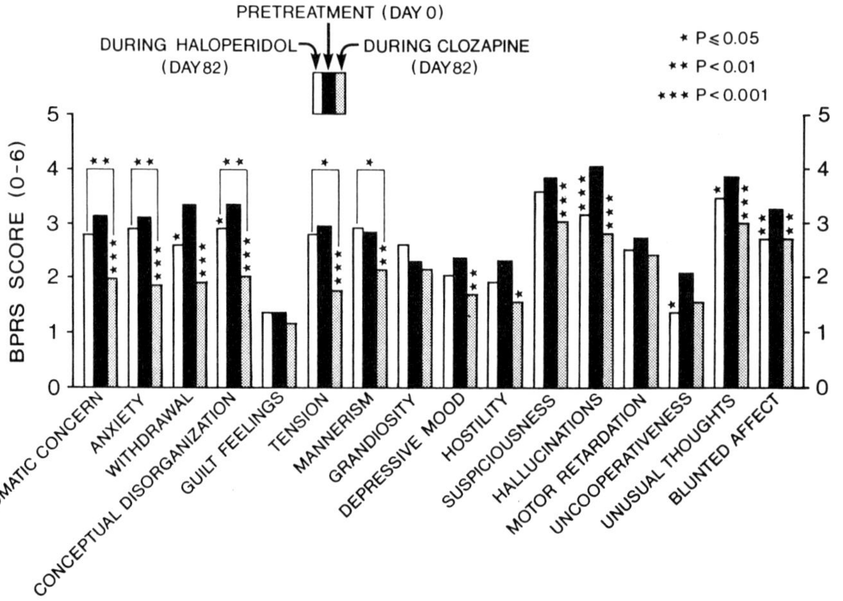

Fig. 2. Mean BPRS scores before and following treatment with clozapine (100–800 mg/day) and haloperidol (3–32 mg/day) ($n = 20$). The drugs were given in randomised order in two 12-week periods, each preceded by drug-free periods (until relapse) (GERLACH et al. 1974). The significance signs above the bars indicate the difference between ratings at day 0 and day 82 (week 12): *$p<0.05$; **$p<0.01$; ***$p<0.001$). In five items, a significant difference was found between clozapine and haloperidol

comparable effects with other neuroleptics like chlorpromazine, levomepromazine, thioridazine and haloperidol (ANGST et al. 1971; GERLACH et al. 1974). It caused a highly significant reduction not only in the productive schizophrenic symptoms, but in anxiety and tension as well. In addition, significant effects were noted on negative symptoms of emotional withdrawal and blunted affect (see Fig. 2). The therapeutic advantage of clozapine appeared to be most pronounced in the severely disturbed patients who, in addition to their schizophrenic symptoms, suffered from anxiety, tension and psychomotor restlessness. Clozapine brought about an often desirable relaxation and sedation, whereas traditional neuroleptics like haloperidol might have caused akathisia, often associated with anxiety and tension. At the recommended dose level (up to 600 mg/day), clozapine does not induce extrapyramidal side effects, although some slowing of movements and reduced facial expression may be related to the sedative effect. Clozapine may even counteract tremor, not only parkinsonian tremor, but also essential tremor (12.5–75 mg/day) (PAKKENBERG and PAKKENBERG 1986).

Clozapine appears to be useful in the prevention and treatment of TD. Available evidence from monkey and human studies indicates that clozapine is the least likely of all antipsychotics available to induce TD (GERLACH et al. 1986). In developed TD, clozapine in low doses (50–250 mg/day) has no direct dyskinesia-suppressing effect, but may allow a spontaneous recovery of the syndrome without aggravating the primary pathophysiological process underlying the syndrome. In higher doses (400–900 mg/day), clozapine can dampen TD moderately, but in general, due to the side effects, such a high-dose treatment cannot be recommended for elderly TD patients. Only in patients suffering from a combination of severe psychotic symptoms and TD, maybe associated with a brain damage, clozapine in relatively high doses may lead to improvement of all symptoms.

Clozapine strongly influences cardiovascular and autonomic functions. It may cause a fall in orthostatic blood pressure and sinus tachycardia. The ECG often shows a flattening or inversion of the T-waves. In rare cases, bundle branch block may occur. These ECG changes diminish slightly during the treatment period and disappear following the discontinuation of the drug. It appears, but has not been proven, that these cardiovascular effects are a little more pronounced for clozapine than for other high-dose neuroleptics. The most unpleasant autonomic side effects are hypersalivation and constipation, but also weight gain should be remembered.

Since the introduction of increased haematological surveillance and tightly restricted utilization following eight deaths in Finland due to agranulocytosis, there has been a drastic decrease in the number of cases of bone marrow suppression, from 0.4 to below 0.1 per 1000, corresponding to the risk of other neuroleptic drugs (KRUPP and MONKA 1982).

Clozapine represents a unique therapeutic potential in severely psychotic patients suffering from productive symptoms in combination with anxiety and tension. The drug appears to be particularly advantageous in psychotic patients with brain damage (large ventricles) and abnormal involuntary movements, patients who do not respond favourably to a traditional neuroleptic treatment, partly due to disturbing akathisia. However, it should always be kept in mind that the drug may have serious side effects, especially autonomic, cardiovascular, and in rare cases, haematological side effects which necessitate close observation and blood monitoring, especially during the first 3 months.

Other broad-spectrum neuroleptics have been developed in order to follow up the success of clozapine. This applies for example to fluperlapine and BW 234 U which both demonstrated antipsychotic properties and only weak extrapyramidal side effects. Unfortunately, like clozapine, both drugs demonstrated the potential for inducing granulocytopenia, so further clinical development had to be stopped. Hopefully, new drugs in this category will be introduced in the near future.

3 Potential New Antipsychotic Drugs

New drugs acting on the DA system in a way different from the D_2 receptor blockade or drugs influencing other neurotransmitters are under development and have been clinically tested in some cases. Some of these drug and treatment principles will be briefly mentioned in the following sections.

3.1 DA D_1 Antagonists and Agonists

Some neuroleptic drugs, especially the thioxanthenes, block D_1 receptors in addition to the D_2 receptor blockage. According to studies in rodents, the D_1-blocking component counteracts the development of DA supersensitivity and tolerance (CHRISTENSEN et al. 1985). This could be an advantage for an antipsychotic drug. In clinical practice, however, no differences have yet been disclosed between neuroleptics with and without a D_1-blocking component, and in monkeys and rodents, single doses of the pure D_1 antagonist (SCH 23390) causes the same extrapyramidal symptoms (dystonia and catalepsy) as a traditional neuroleptic like haloperidol (CHRISTENSEN et al. 1985; WADDINGTON 1986; GERLACH et al. 1987). However, SCH 23390 in long-term administration seems to induce less extrapyramidal effects (unpublished), so D_1 antagonists may certainly have clinical relevance.

A partial D_1 agonist (SKF 38393) has shown interesting behavioral effects in Cebus monkeys (GERLACH et al. 1987). Thus, SKF 38393 causes slight sedation and counteracts stereotypies induced by a D_2 agonist (LY 171555), and it produces oral dyskinesias. In untreated rodents, SKF 38393 elicits grooming, sniffing, and, more seldom, mouth movements (WADDINGTON 1986), and in catecholamine-depleted animals, it causes hyperactivity and circling behaviour (ARNT and HYTTEL 1986). Although these discrepanies can be explained by the different research methodologies, it may be concluded that experiments with full D_1 agonist are necessary before further speculations on the possibilities of D_1 drugs in schizophrenia.

3.2 Presynaptic Antidopaminergic Drugs

Reserpine and tetrabenazine deplete the catecholamines from nerve terminals, thus reducing availability of DA in the synapse. *α-Methylparatyrosine,* which inhibits the synthesis of DA, has the same principal effect. These drugs can potentiate the effects of a traditional postsynaptic DA receptor blockade, so that the dose of the receptor-blocking drug can be reduced, but they do not add to the qualitative therapeutic effect. Furthermore, reserpine and tetrabenazine cause hypotension and depression, and α-methylparatyrosine causes renal side effects. The conclusion seems to be that there is no or minimal clinical advantage in using such a combined post- and presynaptic treatment.

Another presynaptic strategy is to stimulate the *DA autoreceptor*. This reduces DA synthesis and release, inhibits DA neuronal firing and diminishes DA-mediated animal behaviours. Clinical trials with small doses of DA agonists with preferentially presynaptic effect, especially apomorphine, have shown varying response from a significant antipsychotic effect to no effect and even worsening of psychotic symptoms. And later studies with nonapomorphine DA agonists have all been negative.

The development of 3-(3-hydroxyphenyl-*N*-*n*-propylpiperidine (3-PPP) has renewed the interest in the development of presynaptic-acting antipsychotic drugs. The (−)enantiomer is of special interest because, in small doses, it has a pure presynaptic DA receptor-stimulating effect, and in higher doses, an additional postsynaptic DA receptor-blocking effect (Carlsson 1985). Both should contribute to an antipsychotic effect. (−)3-PPP causes no catalepsy and does not increase prolactin. In normal rats (−)3-PPP inhibits explorative behaviour and antagonises behavioural stimulation by DA agonists. As a possible drawback, it should be added that (−)3-PPP has DA agonistic properties against supersensitive DA receptors (Carlsson 1985).

In a study with one monkey with TD, it was found that (−)3-PPP could dampen the dyskinesias without causing catalepsy or sedation (Häggström et al. 1983). In another study, no significant antidyskinesia effect could be found (Casey and Gerlach, unpublished). There was a slight sedating effect of small doses, but higher doses caused stimulation, shivering and nausea. The mechanisms behind these apparently unpleasant side effects are unclear, but they may counteract a potential therapeutic effect. Thus the principle of the autoreceptor agonist treatment is far from clarified.

3.3 Serotonin and Noradrenaline Antagonism

Two other monoamine transmitter systems, serotonin and norepinephrine, have been considered in the treatment of schizophrenia. The plasma concentration of serotonin has been found elevated in chronic schizophrenic patients (DeLisi et al. 1981), and a serotonin antagonist, fenfluramine, has shown beneficial effect in such patients (Kolakowska et al. 1987). The idea of serotonin receptor antagonists being therapeutically useful in schizophrenia is supported by the observations that clozapine has an unusually strong serotonin antagonistic activity. Maybe the effect of a serotonin antagonist will be too weak for a severe schizophrenia but it may add some valuable qualities to the treatment.

Drugs with an α_1-receptor-blocking effect may produce sedation, but in itself no substantial antipsychotic effect. β-Adrenergic receptor blockers such as propranolol has been shown to have beneficial effect in tremor and heart palpitation associated with occasional anxiety as well as akathisia, but controlled studies have shown that β-blockers have no or minimal effect in schizophrenia.

3.4 Peptidergic Drugs

This section would not be complete without mentioning the peptides. This group of transmitters has raised much enthusiasm over the past 10 years. However, the results obtained until now have only limited implication for practical antipsychotic treatment; the main reason being methodological difficulties, especially the limited penetration through the blood-brain barrier of these compounds and their rapid degradation by plasma and tissue peptidases.

In most cases, pilot studies have shown positive effect in the psychotic state, but later controlled trials have been negative. This applies to the metenkephalin analogue FK 33824, β-endorphin, destyrosine-γ-endorphin, desenkephalin-γ-endorphin, and cholecystokinin-octapeptide (CCK-8) (TAMMINGA et al. 1986). However, until the penetrability problem is solved, it is premature to talk about a potential role of peptides in future treatment in schizophrenia.

4 Improved Use of Available Neuroleptics

It is beyond any doubt that today we have at our disposal powerful antipsychotic drugs which can minimise productive schizophrenic symptoms and thereby lead to improvement in secondary autism, inactivity and social isolation. In spite of 35 years of experience, this type of treatment can still be improved. However, it is outside the scope of this chapter to discuss in detail these practical treatment aspects. Only two principles should be emphasised:

1. *There should be a continuous attempt to reduce the dose.* At the beginning of neuroleptic treatment, it may be necessary to use high doses, but as soon as the productive symptom is suppressed, it is time to start a slow dose reduction. The speed of the dose reduction will always be individual, lasting from 1 month to several years. In chronic cases, it may be relevant to reduce the dose once or twice per year, and even withdraw the neuroleptic drug. Studies have shown that up to 40% of schizophrenic patients can manage without neuroleptic drugs in later stages of their disease. Some of these patients appear to gain some sort of mental stability and resistance, so they can function without the protection of a neuroleptic. Such a continuing attempt at dose reduction will inevitably lead to a lower frequency of disturbing side effects.
2. Controlled clinical studies and practical experience indicate that *depot neuroleptics* are superior to the corresponding oral medication in several cases. This involves a better and more stable therapeutic effect, fewer side effects and, secondarily, a better social life. An average lower and more stable plasma concentration of the neuroleptic may be the main factor underlying the advantage of depot neuroleptic drugs (see JOHNSON, this volume).

5 Nonpharmacological Treatment of Schizophrenia

As mentioned, neuroleptics can suppress or eliminate psychotic symptoms, hallucinations and delusions, as well as the subsequent inactivity and contact problems. These drugs, however, cannot change premorbid features, nor reduce primary autism, anhedonia and lack of social energy. In a way, neuroleptics leave the patient in a mental vacuum, without the psychotic experiences which earlier occupied thoughts and feelings.

With this background it should be emphasised that neuroleptic treatment has to be combined with other forms of therapy, with supporting psychotherapy, socio-, milieu and family therapy, rehabilitation, etc. The patient should be offered a wide spectrum of activity possibilities, so he can choose according to his own abilities and ambitions (and not to his doctor's). Security, reliability, respect and sympathy are elementary values in the doctor-patient relationship. The therapist should with his personality contribute to stabilise the patient's vulnerability and bring pleasure and satisfaction into the chaotic life of the patient.

The same attitude should be provided by the society. The patient needs safe living accomodation, and it should be an elementary right of each schizophrenic patient to have his own "home", a room in a hospital or patient community, or an apartment in the society, all depending on the degree of disease.

Unfortunately, there is still an "underworld" of poorly functioning, disturbed schizophrenic patients, living in miserable conditions. And in hospitals, long-term patients are still living in rooms for two to six people, with no private life. Improvements on this point ought to be an essential goal for the future social treatment of schizophrenia.

References

Angst J, Haenicke U, Padrutt A (1971) Ergebnisse eines Doppelblind-Versuches von HF-1854(8-chlor-11-(4-methyl-1-piperazinyl)-5H-dibenzo(b,e)(1,4)diazepine) im Vergleich zu Levomepromazin. Pharmakopsychiatr Neuropsychopharmakol 4:192–200

Arnt J, Hyttel (1986) Inhibition of SKF 38393- and pergolide-induced circling in rats with unilateral 6-OHDA lesion is correlated to dopamine D-1 and D-2 receptor affinities in vitro. J Neural Transm 67:225–240

Bürki HR, Sayers AC, Ruch W, Asper H (1977) Effects of clozapine and other dibenzo-epines on central dopaminergic and cholinergic systems. Arzneimittelforsch 27:1561–1565

Carlsson A (1985) Pharmacological properties of presynaptic dopamine receptor agonists. In: Casey DE, Chase TN, Christensen AV, Gerlach J (eds) Dyskinesia. Research and treatment. Springer, Berlin Heidelberg New York, pp 31–38

Christensen AV, Arnt J, Svendsen O (1985) Pharmacological differentiation of dopamine D-1 and D-2 antagonists after single and repeated administration. In: Casey DE, Chase TN, Christensen AV, Gerlach J (eds) Dyskinesia. Research and treatment. Springer, Berlin Heidelberg New York, pp 182–190

DeLisi LE, Neckers LM, Weinberger DR, Wyatt RJ (1981) Increased whole blood serotonin concentrations in chronic schizophrenic patients. Arch Gen Psychiatry 38:647–650

Gerlach J, Koppelhus P, Helweg E, Monrad A (1974) Clozapine and haloperidol in a single-blind cross-over trial: therapeutic and biochemical aspects in the treatment of schizophrenia. Acta Psychiatr Scand 50:410–424

Gerlach J, Thorsen K, Fog R (1975) Extrapyramidal reactions and amine metabolites in cerebrospinal fluid during haloperidol and clozapine treatment of schizophrenic patients. Psychopharmacologia (Berlin) 40:341–350

Gerlach J, Behnke K, Heltberg J, Munk-Andersen E, Nielsen H (1985) Sulpiride and haloperidol in schizophrenia: a double-blind cross-over study of therapeutic effect, side effects and plasma concentrations. Br J Psychiatry 147:283–288

Gerlach J, Casey DE, Korsgaard S (1986) Tardive dyskinesia: epidemiology, pathophysiology, and pharmacology. In: Shah NS, Donald AG (eds) Movement disorders. Plenum, New York, pp 119–147

Gerlach J, Kistrup K, Korsgaard S (1987) Effect of selective D-1 and D-2 dopamine receptor antagonists and agonists in cebus monkeys: implications for acute and tardive dyskinesias. In: Dahl SG, Gram LF, Paul SM, Potter WZ (eds) Clinical pharmacology in psychiatry. Selectivity in psychotropic drug action – promises or problems? Springer, Berlin Heidelberg New York, pp 236–247

Häggström JE, Gunne LM, Carlsson A, Wikström H (1983) Antidyskinetic action of 3-PPP, a selective dopaminergic autoreceptor agonist, in cebus monkeys with persistent neuroleptic-induced dyskinesias. J Neural Transm 58:135–142

Hartvig P, Eckernäs SÅ, Lindström L, Ekblom B, Bondesson U, Lundqvist H, Halldin C, Någren K, Långström B (1986) Receptor binding of *N*-(methyl-^{11}C) clozapine in the brain of rhesus monkey studied by positron emission tomography (PET). Psychopharmacology (Berlin) 89:248–252

Hyttel J, Larsen JJ, Christensen AV, Arnt J (1985) Receptor-binding profiles of neuroleptics. In: Casey DE, Chase TN, Christensen AV, Gerlach J (eds) Dyskinesia. Research and treatment. Springer, Berlin Heidelberg New York, pp 9–18

Jenner P, Rupniak NMJ, Marsden CD (1985) Differential alteration of striatal D-1 and D-2 receptors induced by the long-term administration of haloperidol, sulpiride or clozapine to rats. In: Casey DE, Chase TN, Christensen AV, Gerlach J (eds) Dyskinesia. Research and treatment: Springer, Berlin Heidelberg New York, pp 174–181

Kalakowska T, Gadhvi H, Molyneux S (1987) An open clinical trial of fenfluramine in chronic schizophrenia: a pilot study. Int Clin Psychopharmacol 2:83–88

Krupp P, Monka C (1982) Agranulocytosis during Leponex treatment. Situation report, March 31, 1982. Sandoz document

Ögren SO, Hall H, Köhler C, Magnusson O, Sjöstrand S-E (1986) The selective dopamine D-2 receptor antagonist raclopride discriminates between dopamine-mediated motor functions. Psychopharmacology (Berlin) 90:287–292

Pakkenberg H, Pakkenberg B (1986) Clozapine in the treatment of tremor. Acta Neurol Scand 73:295–297

Robertson A, MacDonald C (1984) Atypical neuroleptics clozapine and thioridazine enhance amphetamine-induced stereotypy. Pharmacol Biochem Behav 21:97–101

Sedvall G (1984) The use of substituted benzamides in psychiatry. Acta Psychiatr Scand [Suppl] 69:1–162

Sedvall G, Bjerkenstedt L, Lindström L, Wode-Helgodt B (1978) Clinical assessment of dopamine receptor blockade. Life Sci 23:425–430

Tamminga CA, Littman RL, Alphs Ld, Chase TN, Thaker GK, Wagman AM (1986) Neuronal cholecystokinin and schizophrenia: pathogenic and therapeutic studies. Psychopharmacology (Berlin) 88:387–391

Waddington JL (1986) Behavioral correlates of the action of selective D-1 dopamine receptor antagonists. Biochem Pharmacol 35:3661–3667

A Clinician's Comments on Current Trends in Psychopharmacology of Schizophrenia

S. J. DENCKER

1 Introduction

Let me start with a quotation by LEWIS THOMAS, a New Yorker, physician and writer. It is taken from an essay called "On the need for asylums":

> The overestimation of the value of an advance in medicine can lead to more trouble than anyone can foresee, and a lot of careful thought and analysis ought to be invested before any technology is turned loose on the marketplace.

By "an advance in medicine", THOMAS meant the discovery of the antipsychotic agents. "More trouble than anyone can foresee" referred to the federal bodies responsible for the care of schizophrenics. Overconfidence in the antipsychotics resulted in the community health centre movement in the 1960s and even the closure of mental hospitals. Both actions have caused misery to chronic schizophrenics. As participants of this workshop, we are still working with "careful thought and analysis" because we know that the antipsychotic drugs are no panacea but must be the continued objects of observation and further research by clinicians as well as basic researchers.

2 Agonists Versus Receptors

ARVID CARLSSON has stated that the discovery of the stores of serotonin in the brain and other tissues, and their release by reserpine, meant a breakthrough by breaching, for the first time, the gap between brain biochemistry and psychiatry. Other endogenous agonists soon entered the scene. For some time, dopamine was the poor and bad boy in the transmitter family. It was eventually found that dopamine was an agonist in its own right in the brain. When the neuroleptics appeared, in the early 1950s, a blocking effect on the postsynaptic dopamine receptors, influencing a negative feedback mechanism leading to an increased synthesis, was demonstrated. From then on, dopamine was at the centre of interest and the dopamine hypothesis came to the fore.

It eventually became clear that chemical transmission in the central nervous system involves not only firing but also neuromodulation in a very complicated way. The overall action of the antipsychotic drugs on the dopamine receptors is complicated because of the interaction with other receptors such as α-adrenergic

Department II, Lillhagen Hospital, S-42203 Hisings Backa, Sweden.

and serotonergic neurons. The neurons, the receptors and the transmitters together function as a kind of servo-system, transmission complex or biochemical network. So, from that point of view, we can also speak about sociopharmacology.

We can also place the neuromodulators – transmitters as well as neuropeptides – in a hierarchical model. The components may be arranged in order of relevance to a drug therapy as well as to a mental disease per se. We can postulate that there is an agent – and a corresponding receptor – in the centre of the system, with other agents arranged according to their biochemical importance in a particular situation. The central agent is thus the most relevant, but it needs the outer agents for the role they play in the system – the sociopharmacological aspect. An imbalance in this organisation causes mental symptoms or disease, and psychopharmacological drugs help to restore the organisation or to give positive support. As regards schizophrenia and other psychiatric disorders, we do not know whether the central agent is dopamine or a peptide or maybe both in combination – I will return to this matter later.

We must also consider the regional organisation of single neuromodulators and the receptors, i.e. the accessibility of the receptors to drugs in different areas of the central nervous system. JOSÉE LEYSEN said that it appeared impossible to predict the accessibility of receptors to drugs from the structural and physiochemical properties of the drugs. BRUCE COHEN argued against dopamine blockade as the decisive antipsychotic effect. However, the positron emission tomography (PET) technique, according to LARS FARDE (SEDVALL et al., this volume), has demonstrated a 65%–85% blockade of the D_2 dopamine receptors. This blockade did not differ between typical and atypical neuroleptics, which in turn seems to support the hypothesis that dopamine is in the centre. So far, PET scanning has not demonstrated any receptor up- or down-regulation. The results presented are partly contradictory. It must, however, be stressed that the PET scanning technique is practised on the active human brain and gives a good picture of receptor pharmacology in full action. Let us hope that the present discrepancy between some in vitro and in vivo results will change to allow a consensus to be reached about the best models for problem solution!

3 Drugs and Actions

SVEIN DAHL has indicated that the antipsychotic drugs have mobile pieces. The receptor proteins are also mobile and apparently capable, though we do not know to what extent, of changing their functions in a flexible way, for example, from dopamine D_1 to D_2 activity. This means that receptor pharmacology has now moved from a "solid" to a "liquid" phase and we must now change from a static to a dynamic view. Hopefully, we can look forward to even more advanced techniques, enabling us to study the intimate interaction between the drug and the receptor protein. Will that be a slow foxtrot or a wild jitterbug?

Moreover, the new techniques described here will eventually make it possible to visualise the drug configuration. This, in turn, will make it easier to manipulate models of drugs, to learn how they work in relation to the receptors, and to study the effects of changing the structure. That reminds us of the work that helped CRICK and WATSON to build their model of the double helix.

The steady-state plasma concentrations of antipsychotic drugs show large interpatient variations but they remain relatively stable from day to day in each patient. The discussion about a possible "therapeutic window" in treatment with antipsychotic drugs has been confusing. In schizophrenia, a priori there cannot be such a steady-state window as occurs in depressive states when some antidepressants are used. During the course of a psychosis – be it an acute episode of schizophrenia or a relapse – the amount of antipsychotic drug needed is much higher in earlier than in later phases of the disease. I agree with COHEN, however, that the optimal range of drug plasma levels may be narrow in most cases.

The study of separate and well-defined groups will eventually teach us to use the plasma levels of antipsychotic drugs for better monitoring, even in routine cases. However, the receptor response can vary considerably. Some schizophrenics, even in a symptomatically stable phase, can show total or partial refractoriness to a plasma level that gives a good response in other patients. Such refractory schizophrenics may show a good response on a higher plasma level. Especially in such cases, studies of the relationship between drug dosage and plasma concentrations and of symptom reduction versus unwanted effects can be of considerable help.

The dopamine receptor blocking activity in plasma can be measured with the aid of the receptor binding technique. That seems to be an interesting link between pharmacokinetics and receptor pharmacology for evaluating clinical results. In neurotics, a good correlation has been found in steady-state between the benzodiazepines taken and the plasma concentration of the parent drug and its receptor-active metabolites. However, such correlations have not been observed using neuroleptics in psychotic states. The reason is, apparently, that each drug has its own receptor pharmacology profile and the receptor is a mixture of various subclasses of proteins. Anyhow, the simple receptor binding technique can be used for screening patients for compliance and determining the approximate plasma level of the parent drug and the active metabolites.

4 The Clinical Trend

Clinical psychiatry is now approaching the same research level as the biochemical sciences. Patients with an acute psychosis (those with a good long-term prognosis), as well as those with a chronic diseasee like schizophrenia (usually more or less refractory patients), all show individual variations in their responses to the same dose of an antipsychotic agent. So even apparently rather homogeneous psychotic groups must be more carefully analysed to subclassify them, and there must be studies to determine non-pharmacological antipsychotic factors. Actually, clinical research calls attention not only to the need for homogeneous patient groups but also for a standardised and well-controlled physical environment in which to conduct research. The need for evaluation of compliance, for guaranteeing supply of the drug, and for the definition and measurement of relevant non-pharmacological factors have been stressed. The following cardinal rules were accepted: only one antipsychotic drug should be given at a time, and there should be an individualised dose schedule and careful observation for unwanted effects. The use of a benzodiazepine in addition to neuroleptic treatment in cases of anxiety, agitation and insomnia is to be recommended.

In the maintenance treatment phase – as in subacute or chronic patients like schizophrenics and paranoiacs – the risk–benefit ratio concerning wanted and unwanted effects must be carefully determined. DONALD JOHNSON called our attention to depression as an effect of drugs. There is indeed an increased frequency of depressive symptoms in chronic schizophrenia, be it an inherent trait in schizophrenics or a reaction to a poor social and vocational situation. However, I wish to call attention to the slight but usually constant parkinsonian state – more difficult to diagnose during depot than oral administration – that is drug induced and usually mimics depression. Moreover, the better the rehabilitation, the more often we meet the anhedonic syndrome, i.e. reported feelings of emptiness, communication problems and observed passivity. Without being depressed in the strict sense, the anhedonic patient may be diagnosed incorrectly as suicidal.

We have eventually reached consensus, within broad clinical groups, concerning the advantages and disadvantages of the depot neuroleptics. The great advantage of a depot preparation is guaranteed supply. As Johnson has pointed out, depot injections may have their own compliance problems. The ethical problem involved is, however, very simple. Depot injections cannot be used against the patient's will; this is laid down by law in some countries. The depot method or treatment is now established and recommended in chronic schizophrenia. Actually, almost all schizophrenic patients and their families accept this approach when they are properly informed and know that they are being professionally treated. However, depot administration has several other advantages. It is easier to predict the plasma concentration of the drug and by and large easier to monitor the overall drug treatment. Moreover, in comparison with oral administration, the parenteral form means that we bypass the initial biotransformation, increase the bioavailability, and reduce the total drug dose per unit time. The problem with depot administration is the need for more professional management. Correctly used, depot administration does not give more unwanted effects than oral treatment. It should be noted that depot medication cannot replace other treatments in chronic schizophrenia but is only one part – albeit the most important one – of the complete rehabilitation and/or social support programme.

There is a strong trend in current clinical research to use relapse figures as a measure of the efficacy of antipsychotic treatment. Relapse, however, is only one follow-up factor. It seems to me relevant to study social factors as well, such as housing, work, leisure activities and other aspects of quality of life, in relation to the treatment given. The lowest drug plasma level for prevention of relapse may be too low for an optimal life in society. Here, too, the relationships between the optimal plasma concentration of the antipsychotic drug and non-pharmacological factors must be more carefully studied.

5 Side Effects and the Future

All antipsychotic agents cause unwanted effects, especially when they are used in high doses. Dyskinesias are usually considered to be the most dangerous side effects of neuroleptic treatment. An extensive Nordic study of almost 2500 patients on neuroleptics for at least 1 month – in fact almost half the patients had been on neuroleptics for 5–10 years – showed tardive dyskinesia, including initial dyskinesias, to be present in 17%. The Nordic study also demonstrated only a non-significant tendency to an increased frequency of dys- or hyperkinesia beyond 5 years of treatment with neuroleptics. These results are in agreement with those of DANIEL CASEY. We also agree concerning the strategy for further treatment with neuroleptics: if the patient needs the antipsychotic drug for symptom reduction, one should not worry about continuous antipsychotic drug treatment, even if symptoms of tardive dyskinesia have appeared. However, the patient should be followed up more carefully from a clinical point of view.

JES GERLACH gave us his views on the future treatment of schizophrenia; a cloudy landscape. Actually, the present social situation is not good for chronic schizophrenics even if they are offered a rehabilitation programme with a depot neuroleptic, social-skills training and psychotherapy. In a follow-up study from my department, only 6% demonstrated clinical remission. Even though most patients – 96% in this study – were living in the community after the rehabilitation programme, the social remission was usually only partial.

As I see it, there are three ways of helping refractory schizophrenics, and these can be analysed in terms of basic research, and clinical and nursing aspects:

1. By developing drug therapy hierarchies by adding to the neuroleptics or replacing them with clozapine, lithium or benzodiazepines, for example. Only vague basic research hypotheses can be used when trying such treatment strategies. However, there is a lot of clinical evidence of an anecdotal type in favour of combination and variation of the psychopharmacological treatment for better symptom reduction in refractory schizophrenics. There is little, if any, scientific documentation for such alternative treatment. From a nursing point of view, combined drug treatment usually seems to be a good alternative.
2. By increasing the quality of life for those not responding optimally to antipsychotic drug treatment, rehabilitation efforts, and/or social support strategies, and where a careful biochemical examination has not shown any abnormalities. This brings us back to LEWIS THOMAS and his criticism of the administrative bodies and their abuse of basic research innovations. In his essay, he wrote:

   > We should restore the state hospital system, improve it, expand it if necessary, and spend enough money to ensure that the patients who must live in these institutions will be able to come in off the streets and live in decency and warmth, under the care of adequately paid, competent professionals and compassionate surrogate friends.

   An acceptable alternative would be to create some type of Fountain House organisation. However, summing up the discussion so far, it can be said that overoptimistic expectations of the antipsychotic drugs made the overall situation even worse for chronic schizophrenics in many places.

3. By finding out what the real causes of psychosis are, the real future. Maybe dopamine will be found to be more important than ever. Those schizophrenics who respond very well to antipsychotic drugs and/or to a professional rehabilitation programme have no hallucinations, delusions or autistic behaviour but do have anhedonic personalities. Actually, the central dopaminergic system stands out as essential for creativity and thus is of high adaptive value (see CARLSSON, this volume). Anhedonic behaviour might be linked to such traits. We are thus now back to the importance of dopamine.

This means that we need intensified basic biochemical research – the clinical approach has reached an end-point, as already described – in order to help the chronic schizophrenic by more efficient symptom reduction, less disturbing unwanted effects and a better quality of life. This will, by and large, also solve the nursing problem and give society a better conscience.

Affective Disorders

Treating Depression in Acute Stage: Biochemical and Clinical Aspects

O. J. RAFAELSEN and A. GJERRIS

Abstract

The treatment of depression has advanced dramatically over the last 50 years: electroconvulsion, monoamine oxidase inhibitors (MAOIs), cyclic antidepressants – in chronological order. The amine theories have been giving guidance in the development of new antidepressant drugs and have thus been important in the selectivity of drugs acting, for example, primarily on 5-hydroxytryptamine (5-HT) reuptake. Drugs like citalopram, fluoxetine, fluvoxamine, and paroxetine are very selective in their 5-HT reuptake inhibition, so that in clinical practice they can be tested for the specific importance of this system in depression.

Research on cerebrospinal fluid (CSF) has for many years been restricted to amine metabolites, but we have now been able to measure the parent neurotransmitters, thanks to international cooperation. CSF adrenaline was low, noradrenaline normal, and serotonin and dopamine increased in untreated depression. This calls for major revision of the amine theories.

In addition, our animal studies have shown marked increase in CSF adrenaline after MAOIs, and long-term effect of citalopram on CSF noradrenaline. This indicates the need for enlargement of the number of transmitters in the elucidation of the biology of depression and its treatment, and that interactive counterregulations may lessen the initial selectivity of antidepressant drugs.

1 Introduction

Fifty years ago convulsive therapy started a revolution in the somatic treatment of depression. Thirty-five years ago monoamineoxidase inhibitors (MAOIs) started a revolution in the pharmacological treatment of depression. Thirty years ago tricyclic antidepressants opened an era of treatment of all sorts and grades of depression, not only in psychiatric institutions and by psychiatrists, but for the huge numbers of patients seen in every-day life by general practitioners. Revolutions stand out so clearly in the history of man, especially their first-generation effects. It is much more difficult with the second generation. Patients take the wanted effects for granted and, spoiled as they are, grumble about the unwanted effects.

This chapter will discuss to what extent animal experimentation and hypothesis formation have helped to guide us in the clinical use of antidepressants up to the present day. We shall only be concerned with the various antidepressant drugs and not with electroconvulsive therapy (ECT). We can all agree that ECT is still unchallenged as the most active antidepressive principle; but even if important progress in the understanding of the mode of action of ECT in depressive illness

Department of Psychiatry, Rigshospitalet, 9 Blegdamsvej, DK-2100 Copenhagen, Denmark.

has been seen in recent years due to researchers like BOLWIG, FINK, GREEN-SMITH, D'ELIA and OTTOSSON, there is still some way to go before we can form a solid theory unifying the findings from ECT, lithium prophylaxis, MAOIs, and old and new cyclic antidepressants. We shall discuss some of our own CSF studies in man and animals to illustrate where this type of research has led us and others.

In the search for a possible deficiency in the monoaminergic systems in depressive illness, most interest has been concentrated on the amine metabolites 5-hydroxyindoleacetic acid (5-HIAA), 3-hydroxy-4-methoxyphenyl glycol (MHPG) and to a lesser extent on homovanillic acid (HVA) in cerebrospinal fluid (CSF). The reason for measuring the metabolites and not the amines themselves was the lack of proper analytical methods.

2 Amine Metabolites in CSF

As described in a review by POST et al. (1980), the results reported on CSF amine metabolites measured in depressed patients have often been inconsistent. Low, normal or even high concentrations of CSF 5-HIAA, MHPG and HVA have been described in melancholia and in subgroups of depressed patients when compared with controls (VESTERGAARD et al. 1978; ÅGREN 1980; TRÄSKMAN et al. 1981; VAN PRAAG 1982; KOSLOW et al. 1983; ÅSBERG et al. 1984).

3 The "Parent" Amines in CSF

As methods have now been developed which enable us to measure the amines themselves in tissue and CSF, we have at last got the tools for a more exact and also more dynamic investigation of possible amine dysfunctions in depression. POST et al. (1978), CHRISTENSEN et al. (1980) and GJERRIS et al. (1987b) found no differences in CSF concentrations of noradrenaline (NA) when comparing depressed patients with controls. CHRISTENSEN et al. (1980), and GJERRIS et al. (1987b) described a significant reduction in CSF adrenaline (A) in depressed patients. Moreover, supporting the study by BERGER et al. (1984), GJERRIS et al. (1987b) found significantly negative correlations between single items on the Hamilton depression scale (HDS), "somatic anxiety", "somatisation" and CSF-A levels.

Until now CSF concentrations of 5-hydroxytryptamine (5-HT) in depressive patients have only been reported in one study (GJERRIS et al. 1987c). In this study patients with endogenous depression classified according to the Newcastle rating scale for depression had significantly higher concentrations of CSF-5-HT than controls. This finding does not contradict the possible reduction in CSF-5-HIAA in depression described in some studies (ÅSBERG et al. 1984), as high levels of the amine itself and low levels of the main metabolite may express a decrease in rate of metabolism. Our finding (GJERRIS, et al. 1987d) of increased levels of total CSF dopamine (DA) and some reports of reduced levels of CSF-HVA in depression (ÅSBERG et al. 1984) may be explained in the same way. Supporting the findings by KING et al. (1986), who measured free CSF-DA in depressed patients, we found a relationship between "acceptable social function" and high levels of CSF-DA.

4 Antidepressant Treatment – Influence on CSF Amines

A rather consistent finding, contradicting the logic in low CSF-5-HIAA being causal for depression, is that tricyclic antidepressants as well as MAOIs further reduce the level of 5-HIAA in CSF (POST and GOODWIN 1974; MENDLEWICZ et al. 1982; POTTER et al. 1985). Not less confusing is the finding that clinical recovery from depression occurred independently of whether CSF concentrations of 5-HT were increased (MAOI treatment) or decreased (amitriptyline) after clinical recovery. The ratio 5-HIAA/5-HT was evaluated before and after treatment, showing that isocarboxazide and ECT treatment reduced the ratio, whereas amitriptyline increased the ratio (GJERRIS et al. 1987c).

In the study by CHRISTENSEN et al. (1980), patients who had recovered had significantly higher levels of CSF-A after depression than during depression. The character of antidepressant treatment was not standardised in the above-mentioned paper. In the study by GJERRIS et al. 1987b) CSF-A was not measured after clinical recovery, but the finding of low CSF-A in "somatising depression" brings up the question of whether this type of depression responds specifically to treatment with MAOI (isocarboxazide), which has been shown to induce a marked increase in CSF-A in rats, also after long-term treatment (GJERRIS et al. 1984).

5 Amine Turnover

As an expression of amine turnover, ratios of 5-HIAA/5-HT, HVA/DA and MHPG/NA have been calculated and these show no differences when comparing depressed patients with controls. The negative finding might be explained by possible differences in the ventriculo-lumbar gradient between the "parent" amine and its metabolite.

6 Methodological Problems

The interpretation of results from CSF concentration studies is problematic. First, the origin of the substances measured in CSF is not quite clear (POST et al. 1980). Thus, a ventriculo-lumbar gradient influencing the concentrations measured at the lumbar level has been described for 5-HIAA and HVA (GJERRIS et al. 1987a). For NA a similar gradient has been described in one study (ZIEGLER et al. 1977), but for A, DA and 5-HT, results from such gradient studies have not yet been reported. Secondly, other factors such as diurnal and seasonal variation have been described for some of the transmitters, although consensus has not yet been obtained (ÅSBERG et al. 1984; GJERRIS et al. 1987a). Thirdly, physical activity, food intake and level of anxiety have been also described as influencing the amine concentrations measured in CSF (POST et al. 1980).

7 MAO Inhibitors

Our animal studies give rise to some interesting considerations. We chose isocarboxazide, as the only old MAOI with which we have considerable clinical experience, and moclobemide, as the most clinically tested of the new MAOIs that are selective for the MAO-A type and reversible. Rats were treated with daily injections for 6 weeks. Isocarboxazide led to very considerable increases in rat CSF-NA and even more so in CSF-A. Moclobemide showed the same trend, but quantitative changes were more moderate. DaPrada studied the effect of moclobemide on hypothalamus NA and A, and concluded that the effect of moclobemide on A (compared to that on NA) came faster and was more pronounced.

8 Cyclic Antidepressants

In a parallel series of experiments, rats were treated for 6 weeks with either maprotiline, amitriptyline or citalopram in order to cover the spectrum of effects on the adrenergic and the noradrenergic system. It is noteworthy that after 1 week the effect of amitriptyline tended towards a reduction in NA/A values; and it may be even more noteworthy that after 6 weeks citalopram led to a slight, but significant, increase in the NA levels. Our point is that the reputed specificity or lack of it in acute studies may in the long – clinically important – perspective be under the law of change due to interactive readjustments between the various neurotransmitter and neuromodulator systems.

References

Ågren H (1980) Symptom patterns in unipolar and bipolar depression correlating with monoamine metabolites in the cerebrospinal fluid. II. Suicide. Psychiatry Res 3:225–236

Åsberg M, Bertilsson L, Mårtensson B, Scalia-Tomba G-P, Thorén, Träskman-Bendtz L (1984) CSF monoamine metabolites in melancholia. Acta Psychiatr Scand 69:201–219

Berger PA, King R, Lemoine P, Mefford IN, Barchas JD (1984) Cerebrospinal fluid epinephrine concentrations: discrimination of subtypes of depression and schizophrenia. Pharmacol Bull 20:412–415

Christensen NJ, Vestergaard P, Sørensen T, Rafaelsen OJ (1980) Cerebrospinal fluid adrenaline and noradrenaline in depressed patients. Acta Psychiatr Scand 61:178–185

Gjerris A, Barry DI, Christensen NJ, Rafaelsen OJ (1984) Brain and cerebrospinal fluid epinephrine in isocarboxazide and zimeldine-treated rats. In: Usdin E, Carlsson A, Dahlström A, Engel J (eds) Catecholamines, part C: Neuropharmacology and central nervous system – therapeutic aspects. Liss, New York, pp 139–142

Gjerris A, Werdelin L, Gjerris F, Sørensen PS, Rafaelsen OJ, Alling C (1987a) CSF-amine metabolites in depression, dementia and in controls. Acta Psychiatr Scand 75:619–628

Gjerris A, Rafaelsen OJ, Christensen NJ (1987b) CSF-adrenaline – low in "somatizing depression". Acta Psychiatr Scand 75:516–520

Gjerris A, Sørensen AS, Rafaelsen OJ, Werdelin L, Alling C, Linnoila M (1987c) 5-HT and 5-HIAA in cerebrospinal fluid in depression. J Affective Disord 12:13–22

Gjerris A, Werdelin L, Rafaelsen OJ, Alling C, Christensen NJ (1987d) CSF dopamine increased in depression: CSF dopamine, noradrenaline and their metabolites in depressend patients and in controls. J Affective Disord 13:279–286

King RJ, Mefford IN, Wang C, Murchinson A, Caligari EJ, Berger PA (1986) CSF dopamine levels correlated with extraversion in depressed patients. Psychiatry Res 305–310

Koslow SH, Maas JW, Bowden CL, Davis JM, Hanin I, Javaid J (1983) CSF and urinary biogenic amines and metabolites in depression and mania. Arch Gen Psychiatry 40:999–1010

Mendlewicz J, Pinder RM, Stulemeijer SM, van Dorth R (1982) Monoamine metabolites in cerebrospinal fluid of depressed patients during treatment with mianserin or amitriptyline. J Affective Disord 4:219–226

Post RM, Goodwin FK (1974) Effects of amitriptyline and imipramine on amine metabolites in the cerebrospinal fluid of depressed patients. Arch Gen Psychiatry 30:234–239

Post RM, Lake CR, Jimerson DC, Bunney WE, Wood JH, Ziegler MG, Goodwin FK (1978) Cerebrospinal fluid norepinephrine in affective illness. Am J Psychiatry 135:907–912

Post RM, Ballenger JC, Goodwin FK (1980) Cerebrospinal fluid studies of neurotransmitter function in manic and depressive illness. In: Wood JH (ed) Neurobiology of cerebrospinal fluid 1. Plenum, New York, pp 685–717

Potter WZ, Scheinen M, Golden RW, Rudorfor MW, Cowdry RW, Calil HM, Ross RW, Linnoila M (1985) Selective antidepressants and cerebrospinal fluid. Arch Gen Psychiatry 42:1171–1177

Träskmann L, Åsberg M, Bertilsson L, Sjöstrand L (1981) Monoamine metabolites in CSF and suicidal behavior. Arch Gen Psychiatry 38:631–636

van Praag HM (1982) Depression, suicide and the metabolism of serotonin in the brain. J Affective Disord 4:275–290

Vestergaard P, Sørensen T, Hoppe E, Rafaelsen OJ, Yates CM, Nicolaou N (1978) Biogenic amine metabolites in cerebrospinal fluid of patients with affective disorders. Acta Psychiatr Scand 58:88–95

Ziegler MG, Wood JH, Lake CR, Kopin IJ (1977) Norepinephrine and 3-methoxy-4-hydroxyphenyl glycol gradients in human cerebrospinal fluid. Am J Psychiatry 134:565–568

Pharmacological Management of Treatment-Resistant Depression

D. M. SHAW

Abstract

Treatment-resistant depression might be considered as the failure of two families of antidepressant therapy given sequentially at sufficient dosage, for an adequate length of time and with continuous compliance. Patients with treatment-resistant depression should be assessed as though they were new referrals, and factors which may be contributing should be dealt with whenever possible. A sequence of therapies based on a tricyclic antidepressant and a monoamine oxidase inhibitor, each combined with putative adjuvant therapies, is proposed as a working model pending further studies and developments.

1 Introduction

"Treatment-resistant depression" is a widely used term which lacks agreed definition. What is being discussed here is depression in the context of affective psychosis, either in manic depressive illness, depressed type (296.1) or circular type, currently depressed (296.3). Of these, 10%–29% do not respond readily to therapy according to POST (1972), MURPHY (1983), KELLER et al. (1984), BALDWIN and JOLLEY (1986), and VON FAUST et al. (1986). These estimates depend on how this failure to recover is determined and there is no generally accepted agreement on how this should be done. Given that most effective antidepressant therapies give recovery rates of 55%–70%, a reasonable definition of treatment-resistant depression might be those illnesses which have failed to respond to two families of antidepressant treatment given sequentially, for sufficient time, at adequate dosage for that individual and with continuous compliance. This definition would include those patients where the problem is that of a "fixed" depressive episode and would exclude those individuals where the difficulty is rather that of mood instability and rapidly cycling illness, where the main thrust of therapy is prophylactic, the damping down or prevention of mood fluctuation.

2 Apparent Resistance

Some patients are apparently rather than being truly treatment-resistant. Many antidepressants have unpleasant side effects, some patients lose faith in them

Department of Psychological Medicine, University of Wales College of Medicine, Whitchurch Hospital, Cardiff CF4 7XB, UK.

when their mood fails to lift instantly, and others do not accept drug therapy for a whole variety of reasons. Forgetfulness, general cognitive impairment and the distractibility associated with the illness contribute to the overall low compliance with these drugs. So an important area in failure to respond is the willingness and ability of the patient to take the drugs and to do so with continuity.

We also have a responsibility. Sometimes we forget how variable the metabolism of different individuals is, and therefore how important it is to match the dosage to the particular metabolic characteristics of that person. If a set, often low, dose is presented, those who for genetic or environmental reasons have an enhanced capacity for metabolising the drug, may not achieve adequate levels. It is important therefore that we should remember to both tailor dosage to the individual and modify the dosage with time as metabolic processes adapt to the presence of the drug.

In the working definition of treatment resistance by "different families of antidepressant therapy" is meant the tricyclics, monoamine oxidase inhibitors, electroconvulsive therapy and second generation antidepressants. For the time being, and in this context only, perhaps specific amine reuptake blockers like citalopram and fluvoxamine should be included in the tricyclic family.

3 Factors Contributing to Treatment Resistance

The initiation of recovery from affective illness may be hindered by a number of circumstances. Some of these will be amenable to modification. Often, unfortunately, they are not, or the only way they can be modified is by the person becoming well.

3.1 Psychological Factors

Major depressive illness is a highly traumatic life event in its own right. It will be exerting its own form of stress on the patient, to which may be added shame at having what may be regarded as a socially unacceptable condition for which they have "nothing to show". Then there are the additional stresses from spouse, children, other relatives, employers, employees, etc. arising from the failure to function in one way or another.

Many of these problems will not "go away" and cannot therefore be altered at that point in time. However, in addition, depressed patients experience a particular burden in that they impose on themselves the stress of "putting on a front" or of appearing to be normal, often with a forced level of activity. The author has observed partially recovered patients doing this, relapsing repeatedly and only moving into a more progressive process of recovery when they "let go", allow themselves the luxury of "being ill" and just accept what is happening.

Those patients who have major psychological difficulties and who develop a depressive illness and/or who develop a depressive psychotic state during psychotherapy may appear treatment resistant and require a style of management which is outside the scope of this chapter.

Table 1. Some of the physical illnesses associated with depression

System	Condition
CNS	Parkinson's disease, dementia, stroke, multiple sclerosis tumours, trauma Epilepsy
Nutritional	Anaemia, B_{12} or folate deficiency
Endocrine	Hyper- or hypothyroidism Cushing's and Addison's diseases Hypoglycaemia
Metabolic	Porphyria Hyper- or hypokalaemia
Infective	Variety of infections
Cardiorespiratory	There is a possibility that cardiovascular disease in general and obstructive airway disease may be associated with enhanced risk of depression
General	Malignancy

3.2 Physical Illness

Physical illness appears as a complicating factor in this context in two guises. In itself acute or chronic physical illness is associated with increased risk of major depressive illness. This is true at all ages but in the elderly it becomes of particular significance (MURPHY 1983). In addition some physical illnesses seem to be particularly prone to be associated with disturbance of mood (Table 1).

3.3 Drugs

There have been many reports of an association between drugs and depression, possibly clouded at times by chance and by the causal links between depression

Table 2. Drugs possibly inducing depression

Alcohol
Amantadine
Antihypertensive drugs (clonidine, guanethidine, methyldopa, pindolol, propanolol, reserpine)
Chloroquine
Cimetidine
Corticosteroids
Cytotoxic agents
Digoxin
Fenfluramine (rebound)
Immunosuppressive drugs
Indomethazin
Minor tranquillisers (rebound)
Phenobarbitone
Phenytoin
Theophylline

and physical disease. With some drugs the connection is established with greater or lesser degrees of certainty, and some of these are listed in Table 2 (KING 1986; GOFF and JENIKE 1986; GERNER 1984). Often when a patient is taking one of these drugs it can be omitted temporarily or another substance can be substituted. Note that alcohol has been included as a "depressogenic drug".

4 Principles of Management

In approaching the management of treatment-resistant depression, it is suggested that the following principles be applied:

1. – Make sure that the diagnosis is correct and that the condition is not one of apparent resistance
   – Eliminate contributing factors whenever possible
   – Reassess patients in detail: treat them as though they were new referrals: take a new history and repeat the physical and laboratory examinations
2. – Single drugs have proved ineffective – polypharmacy becomes a necessary evil
   – Where possible, drugs have to be taken to their optimal levels; the dosages and regimes have to be flexible and altered to suit the individual
   – Sufficient time must be allowed at optimal dosage levels for a response, but these levels must not be continued interminably when they have proved themselves ineffective
   – Check compliance
   – Pending further knowledge, "adjuvant drugs" claimed to enhance antidepressant drugs will be used even though full proof of their efficacy has yet to be established in some cases.

Most of these points do not require further explanation. Diagnosis after a prolonged period in affective illness can be taxing. As Sir MARTIN ROTH has said, neurotic patients do not have psychotic features, but all psychotic patients do not have psychotic features, but all psychotic patients have neurotic symptoms. This aphorism is apt, particularly if the term "psychotic" is not restricted to "psychotic features" as in DSMIII but is taken to encompass the whole syndrome of depressive illness with its biological features, etc.

So we can anticipate that someone with major depressive illness will have neurotic symptoms, and that the whole picture will be confusing after what has become a prolonged traumatic and destructive experience. It takes very careful interviewing and patient listening to seek out and identify the diagnostic features amongst all the "noise" which is likely to be present in such an individual. The exercise has to be carried out, and if at the end there is still some remaining doubt, it is safer to assume that affective illness is the primary pathology and to treat according, rather than to attach the label of, for instance, "neurotic depression" or "anxiety state" prematurely.

Once the diagnostic features have been identified, they must be recorded carefully and in detail, so that if "diagnostic doubt" returns to the team, the evidence is there at least for that point in time.

5 Choice of Drugs and Taking Them to Their Optimal Dosage

We are at a point of transition in our choice of drugs as new compounds with more specific and selective pharmacological properties are introduced. At the present time, however, most of the existing evidence on the treatment of refractory depression (such as it is and with all its limitations) is with the "older" drugs. Most clinicians will, therefore, prefer to retain these more familiar remedies for the group of patients under discussion, at least until more research has been done. So the question is: how do we produce optimal levels of drugs matched to the patients needs? For many antidepressants it is a matter of chance, experience or even luck. We do not have sufficient experience with the newer antidepressants to know how their administration should be managed and if dose/response is within a range or linear.

Leaving aside the possibility that some drugs may have a therapeutic window, it has been assumed here that treatment failure is more likely to be because of inadequate dosage than that one has overreached some maximum for that compound. For instance, WATT et al. (1972) and SIMPSON et al. (1976) have demonstrated the superiority of a dose of 300 mg over that of 150 mg for imipramine. It may be that for drugs like imipramine and possibly dothiepin (without encouraging such rigidity as might be implied by doses of 150 or 300 mg), a more enterprising and open-ended attitude to the amounts prescribed might have beneficial effects on outcome.

There are some drugs where side effects are a practical ceiling. Of course, there is no guarantee that such a ceiling will correspond to the most effective therapeu-

Table 3. Some of the drugs which may be titrated to an end point

Drug	End point		Comment
	The presence of *mild* orthostatic hypotension	Slight sedation which does not "habituate" after 4–5 days	
Clomipramine	√	–	Sedation may be part of the side effect profile but is not relevant in this context
Amitriptyline	√	–	
Phenelzine	√	√	Orthostatic hypotension is the more frequent end point
Tranylcypromine	√	–	
Mianserin	–	√	The early dosage ranges proposed may have been too low. Slight sedations seem to be a useful "marker" for this compound

tic range, and indeed for many the side effects have no relevance in this respect. It is a personal opinion that with some drugs it may be possible to titrate the dose upwards every 5 days or so and reach a particular side effect end point which may have some significance for therapeutic response (Table 3). The dosage required to reach this end point may not be that required to keep patients there as conditions change with time. So to keep patients at this point requires readjustments of dosage and, again, a flexible approach.

Since we lack consensus about theoretical therapeutic windows, an alternative policy can be to use "safe" compounds with low side effect profiles and start in what is generally thought of as the normal therapeutic dosage. The dose is edged up at rather longer intervals (weeks rather than days) than the 5-day periods suggested for clomipramine, amitriptyline, mianserin and the monoamine oxidase inhibitors (MAOIs) (Table 3). This will show if an "unusual" dosage is suitable for that individual, and the demonstration that this is so may be the appearance of the beginnings of recovery.

6 Flexibility of Regimes

This topic has been mentioned several times already as regards flexibility in dosage in the induction period and throughout the subsequent weeks to allow for metabolic adjustment to the continuing presence of the drug. How long should the regime be continued, how flexible should the time scale of therapy be? In general, once a programme has been brought to its peak, then some change – or at least the beginnings of change – should be expected within 4–6 weeks. The statistical likelihood of subsequent benefit is small if the first signs of improvement have not appeared by this time and there is no point in continuing after 8 weeks at the most. In general therefore, "aliquots of therapy" should occupy about 6 weeks (QUITKIN et al. 1984) from the time the regime has been fully established.

7 Attempts to Enhance the Activity of Antidepressant Drugs

Trials in treatment-resistant illness are not the easiest to perform, and some of the suggested ways of increasing the efficacy of antidepressant therapy have been incompletely researched.

The antidepressant activity of lithium used by itself is questionable, but there have been favourable reports on its ability to potentiate tricyclic drugs (NEUBAUER and BERMINGHAM 1976; DEMONTIGNY et al. 1981, 1983; HENINGER et al. 1983) and also iprindole (DEMONTIGNY et al. 1985).

The early reports suggested that lithium induced improvement very rapidly, in a matter of days. This was not found by PRICE et al. (1986) who showed that in those whom lithium appeared to help, the process took place in about 3 weeks.

ECCLESTON (1984) and BARKER and ECCLESTON (1984) have proposed the addition of lithium to therapy with MAOI, and this has been included in the pro-

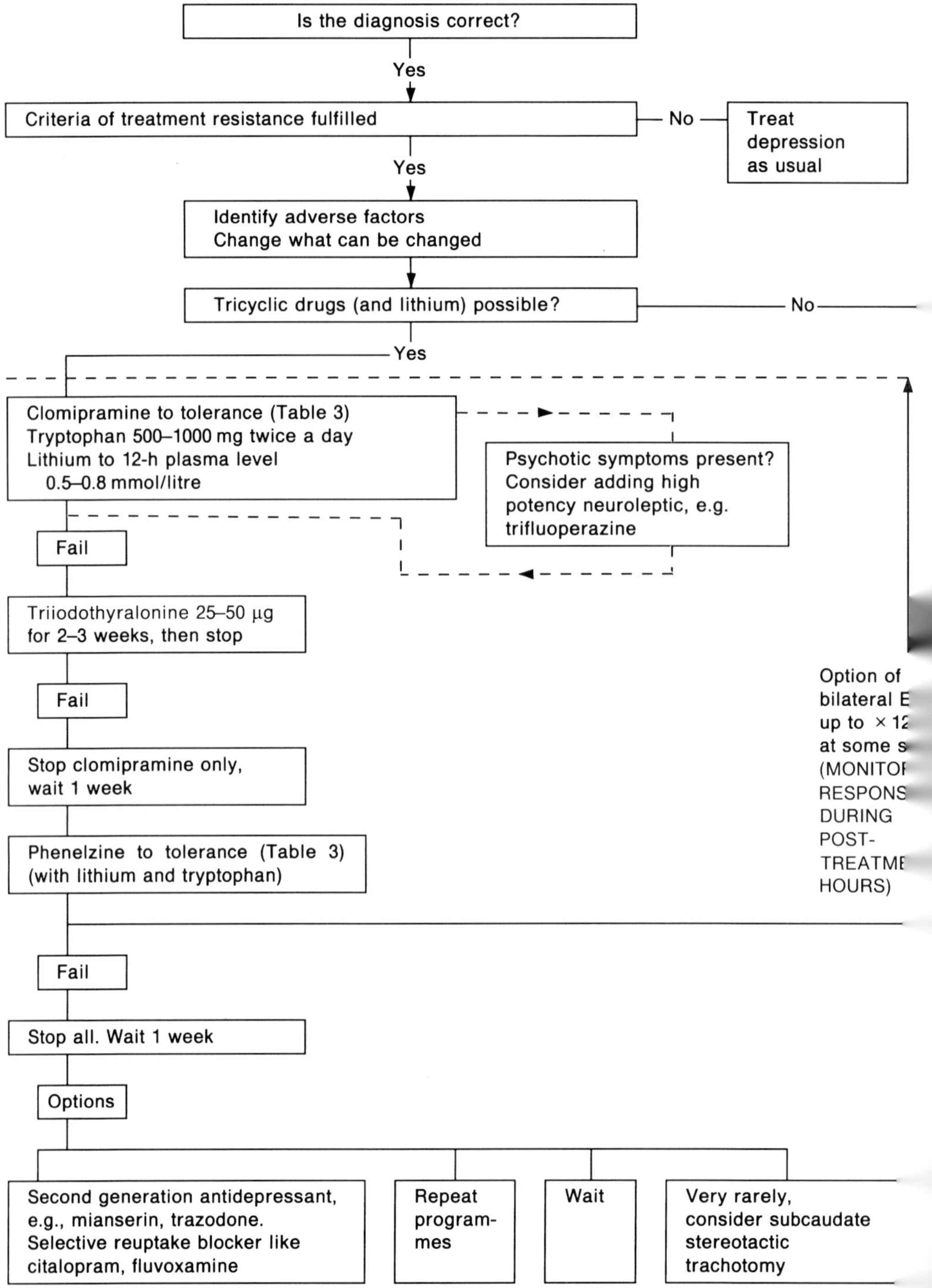

Is the diagnosis correct?
Yes
Criteria of treatment resistance fulfilled
No
Treat depression as usual
Yes
Identify adverse factors
Change what can be changed
Tricyclic drugs (and lithium) possible?
No
Yes
Clomipramine to tolerance (Table 3)
Tryptophan 500–1000 mg twice a day
Lithium to 12-h plasma level 0.5–0.8 mmol/litre
Psychotic symptoms present? Consider adding high potency neuroleptic, e.g. trifluoperazine
Fail
Triiodothyralonine 25–50 μg for 2–3 weeks, then stop
Fail
Stop clomipramine only, wait 1 week
Phenelzine to tolerance (Table 3) (with lithium and tryptophan)
Fail
Stop all. Wait 1 week
Options
Second generation antidepressant, e.g., mianserin, trazodone. Selective reuptake blocker like citalopram, fluvoxamine
Repeat programmes
Wait
Very rarely, consider subcaudate stereotactic trachotomy

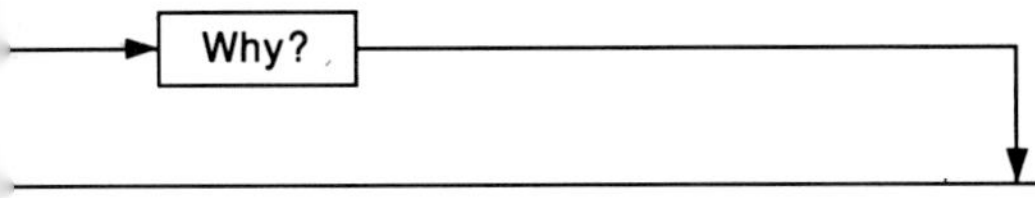

erapy	Antocholin-ergic side effects a problem	Acute/chronic heart disease heart failure	Marked hyper-tension recent stroke; conditions where change in BP a problem	Epilepsy, low convulsive threshold	Sensitivity or other intolerance to tricyclics	Suicidal risk
T	+	Doubtful	Each case on its merits	+	+	+
nserin	+	+	+		+	−
zodone	+	+	+	Possible	+	−
OI	+	+	−	−	+	−
xazine	−	−	−	+	−	−
T reuptake blocker .g. fluvoxamine italopram	+	+	+	+	+	+

g: With the exception of MAOIs which are potentiated by tryptophan, we know little about adjuvant activity these drugs

Fig. 1. Flow diagram of proposed treatment programme for treatment-resistant depression and availability of drugs for "problem" patients

gramme plan suggested here (Fig. 1). However, it must be recognised that the work to date by authors such as NELSON and BYCK (1982), HIMMELHOCH et al. (1972), and PRICE et al. 1985) needs expanding.

Several groups (COPPEN et al. 1963; PARE 1963; GLASSMAN and PLATMAN 1969 and others) have demonstrated potentiation of MAOIs by tryptophan in depression, and this has led to the incorporation of this amino acid with MAOIs in the attempted treatment of resistant illness.

Similar studies of tryptophan and tricyclics – again with nonresistant patients – have been inconsistent in their findings. ROOS (1976) and WALINDER et al. (1976, 1981) found that giving the two drugs together was advantageous but clear additional benefit from combining tricyclics with tryptophan was not demonstrated by SHAW et al. (1975), CHOUINARD et al. (1979), and THOMSON et al. (1982). The question of the tricyclic tryptophan combinations remains open.

Initially, triiodothyronine (T3) was tried with tricyclics as a means of increasing the rate of recovery (PRANGE et al. 1969), and in parallel with this, and later, in treatment-resistant individuals (EARLE 1970; GOODWIN et al. 1982). These studies gave positive results, but others have found supplements of T3 with tricyclic drugs less useful (AKISKAL 1985; GARBUTT et al. 1986). Once again the matter is unclear.

Among what are perhaps the less popular ways of enhancing recovery from depressive illness has been to give tricyclic drugs and add methyl phenidate or dextroamphetamine (KATON and RASKIND 1980; KAUFMANN et al. 1984; DRIMMER et al. 1983). A study in tricyclic-resistant patients in a small group of unipolar patients was promising (WHARTON et al. 1971). They were suffering from delusional depression – a group of patients who should perhaps be considered as drug resistant rather than treatment resistant.

Reserpine is of interest in that it releases from and blocks storage of transmitters in aminergic neurones, and it was perhaps a bold step to try to enhance antidepressant therapy in patients on tricyclic drugs (POLDINGER 1963). Subsequent studies have supported its value in therapy-resistant patients (HASCOVEC 1967; HOPKINSON and KENNY 1975; MOSKOVICH and MESTER 1984), and this is a procedure which well deserves further investigation.

A possible role of carbamazepine as an adjuvant therapy has yet to be assessed in resistant depression even though its function as a prophylactic agent seems to be reasonably well established.

Finally, there is the question of whether or not, when a tricyclic antidepressant has failed, it is worthwhile switching to an alternative drug of the same family. Some clinicians favour changing from one drug which acts predominantly on, say, serotoninergic systems to another which acts mostly on noradrenergic neurones, and vice versa. There is no actual evidence demonstrating that this is a beneficial manoeuvre. However, in some individuals it is worth considering from two points of view. Patients vary considerably in their reaction to drugs and their preferences. One may experience the sedative effects of, say, amitriptyline as intolerable and may be able to take imipramine or a secondary amine tricyclic in larger doses and in a more flexible way. The converse may be true, a sedating amine reuptake blocker may be preferred.

Another reason for switching is the introduction of more specific amine reuptake blockers (e.g. citalopram and fluvoxamine) where the presence of anticholinergic side effects, lack of induction of postural hypotension or interference with psychomotor performance may limit the administration of the classical tricyclic drugs.

The simultaneous giving of MAOIs and tricyclics has had a checkered career largely because this manoeuvre is safe only if the underlying pharmacology and the rules it imposes are fully understood. However, there is little evidence that combining drugs of this type in this way offers any advantage over the same compounds given sequentially at adequate dose and for sufficient time. Certainly, the studies of RAZANI et al. (1983), YOUNG et al. (1979) and WHITE and SIMPSON (1984) do not support the use of "combined antidepressants".

8 Treatment Programmes

It has been assumed that individual treatments, having been brought to "their best" will be run for about 6 weeks or a little more, and that what will be assessed then is not whether they have worked, but whether there are the beginnings of movement in the right direction. Thereafter most patients will require antidepressant treatment for 6 months and some will be moved over to prophylactic programmes. It is appreciated that people have preferences, and that the author's preferences and prejudices have decided some of the drugs chosen. It is also acknowledged that in no way is it possible to cover all clinical contingencies.

The flow diagram (Fig. 1) starts after the exclusion of patients who do not meet the criteria of treatment resistance because of noncompliance or inadequate therapies of other origin, but includes the starting questions: is the diagnosis right or is the diagnosis still right?

A pertinent question would be to ask why the particular combinations were chosen for the proposed flow diagram for the mangement of treatment-resistant depression. It is in part based on unpublished observations by ECCLESTON, LOUDON, and ASHCROFT. In addition, each half combines one fairly well recognised adjuvant therapy (tricyclic plus lithium, MAOIs plus tryptophan) with a second less well-demonstrated pairing (tricyclic plus tryptophan, MAOI plus lithium).

Perhaps some clinicians would prefer to end the tricyclic phase by keeping the tricyclic drug, discontinuing lithium and tryptophan, and trying reserpine with the tricyclic drug. This would be a potentially useful addition, particularly if there is a particular need to avoid MAOIs, but in the author's experience very few patients fail to respond to the grouping of treatments as set out in Fig. 1.

Acknowledgement. I would like to thank G. BALLARD for her help in the preparation of this manuscript.

References

Akiskal HS (1985) A proposed clinical approach to chronic and "resistant" depressions: evaluation and management. J Clin Psychiatry 46:32–36

Baldwin RC, Jolley DJ 81986) The prognosis of depression in old age. Br J Psychiatry 149:574–583

Barker WA, Eccleston D (1984) The treatment of chronic depression: an illustrative case. Br J Psychiatry 147:317–319

Chouinard G, Young SN, Annable L, Sourkes TL (1979) Tryptophan-nicotinamide, imipramine and their combination in depression: a controlled study. Acta Psychiatr Scand 59:395–414

Coppen A, Shaw DM, Farrell JP (1963) Potentiation of the antidepressive effects of a monoamine oxidase inhibitor by tryptophan. Lancet I:79–81

DeMontigny C, Grunberg F, Mayer A, Deschenes J-P (1981) Lithium induced rapid relief of depression in tricyclic and antidepressant drug non-responders. Br J Psychiatry 138:252–256

DeMontigny C, Cournoyer G, Morissette R, Langlois R, Caille G (1983) Lithium carbonate addition in tricyclic antidepressant-resistant unpolar depression. Arch Gen Psychiatry 40:1327–1334

DeMontigny C, Elie R, Caille G (1985) Rapid response to the addition of lithium in iprindole-resistant unipolar depression: a pilot study. Am J Psychiatry 142:220–223

Drimmer EJ, Gitlin MJ, Gwirtsman HE (1983) Desimipramine and methylphenidate combination treatment for depression. Am J Psychiatry 140:241–242
Earle BV (1970) Thyroid hormone and tricyclic antidepressants in resistant depressions. Am J Psychiatry 126:1667–1669
Eccleston D (1984) Evaluation and treatment of chronic depressive illness. Hosp Update 10:517–523
Garbutt JC, Mayo JP, Gillette GM, Little KY, Mason GA (1986) Lithium potentiation of tricyclic antidepressants following lack of T3 potentiation. Am J Psychiatr 143:1038–1039
Gerner RH (1984) Antidepressant selection in the elderly. Psychosomatics 25(7):528–535
Glassman AH, Platman SR (1969) Potentiation of a monoamine oxidase inhibitor by tryptophan. J Psychiatr Res 7:83–88
Goff DC, Jenike MA (1986) Treatment-resistant depression in the elderly. J Am Geriatr Soc 34:63–70
Goodwin FK, Prange AJ, Post RM, Muscettola GE, Lipton MA (1982) Potentiation of antidepressant effects by 1-triiodothyronine in tricyclic non-responders. Am J Psychiatr 139:34–38
Haskovec L (1967) The action of reserpine on imipramine-resistant depressive patients: clinical and biochemical study. Psychopharmacologie (Berlin) 11:18–30
Heninger GR, Charney DS, Sternberg DE (1983) Lithium carbonate augmentation of antidepressant treatment. Arch Gen Psychiatry 40:1335–1342
Himmelhoch JM, Petre T, Kupfer JD, Swartzburg MD, Byck R (1972) Treatment of previously intractible depressions with tranylcypromine and lithium. J Nerv Ment Dis 155:216–220
Hopkinson G, Kenny F (1975) Treatment with reserpine of patients resistant to tricyclic antidepressants. Psychiatr Clin (Basel) 8:109–114
Katon W, Raskin M (1980) Treatment of depression in the medically ill elderly with methylphenidate. Am J Psychiatry 137:963–965
Kaufmann MW, Cassem NH, Murray GB et al. (1984) Use of psychostimulants in medically ill patients with neurological disease and major depression. Can J Psychiatry 29:46
Keller M, Klerman G, Lavori PW, Coryell W, Endicott J, Taylor J (1984) Long-term outcome of episodes of major depression. JAMA 252:788–792
King DJ (1986) Drug-induced psychiatric syndromes. Prescribers J 26(3):50
Moscovich D, Mester R (1984) Tricyclic antidepressive treatment reinforced by reserpine. Isr J Psychiatry Relat Sci 21:283–289
Murphy E (1983) The prognosis of depression in old age. Br J Psychiatry 142:111–119
Nelson JC, Byck R (1982) Rapid response to lithium in phenelzine non-responders. Br J Psychiatry 141:85–86
Neubauer H, Bermingham P (1976) A depressive syndrome responsive to lithium. J Nerv Ment Dis 163:276–281
Pare CMB (1963) Potentiation of a monoamine oxidase inhibitor by tryptophan. Lancet II:527–528
Pöldinger W (1963) Combined administration of desimipramine and reserpine or tetrabenazine in depressive patients. Psychopharmacologie (Berlin) 4:308–310
Post F (1972) The management and nature of depressive illness in late life – a follow through study. Br J Psychiatry 121:393–404
Prange AJ, Wilson IC, Rabon AM, Lipton MA (1969) Enhancement of imipramine antidepressant activity by thyroid hormone. Am J Psychiatry 126:457–469
Price LH, Conwell Y, Nelson JC (1983) Lithium augmentation of combined neuroleptic-tricyclic treatment in delusional depression. Am J Psychiatry 140:318–322
Price LH, Charney DS, Heninger GR (1985) Efficacy of lithium-tranylcypromine treatment in refractory depression. Am J Psychiatry 142:619–623
Quitkin FM, Rabkin JG, Ross D, McGrath PJ (1984) Duration of antidepressant drug treatment. Arch Gen Psychiatry 41:238–245
Razani J, White KL, White J, Simpson G, Sloane RB, Rebal R, Palmer R (1983) The safety and efficacy of combined amitriptyline and tranylcypromine antidepressant treatment. Arch Gen Psychiatry 40:657–661
Roos B-E (1976) Tryptophan, 5-hydroxytryptophan and tricyclic antidepressants in the treatment of depression. Monogr Neural Sci 3:23–25

Shaw DM, MacSweeney DA, Hewland R, Johnson L (1975) Tricyclic antidepressants and tryptophan in unipolar depression. Psychol Med 5:276–278

Simpson GM, Lee JM, Cuculica A, Kellner R (1976) Two dosages of imipramine in hospitalised endogenous and neurotic depressives. Arch Gen Psychiatry 33:1093–1102

Thomson J, Rankin H, Ashcroft GW, Yates CM, McQueen JK, Cummings SW (1982) The treatment of depression in general practice: a comparison of l-tryptophan, amitriptyline, and a combination of l-tryptophan and amitriptyline with placebo. Psychol Med 12:741–751

von Faust V, Hole G, Wolfesdorf M (1986) Die sogenannte therapieresistente Depression. Fortschr Med 104:23–24

Walinder J, Skott A, Carlsson A, Nagy A, Roos B-E (1976) Potentiation of the antidepressant action of clomipramine by tryptophan. Arch Gen Psychiatry 33:1384–1389

Walinder J, Carlsson A, Persson R (1981) 5HT reuptake inhibitors plus tryptophan in endogenous depression. Acta Psychiatr Scand 63 (Suppl 290):179–190

Watt DC, Crammer JL, Elkes A (1972) Metabolism, anticholinergic effects and therapeutic effects on outcome of desmethylimipramine in depressive illness. Psychol Med 2:397–405

Wharton RN, Perel JM, Dayton PG, Malitz S (1971) A potential clinical use for methylphenidate with tricyclic antidepressants. Am J Psychiatry 127:1619–1625

White K, Simpson G (1984) The combined use of MAOIs and tricyclics. J Clin Psychiatry 457(2):67–69

Young JPR, Lader MH, Hughes MC (1979) Controlled trial of trimipramine, monoamine oxidase inhibitors, and combined treatment in depressed outpatients. Br Med J 2:1315–1317

Is There a Long-Term Protective Effect of Mood-Altering Agents in Unipolar Depressive Disorder?

R. J. BALDESSARINI [1] and M. TOHEN [2]

Abstract

Major depression is common, often severe, and usually recurrent, and it carries an excess risk of mortality due to medical illness as well as suicide. At referral centers, recurrence risk averages 85% within 2–3 years of full recovery from an acute episode. The natural history of major depression is highly variable, but typically episodes last ca. 6 months, with cycles of ca. 2 years. Yet, most long-term treatment studies are limited to the year or two following recovery from an acute episode. Accordingly, available evidence best supports a *relapse*-preventing effect of tricyclic antidepressants or lithium within the first months after apparent recovery but is less compelling regarding prevention of later *recurrences* of new episodes. Other treatments have not been evaluated systematically. The hypothesis that bipolarlike, but apparently unipolar, patients might respond selectively to lithium maintenance requires further testing. Knowledge of long-term dose-benefit and dose-risk relationships is starting to emerge for lithium, but these relationships remain inadequately tested for antidepressants. Actual levels of clinical treatment of major depression appear to fall short of the ideal, and much additional research and education is required to improve care in this very common disorder.

1 Introduction

Major affective disorders continue to be leading causes of psychiatric disability, loss of productivity, consumption of health services, and human suffering (BALDESSARINI 1983; PRIEN and KUPFER 1986). Major depression affects more than ten of every 100 persons at some time. It is associated with an excess of mortality, due not only to suicide or other violent causes but probably also to medical diseases. The risk of suicide, at least, can probably be decreased by adequate pharmacological treatment or electroconvulsive therapy (ECT) (AVERY and WINOKUR 1976) although the effect of adequate treatment on nonviolent death risk is less clear due in part to the covariance of prior medical illness and cautious antidepressant therapy (D. W. BLACK, G. WINOKUR, and A. NASRALLAH 1987, unpublished observations).

The great majority of major depressions are recurrent (unipolar, UP, disorder), alternate or mix with excited psychotic states (bipolar manic-depressive illness), or may become chronic. Thus, the need to develop safe, effective, and efficient long-term treatments for this disorder is extraordinarily important. The wide ac-

[1] Mailman Research Center, McLean Division, Massachusetts General Hospital, Belmont, MA 02178, USA.

[2] Departments of Psychiatry and Programs of Neuroscience and Psychiatric Epidemiology of Harvard Medical School, Boston, MA 02115, USA.

ceptance of the antidepressants and lithium salts for the treatment of major affective episodes since 1949–1959 led to their being considered for long-term use. Despite the interest shown in this topic since the early 1960s, the available research basis for current practice and future planning is surprisingly limited, largely inconclusive, and strikingly out of proportion to the magnitude of the public health problem at issue. The state of knowledge of the efficacy and safety of long-term antidepressant or lithium treatment of UP depression has been reviewed in the past decade (Davis 1976; Coppen and Peet 1979; Schou 1979; Baldessarini 1983, 1985; Prien 1983). The present overview highlights some emerging impressions from the available research on this topic and provides suggestions for further inquiry.

2 Natural History of Unipolar Disorder

In order to understand the literature on the long-term treatment of recurrent major depression (UP disorder), it is important to define the characteristics of the disorder, and especially its reported pattern of relapses and recurrences (Table 1). The current impression concerning UP disorder is that most cases of depression followed up for several years reveal a tendency to recur or to show chronic, partial disability with major episodes (Zis and Goodwin 1979; Prien and Kupfer 1986).

Usually, episodes are not sharply defined, and the course of illness in individuals can be highly variable, making the design and interpretation of studies in this field difficult (Murphy et al. 1974). Moreover, it is not known to what extent the treatment of episodes of major depression with ECT or antidepressants may alter

Table 1. Characteristics of recurrent, endogenous unipolar major affective illness (unipolar manicdepressive illness)

Characteristic	Value
Lifetime morbid risk (females higher)	10%–20%
Diagnostic error (later bipolar)	5%–10%
Unipolar (unipolar plus bipolar-II) to all major affective cases	62%
Single-episode cases	5%
Cumulative recurrence risk	
6 months	48%
1 year	58%
2 years	75%
3 years	85%
Episode duration (treatment not controlled)	3–6 months
Episode duration (estimated, without treatment)	4–10 months
Cycle length (start to start of episodes, which tend to shorten ca. 5% per cycle through first 6 cycles)	13 months
Estimated depressing-free interval (cycle length minus 4.5 months episodes)	8.5 months

References are based on reports cited in Zis and Goodwin (1979), Baldessarini (1983), and others.

the natural history of the disorder, perhaps increasing the proportion of briefer or milder episodes. Most of the data summarized in Table 1 come from patients evaluated between the 1940s and the early 1970s, before long-term up maintenance treatments were common. Nevertheless, some long-term use of lithium in UP disorder was starting in the 1960s, and it has been usual to continue antidepressant treatment for 6–12 months after recovery from an episode of depression since the 1960s as well. The long-term treatment literature is heavily biased toward the continuation of treatment after recovery from an acute episode of depression, and only sometimes after an interval of stability of several months. This choice of study design is predisposed to detecting events early in follow-up and probably selects for synchronization of recurrence cycles. Consistent with this prediction is the interval risk of "relapse" at various times on a placebo after the end of a treated acute depressive episode (plus 2 months of stability on an antidepressant): 38%, 6%, 9%, 9%, and 15% at 4, 6, and 8 months, and 1 and 2 years, respectively (PRIEN and KUPFER 1986). However, the additional finding that the episode interval tends to fall with succeeding episodes of recurring major affective illness (GROF et al. 1974) makes it less likely that the risk of a recurrence may be reduced in the year or two after a full recovery from an episode.

Despite these caveats concerning research on the natural history of UP disorder, some features are particularly pertinent to long-term treatment. Thus, single episodes of major depression are now rare (less than 10% of cases), in contrast to the pre-1950 literature (15%–50%; ZIS and GOODWIN 1979), and the risk of diagnostic error due to the late appearance of bipolarity probably averages <10%. Acute depressive episodes now last about 3–6 months, but some cases in the pre-ECT and -psychopharmacology era continued up to a year (ZIS and GOODWIN 1979). More accurate estimates of the contemporary natural history of an acute episode of major depression are unavailable; moreover, it will probably not be studied again due to ethical considerations concerning the withholding of treatment. There is better information concerning the length of UP cycles (interepisode time). Some, but not all, studies have found that this measure tends to shorten with successive recurrences, at least through the first six to eight episodes, and perhaps among patients with late-onset depression; however, depression in the elderly often follows a chronic course, making it difficult to distinguish discrete episodes (GROF et al. 1974). Overall, UP cycle length has averaged about 1 year (Table 1). Accordingly, long-term studies should ideally continue for at least 2–3 years after a period of ca. 6 months to assure full recovery from an index acute episode of depression. Very few long-term treatment trials have approached such a standard. Fewer still have utilized the alternative strategy of treatment discontinuation, as has been more common in long-term, placebo-controlled studies of schizophrenia (BALDESSARINI 1985). These shortcomings in the therapeutics research on depression may be due to ethical considerations concerning the continuation of potentially toxic treatments long after the disappearance of manifest symptoms on the one hand, and impressions concerning the risk of premature discontinuation within the first months after recovery from an acute episode on the other.

3 Research on Long-Term Treatment of Depression

Soon after the introduction of antidepressant agents in the mid-1950s, there was interest in their possible usefulness in the treatment of both late and acute phases of major depression. Clinicians found that following successful termination of an episode of major depression with a tricyclic antidepressant (TCA) or ECT, the discontinuation of TCA treatment led to a high rate of relapse (reemergence of illness in the early postrecovery phase of a depression, during the expected period of risk for an untreated episode). This risk could be limited by continued treatment. Following slow acceptance of the indubitable antimanic effects of lithium salts during the 1950s and 1960s, attention turned toward their possibly even greater clinical importance in the long-term prevention of relapses and recurrences of bipolar disorder. Despite early skepticism about the ability of lithium to reduce morbidity due to depression as well as mania, a few enthusiastic European investigators considered whether lithium might have a protective effect in UP as well as bipolar disorder.

In one of the earliest studies of an apparent long-term protective action of lithium in recurrent major depression, HARTIGAN (1963) reported that only one of seven UP patients with previously frequent severe depressions had a major episode over 3–4 years of treatment with lithium. Soon thereafter, BAASTRUP and SCHOU (1967) presented life histories of a large series of manic-depressive patients before and during lithium treatment. Their analysis of 22 unequivocally UP cases indicated that the incidence of relapses was 1.6 per person-year before, and only 0.4 during, lithium treatment lasting several years ($p < 0.001$). In a similar early retrospective study, ANGST et al. (1970) reported on comparisons of 2.2-year-average follow-up and equally long past history that included 58 UP cases, in whom the morbidity (months depressed per person-year) was reduced four fold from 1.2–0.3 during lithium treatment ($p < 0.001$); recurrence rates, however, were decreased in only about half of the cases. Although this imperfectly controlled approach to evaluating preventive treatment was criticized at the time, the results were highly provocative and led to the establishment of the long-term effectiveness of lithium in bipolar disorder within the next few years (DAVIS 1976; SCHOU, this volume).

Following criticism of these early anecdotal and naturalistic case studies, a series of prospective, placebo-controlled trials of lithium were undertaken in both UP and bipolar patients. The overall results of these studies, as well as of controlled trials of continued use of antidepressants, are summarized in Table 2. Most studies involved relatively brief trials, almost always after recovery from an acute depressive episode. Few studies continued to 2 years, and very few to 3 years, despite the evidence that true preventive effects on recurrence are unlikely to be proved in studies shorter than 2 years. These studies provide good evidence for a sustained, partial protective effect of lithium and TCAs; however, monoamine oxidase (MAO) inhibitors and atypical antidepressants have not been evaluated adequately in this way.

The cumulative risks of relapse and recurrence are high: over 80% on a placebo and 40%–70% on active medication, within 2–3 years. Thus, with all forms of

Table 2. Pooled cumulative rates of relapse or recurrence of unipolar major affective disorder from controlled studies of continuation or maintenance treatment

Treatment	Length			
	0.5	1	2	3
Placebo control[a]				
Risk rate (%)	48	58	85	84
Protection ratio	1.0	1.0	1.0	1.0
No. of studies	14	12	7	4
Lithium salts				
Risk rate (%)	29[b]	32[b]	53[b]	60
Protection ratio	1.8	1.9	1.5	1.2
No. of studies	9	11	7	4
Antidepressants				
Risk rate (%)	22[b]	46	56[b]	68
Protection ratio	2.2	1.4	1.5	1.2
No. of studies	7	4	4	2
Lithium and antidepressant				
Risk rate (%)	19[b]	27[b]	43[b]	63
Protection ratio	2.6	2.1	1.8	1.3
No. of studies	5	4	2	1
Total no. of patients	909	756	634	376

References are from studies cited in SCHOU (1979), BALDESSARINI (1983, 1985), and PRIEN (1983).
[a] Pooled control data from all studies is shown, but the numerator used to compute the protection ratio for each treatment was limited to matched control groups only.
[b] Significance by Yates'-corrected MANTEL-HAENSZEL χ^2 analysis (of studies with complete 2×2 tables only) yielded $p < 0.001$ or less for test of treatment effect.

treatment, a striking proportion of patients eventually relapsed, and drug–placebo differences became somewhat smaller over time. Moreover, the strongest protection was provided in the first 6 months, suggesting that a major proportion of the benefit may involve preventing reemergence of symptoms of an acute episode (relapse) during a limited early period of probably increased risk.

The reasons for the apparent tendency for any treatment effect to be lost over prolonged follow-up periods are not clear; however, the possibility of less efficacy for recurrence than for relapse should be considered. In addition, there may be artifacts due to time-related changes in the nature of the populations remaining under observation or to technical problems, including nonadherence to protocols and the loss of sensitivity of repeated clinical measurements over time.

Several other uncontrolled studies yielded remarkably similar results with respect to 6-month and 1-year lithium prophylaxis; still others, however, gave unreliable and highly variable results at later times (usually 3–4 years), with recurrence rates ranging from 15%–100%. Several other significant controlled studies have been carried out on the 6-month effects of TCAs in patients who may not meet worldwide UP manic-depressive criteria and tended to have features of "neurotic," anxious, mild-to-moderate, and sometimes chronic, depression (therefore not included in Table 1). However, their results are strikingly similar to those tabulated for the 6-month studies of UP disorder. For example, amitriptyline and placebo yielded mean 6-month relapse rates of 21% and 54%, respectively (KLERMAN et al. 1974; STEIN et al. 1980). Additional uncontrolled trials of apparently similar patients have given similar 6-month relapse rates for a TCA (ca. 20%). Perhaps the sharp distinction between the relatively broad current American concept of "major depressive disorder" and the traditional category of UP manic-depressive illness does not hold up with respect to predicting an early relapse-preventing response to an antidepressant.

In the search for more powerfully predictive subcategories among major affective disorders, it has been hypothesized that bipolar disorder may include a broader spectrum than has commonly been accepted, and that a "true UP manic-depressive" or subtly bipolar ("pseudounipolar") group may share a bipolar genotype and have a selective long-term mood-stabilizing response to lithium salts. Such patients might include those with a family history of bipolar or recurrent psychotic disorders and a relatively early age of onset of severe anergic depression, with at least a moderately high recurrence rate of discrete episodes; they may have some cyclothymic or occasional mildly hypomanic features and may become manic when given an antidepressant or ECT (MENDLEWICZ et al. 1973; AKISKAL 1983; GROF et al. 1983). A crucial test of this hypothesis would be the effect of lithium on cases of recurrent depression with only mild, subclinical hypomania, often called bipolar type II (BP-II) disorder. This group may contribute to some of the variance in older studies of lithium for supposedly UP manic-depressives, but among the few who have been studied (ca. 30–40 cases that appear in several reports), the results of lithium treatment are disappointing. Recurrence rates have been similar (about 40%–50% at 16 months and about 60% at 2–3 years of treatment with placebo or lithium), with only limited reduction in morbidity from depression and trends toward less total time hypomanic (DUNNER et al. 1982). An emerging view is that BP-II disorder may not simply be a mild form or precursor of bipolar disorder since it tends to have a stable course and to appear excessively among first-degree relatives of index cases (CORYELL et al. 1987). It is an important entity among clinically UP disorders that requires additional intensive study. In particular, the suggestion that lithium may be especially helpful for the long-term treatment of these or other phenotypically UP, but otherwise bipolarlike, patients requires further scientific testing.

4 Dose-Effect Relationships in Long-Term Treatment of Depression

The matter of establishing dose-effect and dose-risk relationships for psychotropic agents used for long-term treatment has only recently received serious consideration (BALDESSARINI 1985). Yet, there is an extraordinary paucity of data concerning optimal long-term doses or plasma levels of antidepressant drugs. There is somewhat more information concerning lithium, in part reflecting concern about its narrow margin of safety (therapeutic index). Several groups have reviewed their case experience and found a relationship between a less favorable clinical outcome and low average plasma concentrations of lithium (MAJ et al.

1986). In one study of 45 UP patients, a mean plasma lithium level ≤0.7 mEq/L yielded a 2-year failure rate of 56%, whereas higher levels failed in only 6.5% of cases (PRIEN and CAFFEY 1976). A prospective, controlled trial of lithium doses in 69 bipolar patients found a continuous increase in both benefits and side effects of lithium with increasing average plasma levels between 0.3 and 0.9 mEq/L, with corresponding recurrence rates ranging from 65%–25% over 2 years (MAJ et al. 1986). Further studies of this type in UP patients are required.

5 Other Treatments

Long-term treatment of UP disorder with alternatives to TCAs or lithium salts has scarcely been evaluated systematically yet. While MAO inhibitors are sometimes used, we found no controlled, prospective trials of their use in recurrent, endogenous UP depression. Neuroleptics sometimes are added to failing regimens of lithium treatment in bipolar patients, even though there is virtually no research support for a recurrence-preventing effect of neuroleptics. There are a few small, partially controlled trials of addition of flupenthixol or haloperidol to lithium; however, none provides encouraging support for a beneficial effect in the depressive aspect of manic-depressive illness, and some patients showed more depressive morbidity even with some sparing of mania. Finally, the recent emergence of interest in anticonvulsants (carbamazepine, valproate, and clonazepam) in the treatment of mania or of bipolar disorder has not yet led to controlled, prospective trials in UP disorder; nor does experience with carbamazepine in bipolar patients provide encouraging support for a sustained antidepressant effect (PLACIDI et al. 1986; FRANKENBURG et al. 1988).

6 Current Practice

Even though the evidence for long-term beneficial effects of lithium or TCAs in recurrent major UP depression is substantial (Table 2), the level of actual clinical usage stands in striking contrast to this evidence. In a recent survey of hospital prescription practices in the use of antidepressants, RISSE et al. (1985) found that only 15% of antidepressant prescriptions were for patients with evidence of major depression (others were anxious, dysphoric, or alcoholic in most cases). Even more remarkably, only 18% of all the prescriptions were for longer than a year, and long-term use of the drugs for UP patients accounted for less than 1% of all prescriptions for antidepressants!

A recent review of treatments given to patients in the community prior to entry into a study sponsored by the USA National Institute of Mental Health of major affective disorders in five leading American university departments of psychiatry indicated that only 12% of 217 UP patients (and the same proportion of 73 suicidal cases) received what would be considered probably adequate daily doses of an antidepressant (at least 150 mg imipramine or its equivalent), although 86%

were given some form of psychotherapy or an anxiolytic agent (KELLER et al. 1982). Even more remarkably, the treatment received by these seriously depressed patients within the referral centers was only slightly more vigorous: 55% of inpatients and 73% of outpatients were given less than the equivalent of 200 mg imipramine per day at any time (KELLER et al. 1986). In a 1-year follow-up of some of these patients, CORYELL et al. (1987) recently reported that only about 25% of the UP patients were kept on doses of TCAs of at least 200 mg imipramine per day for 4 weeks at any time, and fewer than 10% ever received lithium for at least 2 weeks.

The reasons for this relatively low level of vigor in the treatment of severely ill depressed patients are not entirely clear. They may include a lack of appreciation of the evidence concerning the benefit-risk ratio pertinent to such treatment, as has been reviewed here, or a lingering suspicion that the efficacy of antidepressants and of lithium for depression is limited, while risks of toxicity are high. It has also been suggested recently that daily doses as low as the equivalent of 75 mg imipramine may be adequate for many depressed patients (WHO 1986). A more likely reason for cautious therapy is that patients are significantly intolerant of the side effects of these agents and may fail to perceive a relationship between drug acceptance and short-term – let alone long-term – benefit, based on their own experience with or without medication (BALDESSARINI 1985). Less commonly, despite vigorous trials of such treatment, responses may fail over time, perhaps as a manifestation of drug tolerance, as evidenced by the responsiveness of some patients to increasing doses of an antidepressant or to another type of agent following loss of benefit with a previously successful antidepressant regimen (COHEN and BALDESSARINI 1985).

7 Conclusions and Recommendations

Major depression is one of the most significant public health problems which psychiatrists are responsible for dealing with and contributes importantly to severe morbidity, consumption of resources, impairment of function of potentially productive persons, and increased mortality due at least to suicide and accidents. The great majority of major UP depressions occur episodically, and many involve a degree of chronic disability as well; as many as 85% recur within 2–3 years following apparently full recovery from an index episode. Typical cycles of recurrence average about 2 years, and single episodes last about 6 months (less with treatment). Despite this natural history, surprisingly few long-term studies of maintenance antidepressant or mood-stabilization therapy have persisted for more than a year after recovery from an acute episode. These studies provide strong evidence for a partial protective effect of lithium or of a few imipramine like agents for several months after apparent recovery from an acute episode of major depression. This effect is perhaps due to their preventing overt relapse during a period of particular vulnerability, the basis of which remains unknown and not yet defined by biological characteristics (BALDESSARINI 1983). The evidence for a longer-lasting average protective effect against major recurrences (Table 2) and for reduced morbidity as time spent in depression (COPPEN and PEET 1979) over 1–2 years is good for lithium alone or in combination with a TCA, but not as strong for a TCA alone. Evidence for all such treatments is weaker at later times of follow-up, and controlled studies longer than 2 years are rare.

Realistically, it will be difficult to justify very long-term prospective studies of UP disorder with a placebo group in the future. Choices include comparative studies of innovative treatments with currently available, partially evaluated standard agents. It may also be feasible to design ethical placebo substitution studies at late times following full recovery from an acute episode to separate protection from relapses and recurrences without synchronization by starting treatment after an acute episode. Further evaluations of dose-related benefit-risk ratios are required to define the best compromises between inadequate protection and excessive toxicity or failure of compliance.

It would also be helpful if all studies on this topic would be more forthcoming about matters that tend to remain obscure in the literature, including analyses of the distribution of episode recurrence rates by time and by person, as well as measures of illness severity and of the duration and timing of all depressive morbidity. For example, it is not clear how many UP patients respond or in what way at various times. Do a minority of excellent responders contribute disproportionately to mean trends? Do some patients suffer more moderate morbidity over a longer time? The present analysis (Table 2) dealt with rates of purportedly discrete episodes since they have been a commonly employed measure. Much more work is required to evaluate better-defined subgroups, particularly within the currently broad American concept of "major depression." In the meantime, in addition to the research reviewed here, clinical experience teaches that many depressed patients do poorly when antidepressant or mood-stabilizing treatment is withdrawn, but also that drugs of this kind are underused in current medical practice. Correction of the latter problem requires vigorous dissemination of available information to patients and physicians while urgently needed further research continues.

Acknowledgments. This work was supported, in part, by NIMH awards and grants MH-47370, MH-31154, and MH-36224. Bibliographic assistance was provided by Mrs. LYNN DIETRICH of the McLean Mental Health Science Library computer-search division, by the Psychiatric Library of the Clarke Psychiatric Institute in Toronto, and by Mrs. MILA CASON, who also prepared the manuscript. We also thank Dr. GEORGE WINOKUR for providing unpublished results of recent epidemiological studies on mortality rates in Iowa.

References

Akiskal HS (1978) Diagnosis and classification of affective disorders: new insights from clinical and laboratory approaches. Psychiatr Dev 2:123–160

Angst J, Weis P, Grof P, Baastrup PC, Schou M (1970) Lithium prophylaxis in recurrent affective disorders. Br J Psychiatry 116:604–614

Avery D, Winokur G (1976) Mortality in depressed patients treated with electroconvulsive therapy and antidepressants. Arch Gen Psychiatry 33:1029–1037

Baastrup PC, Schou M (1967) Lithium as a prophylactic agent. Its effectiveness against recurrent depressions and manic depressive psychosis. Arch Gen Psychiatry 16:162–172

Baldessarini RJ (1983) Biomedical aspects of depression and its treatment. American Psychiatric Press, Washington
Baldessarini RJ (1985) Chemotherapy in psychiatry: principles and practice. Harvard University Press, Cambridge
Cohen BM, Baldessarini RJ (1985) Tolerance to therapeutic effects of antidepressants. Am J Psychiatry 142:489–492
Coppen A, Peet M (1979) The long-term management of patients with affective disorders. In: Paykel ES, Coppen A (eds) Psychopharmacology of affective disorders. Oxford University Press, New York, pp 248–256
Coryell W, Andreasen NC, Endicott J, Keller M (1987) The significance of past mania or hypomania in the course and outcome of major depression. Am J Psychiatry 144:309–315
Davis JM (1976) Overview: Maintenance therapy in psychiatry. II. Affective disorders. Am J Psychiatry 133:1–13
Dunner DL, Stallone F, Fieve RR (1982) Prophylaxis with lithium carbonate: an update. Arch Gen Psychiatry 39:1344–1345
Frankenburg F, Tohen M, Cohen BM, Lipinski JF (1988) Long-term response to carbamazepine: a retrospective study. J Clin Psychopharmacol 8:130–132
Grof P, Angst J, Haines T (1974) The clinical course of depression: practical issues. In: Angst J (ed) Classification and prediction of outcome in depression. Springer, Berlin Heidelberg New York, pp 141–147
Grof P, Hux M, Grof E, Arato M (1983) Prediction of response to stabilizing lithium treatment. Pharmacopsychiatry 16:195–200
Hartigan GP (1963) The use of lithium salts in affective disorders. Br J Psychiatry 109:810–814
Keller MB, Klerman GL, Lavori PW, Fawcett JA, Coryell W, Endicott J (1982) Treatment received by depressed patients. JAMA 248:1848–1855
Keller MB, Lavori PW, Klerman GL, Andreasen NC, Endicott J, Coryell W, Fawcett J, Rice JP, Hirschfeld RMA (1986) Low levels and lack of predictors of somatotherapy and psychotherapy received by depressed patients. Arch Gen Psychiatry 43:458–466
Klerman GL, DiMascio A, Weissman M, Prusoff B, Paykel ES (1974) Treatment of depression by drugs and psychotherapy. Am J Psychiatry 131:186–191
Maj M, Starace F, Nolfe G, Kemali D (1986) Minimum plasma lithium levels required for effective prophylaxis in DSM III bipolar disorder: a prospective study. Pharmacopsychiatry 19:420–423
Mendlewicz J, Fieve R, Stallone F (1973) Relationship between effectiveness of lithium therapy and family history. Am J Psychiatry 130:1011–1013
Murphy GE, Woodruff RA, Herjanic M, Super G (1974) Variability of the clinical course of primary affective disorder. Arch Gen Psychiatry 30:757–761
Placidi GF, Lenzi A, Lazzerini F, Cassano G, Akiskal HS (1986) The comparative efficacy and safety of carbamazepine vs. lithium: a randomized, double-blind 3-year trial in 83 patients. J Clin Psychiatry 47:490–494
Prien RF (1983) Long-term maintenance therapy in affective disorders. In: Rifkin A (ed) Schizophrenia and affective disorders: biology and drug treatment. Wright-PSG, Littleton, MA pp 95–115
Prien RF, Caffey EM Jr (1976) Relationship between dosage and response to lithium prophylaxis in recurrent depression. Am J Psychiatry 133:567–570
Prien RF, Kupfer DJ (1986) Continuation drug therapy for major depressive episodes: how long should it be maintained? Am J Psychiatry 143:18–23
Risse SC, Beitman BD, Brinkley JR (1985) Evaluation of long-term of antidepressant medication. Hosp Community Psychiatry 36:1215–1216
Schou M (1979) Lithium as a prophylactic agent in unipolar affective illness: comparison with cyclic antidepressants. Arch Gen Psychiatry 36:849–851
Stein MK, Rickels K, Weiss CC (1980) Maintenance therapy with amitriptyline: a controlled trial. Am J Psychiatry 137:370–371
World Health Organization (WHO) Collaborative Study Group (1986) Dose effects of antidepressant medication in different populations. J Affect Dis 2 [Suppl]:S1–S67
Zis AP, Goodwin FK (1979) Major affective disorder as a recurrent illness: a critical review. Arch Gen Psychiatry 36:835–839

Lithium in Manic-Depressive Illness: Plusses, Pitfalls, and Perspectives

M. Schou

Abstract

Prophylactic lithium treatment of manic-depressive illness offers advantages to patient and family, to society, to the psychiatrist, and to research. The treatment must be administered in accordance with certain guidelines in order to provide maximal efficacy and minimal risk. Research on the mode of action of lithium and its prophylactic alternatives may serve to elucidate metabolic disturbances in the brains of manic-depressive patients. It might also one day reveal biological factors which govern mood, activity and mental speed. Could such knowledge be misused to manipulate mood, one's own or that of others?

1 Introduction

A medical student with preconceived notions about the purely social and psychological origin of mental disorders started clinical service at a psychiatric hospital. He scorned the use of sedative and "motivation inhibiting" drugs, but when he heard patients report how lithium had stopped a disease that was characterized by fierce and frequent manic-depressive recurrences that previously had resisted all social and psychological interventions, he conceded that biological factors might play some role in some mental illnesses.

Had he learned the truth? Had he learned the whole truth? Let us look at another example.

In 1969 we carried out a double-blind discontinuation trial in order to test the prophylactic effect of lithium (Baastrup et al. 1970). About 100 patients who had been receiving lithium treatment for more than a year were transferred double-blind to placebo or to continued lithium treatment. Within 6 months, more than half of the placebo patients relapsed; none of the lithium patients did so. The trial accordingly documented the prophylactic efficacy of lithium.

What is relevant in this connection is, however, that the patients, who did not know they were participating in an experiment, all had a valid psychological explanation of why a relapse had occurred at just that time: marital conflicts, financial difficulties, or moving into a new apartment. The relapses led to hospital admission, and the ward personnel, who apart from a few initiates did not know about the discontinuation trial, accepted fully the patients' psychological explanations of the causes of the relapses.

The Psychopharmacology Research Unit, Aarhus University Institute of Psychiatry and The Psychiatric Hospital, Skovagervej 2, DK-8240 Risskov, Denmark.

These experiences can be viewed in two ways. One can assume that lithium corrected the biochemical disturbance underlying the manic-depressive illness, that the development of relapses in the placebo group was determined exclusively by this disturbance, and that the subjectively convincing psychological explanations represented a rationalization. It is, however, also conceivable that the relapses in the placebo group were in fact provoked by environmental stress in persons of a particular disposition, and that the effect of lithium in the treated group was to raise the threshold for environment-induced relapses.

I do not care to choose between these interpretations, and the truth is presumably a both/and rather than an either/or. One cannot crumple one side of a piece of paper without also crumpling the other. That is how I view psyche and brain.

Having given this scientific credo, I shall outline some of the particular benefits or plusses that characterize lithium as a pharmacotherapeutic agent in manic-depressive illness.

2 Plusses for Patient and Family

Quantitatively, one obtains an impression of the efficacy of lithium prophylaxis from Tables 1 and 2. Table 1 shows data from a review in which observations were pooled from a number of double-blind, placebo-controlled prophylactic studies (Schou 1978). As a measure of efficacy I used the percentage of patients falling ill within 1 year after the start of treatment. This is admittedly a crude yardstick since it does not distinguish between patients who suffered only one relapse and patients who suffered more, but it was the only measure that could be used for pooling data from different studies.

Table 1 shows that patients given dummy tablets were at high risk of recurrences: more than half suffered relapse within a year. Maintenance treatment with lithium led to a marked reduction in the risk of falling ill, almost the same in bipolar and unipolar cases. Treatment with antidepressant drugs led to similar re-

Table 1. Lithium versus placebo, and antidepressants versus placebo: weighted means of calculated percentages of patients relapsing within 1 year after start of treatment (pooled data from 14 studies)

Diagnostic group	Medication	No. of patients	Patients relapsing within one year (%)
Bipolar	Placebo	187	73
	Lithium	186	20
Unipolar	Placebo	77	65
	Lithium	76	22
Bipolar	Placebo	10	(68)
	Antidepressant	11	(59)
Unipolar	Placebo	187	67
	Antidepressant	187	35

Table 2. Outcome of prophylactic lithium treatment of manic-depressive illness in the German Democratic Republic in the years 1967–1977 (number of patients = 623)

	Before lithium	During lithium	During/before lithium
Mean episode frequency (starts per year)	1.59	0.25	0.16
Mean time ill (months per year)	4.12	2.06	0.50
Patients requiring other drugs in more than minimal dosage (%)	45	14	0.31

sults in the unipolar patients, whereas too few bipolar patients completed the trials to permit any conclusions. They dropped out because they suffered manic relapses during administration of the antidepressant drugs.

However, efficacy of treatment given in a research setting is not always the same as efficacy of treatment given under everyday clinical conditions. The quantitative outcome of long-term lithium treatment under the latter circumstances has been revealed by information collected from the psychiatric clinics of a whole country, namely the German Democratic Republic (FELBER 1981). The data were obtained over a period of about 10 years, between 1967 and 1977, and the study incorporated patients from 31 psychiatric clinics and hospitals. For 623 patients sufficient information was available to permit intraindividual comparison of episode frequency and length of time ill over equally long periods before and during lithium treatment. Table 2 shows a marked reduction in episode frequency. Bipolar and unipolar patients responded best, schizoaffective patients less well. Time ill was reduced by half, and there was less need for other drugs during lithium than before lithium.

It is worth emphasizing that successful relapse prevention involves gains in addition to those which can be expressed quantitatively. Such benefits include reduced human suffering, increased stability of mood during intervals, regained self-confidence, renewed trust in the future, and improved marital and family relations. These gains are of central importance for the patients and their family. Successful prophylactic treatment of frequently recurring manic-depressive illness may improve the quality of life miraculously.

3 Plusses for Society

Various authors have calculated the economic gains of lithium prophylaxis for society. In the East German study the savings amounted to about one million East German Marks for the 623 patients for 1 year (FELBER and KÖNIG 1979). Related calculations for the United States showed in one study (CUSANO et al. 1977) an estimated saving of hospital expenses of 1000 dollars per patient per year, to which should be added savings due to preserved working capacity. Another study calculated the total savings in hospital costs for the United States over 10 years to be 2.9 billion dollars, to which should be added 1.3 billion gained in production (REIFMAN and WYATT 1980). That was in 1980; prices have not fallen since then.

4 Plusses for the Psychiatrist

It is always gratifying to administer an effective treatment, and in most cases prophylactic lithium treatment gives great satisfaction to both patient and physician. In countries with private practice some psychiatrists may have misgivings about a therapy which is so effective that the doctor is rarely needed, but I believe that the gratification of having provided substantial help far outweighs such considerations.

Moreover, it would be wrong to assume that lithium treatment, effective as it is, makes psychological support and human interest superfluous. On the contrary, lithium may make psychotherapy of manic-depressive patients feasible and meaningful, and if long-term maintenance treatment of any kind is to give satisfactory results, it must be based on close and confident cooperation between physician, patient, and family. Continued support reduces noncompliance and increases efficacy. If prophylactic trials of recent years have sometimes had poorer outcomes than the early trials, the explanation may be that more patients are treated outside hospital and fewer admitted, so that other populations are now tested. However, one cannot exclude the possibility that attention to infrastructure and care has slackened now that pharmacological prophylaxis is more or less taken for granted.

Not only must dosages, side effects, and signs of relapse be under supervision. The unavoidable personal and social problems associated with long-term treatment must be attended to through appropriate psychological support, and it is essential that patients be carefully informed and instructed, both verbally and in written form. Books written specifically for patients and relatives are available in several languages (SCHOU 1983, 1984a, b, 1986a–c); they may serve as a basis for discussions between physician, patient, and family.

5 Plusses for Research

The use of lithium for manic-depressive illness has, as a by-product, led to discoveries that are useful in other branches of science. As an example the so-called lithium clearance method for the determination of V_{prox}, i.e., the output of water and sodium from the proximal tubules, may be mentioned. The method has been elaborated by KLAUS THOMSEN in our institute (THOMSEN 1984; THOMSEN and SCHOU 1986). Lithium is filtered freely through the glomerular membrane and is reabsorbed in the proximal tubules together with, and to the same extent as, water and sodium. However, under almost all circumstances lithium passes unreabsorbed through the loop of Henle, the distal tubules and the collecting ducts, so that the renal lithium clearance is identical with, and can be used as a measure of, V_{prox}. The method consists in determining the lithium clearance after administration of a small test dose of lithium to the animals or subjects under investigation, a dose so small that it does not affect kidney function.

It is accordingly now possible, for the first time, to determine V_{prox} without performing micropuncture, without the use of anesthesia and surgery, and repeatedly in the same individual, in normal subjects and in patients suffering from various diseases, under varying dietary conditions, and under the influence of different agents. After some initial hesitation about accepting something that came from psychiatry, kidney physiologists, internists, and nephrologists have greeted the method enthusiastically, and it is now being used extensively and with interesting results.

6 Pitfalls and Precautions

Fears have at times been expressed that when lithium treatment is given over many years it might lead to progressive destruction of the patients' brains, thyroids or kidneys. These fears can be set at rest: it does not. If lithium therapy is administered according to a limited number of guidelines and precautions, it is a safe treatment as well as an effective one.

But it is important that the guidelines and precautions *are* respected. If they are not, severe lithium intoxication can develop which may lead to death or long-lasting cerebellar damage. It is important to note, however, that lithium intoxication does not develop suddenly and does not occur capriciously. There are warning signs and symptoms that herald impending intoxication, and accumulation of lithium takes place in special risk situations, which physicians and patients would be wise to memorize and avoid. These situations are characterized by dehydration and sodium deficiency, and they include conditions with loss of fluid or salt, low-salt diet, abrupt slimming regimens, and treatment with diuretics or nonsteroidal antirheumatics. Particularly important, while particularly frequent, is physical illness with fever, for example influenza. Under all these circumstances lithium treatment should temporarily be discontinued or the dosage reduced (Schou 1984c).

Since some lithium-treated patients have a reduced capacity for concentrating urine, they are at an increased risk of becoming dehydrated, and fluid should be administered parenterally to patients who vomit massively or are unconscious for many hours, as well as during the night before operation with narcosis when oral fluid intake is forbidden.

7 Perspectives

Neither for lithium nor for its alternatives does one know the biological mechanism which is responsible for the effects on manic-depressive illness, but research in the area is very active. Lithium influences many systems, and it is difficult to decide which effects are relevant for the therapeutic and prophylactic actions. It is to be hoped that the appearance of alternatives to lithium may facilitate the sorting of observations and hypotheses. Lithium acts on enzymes, hormones, and membranes, with consequent effects on, for example, electrolyte transport, transmitter release, and receptor sensitivity. Because the key is so small, it fits into many locks. It is presumably not farfetched to assume that some of the special effects of lithium are caused by similarities to or dissimilarities from the naturally occurring cations sodium, potassium, calcium, and magnesium.

In recent years interest has focused on the limbic system, GABA-ergic functions, cerebral adenosine receptors, cyclic nucleotides, phosphoinositol as a messenger, and the action of calcium on neurotransmission. Effects have also been observed on the regulation of chronobiological functions.

Lithium offers a number of research advantages: (a) it exerts a more specific action on manic-depressive illness than the conventional neuroleptics and antidepressants; (b) it acts against both manias and depressions, prophylactically and therapeutically against the former, prophylactically and to some extent therapeutically against the latter; (c) it is not metabolized in the organism, and problems of active or inactive metabolites do not exist; and (d) the quantitative determination of lithium in tissues and tissue fluids is rapid, specific, and accurate. As an important further advantage it may be mentioned that (e) although lithium counteracts *abnormal* mood changes with considerable efficacy, it interferes to a remarkably low extent with *normal* mood level and mood changes.

Since lithium treatment prevents both manic and depressive relapses, one may visualize lithium as exerting a regulating or stabilizing effect on those cerebral processes that govern the mood and which presumably are out of balance in the affective psychoses. The day will presumably come when we succeed in finding out how lithium and its alternatives do what they do in manic-depressive illness. This may lead to treatments with a larger therapeutic range and still greater specificity.

And what about the more distant future? If research should at some time succeed in clarifying the cerebral mechanisms which govern the levels of mood, activity, and mental speed, this would seem to open up possibilities of not only *normalizing* but also *manipulating* mood. It might, for example, be possible through chemical or electrical procedures to adjust the mood to a particular level, one's own mood or that of others. One may perhaps become able to choose a life in light chronic mania, subjectively more attractive than even the most pleasant hash or alcohol euphoria. A happy vision? Or a frightening one? It is at any rate a possibility which has wide perspectives and which forces us to ponder the central issue: Should scientists under all circumstances reveal the secrets of nature, or are there doors which they should abstain from opening because of the possible consequences?

References

Baastrup PC, Poulsen JC, Schou M, Thomsen K, Amdisen A (1970) Prophylactic lithium: Double-blind discontinuation in manic-depressive and recurrent-depressive disorders. Lancet II:326–330

Cusano PP, Mayo J, O'Connell RA (1977) The medical economics of lithium treatment for manic-depressives. Hosp Community Psychiatry 28:169–173

Felber W (1981) Rezidivprophylaxe affektiver Erkrankungen mit Lithium und ihre Auswirkungen. Psychiatr Clin (Basel) 14:161–166

Felber W, König L (1979) Fünfjähriges Lithium-Erprobungsprogramm – Auswertung von 850 Behandlungsunterlagen. In: Schulze HAF, Biersack W (eds) Konzeptionen und Modelle der langfristigen Betreuung in der Nervenheilkunde. Hirzel, Leipzig, S. 86–91

Reifman A, Wyatt RJ (1980) Lithium: a brake in the rising cost of mental illness. Arch Gen Psychiatry 37:385–388

Schou M (1978) Lithium for affective disorders: cost and benefit. In: Ayd FJ, Taylor IJ (eds) Mood disorders: the world's major public health problem. Ayd Medical Communications, Baltimore, pp 117–137

Schou M (1983) Lithiumbehandling af manio-depressiv sygdom: en vejledning, 2nd edn. Arkona, Aarhus

Schou M (1984a) Le lithium: guide pratique pour les médecins et les patients. Presses Universitaires de France, Paris

Schou M (1984b) Lithium treatment of manic-depressive illness: a practical guide (in Japanese). Igakushuppan-Sha, Tokyo

Schou M (1984c) Long-lasting neurological sequelae after lithium intoxication. Acta Psychiatr Scand 70:594–602

Schou M (1986a) Lithium treatment of manic-depressive illness: a practical guide, 3rd edn. Karger, Basel

Schou M (1986b) Lithium-Behandlung der manisch-depressiven Krankheit: Information für Arzt und Patienten. 2. Aufl. Thieme, Stuttgart

Schou M (1986c) Il trattamento con litio della malattia maniaco-depressiva: una guida pratica. Athena, Roma

Thomsen K (1984) Lithium clearance: a new method for determining proximal and distal tubular reabsorption of sodium and water. Nephron 37:217–223

Thomsen K, Schou M (1986) Lithium clearance: a new research area. News Physiol Sci 1:126–128

Basic and Clinical Aspects of the Activity of the New Monoamine Oxidase Inhibitors

A. Delini-Stula [1], E. Radeke [1], and P. C. Waldmeier [2]

Abstract

The clinical relevance of the neurobiochemical and pharmacological properties of the new generation of monoamine oxidase inhibitors (MAOIs) is reviewed and discussed. The most distinctive characteristics of these drugs are the selectivity, competitive nature and reversibility of their MAO-inhibiting action. The most selective MAO-A inhibitors are moclobemide and brofaromine, with ratios between their MAO-A and MAO-B inhibiting potency (estimated in in vitro assays) of 1 : ≧1000 and 1 : 500, respectively, whereas the least selective drug is cimoxatone with a ratio of 1 : 66. If in vitro findings are considered, the most potent MAO-A inhibitor seems to be cimoxatone and the least potent toloxatone. After oral administration, however, cimoxatone, brofaromine and moclobemide appear to be about equally effective in inhibiting brain MAO-A. All these drugs are short acting and their MAO-inhibiting action is reversible within 24 h or, in the case of brofaromine, 48 h. Due to the selectivity and reversibility of the MAO-A inhibition, they were found to be less likely to induce large increases in the pressor responses to tyramine, both in animals and in man. In patients treated with 150 mg/day for 4 weeks, brofaromine, which appears to be the best-characterized drug in this respect, produced about a 4-fold increase in sensitivity to tyramine. Although the clinical antidepressant efficacy of these drugs remains to be confirmed in more extensive studies, based on their neurobiochemical and pharmacological properties, clear advantages in respect to their side-effect profiles are to be expected in comparison with the classical MAOIs.

1 Introduction

The discovery of the clinical antidepressant activity of the inhibitors of the enzyme monoamine oxidase (MAOI) was, like the discovery of imipramine, due to serendipity. In the early 1950s, based on the observation that tuberculous patients treated with isoniazid and iproniazid show euphoria and improvement of mood, French psychiatrists suggested the use of these drugs in the treatment of depression. Of these two compounds it was iproniazid, the isopropyl derivative of isoniazid, which became the first clinically employed MAOI antidepressant. The pharmacological rationale for the use of iproniazid was subsequently provided by the discovery that it reversed the immobility, ptosis, and catalepsy of reserpine-treated rats, an effect which was found to be associated with an increase concentration of the monoamines in the brain caused by the inhibition of their deamination by this drug (Brodie et al. 1956).

The first generation of MAOIs introduced into clinical practice in the late 1950s and early 1960s comprised a structurally heterogeneous class of com-

[1] Clinical Research and Development and
[2] Research Laboratories, Pharmaceuticals Division Ciba-Geigy Ltd., Basle, Switzerland.

pounds. Iproniazid represented the MAOIs with hydrazinic moieties and tranylcypromine those with nonhydrazinic structure. However, all these compounds had the one common characteristic of inhibiting irreversibly and nonselectively the activity of intracellular mitochondrial monoamine oxidase. Consequently, they inhibited oxidative deamination of endogenous as well as exogenous amines into inactive degradation products.

The initially widespread and enthusiastic clinical use of the first generation of MAOIs was, however, rather short lived. Soon it became obvious that these drugs induce various and sometimes severe adverse reactions. This led to a great limitation of their clinical application or to their use being almost completely abandoned in most countries. In this respect, apart from hepatotoxic effects, of particular concern were fatal hypertensive crises resulting from the massive increase in the blood levels of tyramine after ingestion of tyramine-containing food ("cheese reaction"). Whereas the hepatotoxic effects were apparently specifically related to the hydrazine structure, enhanced tyramine effects were the consequence of the pharmacodynamic properties of these drugs.

The recent resurgence of interest in MAOIs, as valid alternatives to the therapy of depression with the inhibitors of the monoamine uptake, is based on the discovery that the enzyme monoamine oxidase is present in two distinct forms, known as MAO-A and MAO-B (JOHNSTON 1968; TIPTON et al. 1982; FOWLER and ROSS 1984). The MAO-A form, highly sensitive to low concentrations of clorgyline, preferentially metabolizes serotonin (5-HT), noradrenaline, and dopamine (DA). Conversely, the MAO-B form, predominantly blocked by selegiline (Deprenil) and low doses of pargyline, is responsible for the deamination of benzylamine and phenethylamine (PEA). Amines such as tyramine, tryptamine, and octopamine were found to be the substrates for both enzyme forms. As a consequence of these findings, the possibility emerged that drugs showing clear selectivity for the MAO-A form may retain the antidepressant properties without the deleterious adverse cardiovascular reactions ("cheese effect") caused by inhibition of the deamination of the pressor amines, particularly tyramine. Since tyramine is the substrate for both enzyme forms, in the presence of MAO-A inhibition it could still be alternatively metabolized by the MAO-B enzyme. This assumption led to the development of a number of drugs showing highly selective MAO-A-inhibiting properties. Besides this, the new or "second"-generation MAOIs have another particular characteristic which contrasts with the classical MAOIs: the reversibility of their action.

2 Biochemical and Pharmacological Characteristics of MAO-A Inhibitors

All MAOIs may be classified into different categories according to their principal properties: selectivity and reversibility of their enzyme-inhibiting action. The representative compounds from each group are listed in Table 1.

The selectivity of enzyme-inhibiting action could be well demonstrated by the differences in the potencies of these compounds to prevent the deamination of 5-

Table 1. Biochemical classification of MAOIs

Characteristics of MAO inhibition	Degree of selectivity	Prototypes
Irreversible	Nonselective	Isocarboxazide Iproniazid Phenelzine
Irreversible	Preferential	MAO-A Clorgyline MAO-B Selegiline Pargyline
Partially reversible	Nonselective	Tranylcypromine
Reversible	Selective	MAO-A Moclobemide Brofaromine Toloxatone MAO-B MD 780236

HT or PEA in the presence of tissue MAO. The estimations could be done by in vitro assays using tissue homogenates, as well as in ex vivo or in vivo preparations. Based on the findings reported in the literature (FOWLER and ROSS 1984; STROLIN BENEDETTI et al. 1983; WALDMEIER et al. 1983a, b; DA PRADA et al. 1983), cimoxatone and brofaromine appear from in vitro assays to be the most potent MAO-A inhibitors, but only brofaromine and moclobemide could be considered to be highly selective as well. Among these drugs toloxatone has the weakest MAO-A-inhibiting action, but its selectivity is higher than that of cimoxatone (KAN et al. 1978; KAENE et al. 1979).

After oral administration, however, in ex vivo and in vivo assays the potencies of cimoxatone, brofaromine, and moclobemide on a mg/kg basis are comparable (Tables 2 and 3). The fact that moclobemide and cimoxatone are almost equipotent in in vivo assays but differ by a factor of more than 300 in in vitro assays (DA PRADA et al. 1983) indicates that the MAO-A-inhibiting property of moclobemide resides mainly in an active metabolite (or metabolites). This is, perhaps, also the reason for preferential inhibition of the liver MAO-A enzyme by this drug after its oral administration (ratio of ED_{50} brain/liver = 2:5, WALDMEIER et al. 1983a), a phenomenon which is also observed with classical irreversible MAOIs (WALDMEIER et al. 1981). It is worth mentioning that brofaromine and cimoxatone show 50% inhibition of liver and brain MAO-A at about equipotent oral doses.

The reversibility and the competitive nature of the interaction of the selective MAO-A inhibitors with the active enzyme sites is one of the additional important characteristics of this new generation of MAOIs. This property is well demonstrated by the time-course of their action in in vivo experiments. In contrast to the classical MAOIs and clorgyline, which induce long-lasting inhibition of MAO enzymatic activity in the brain (half-life 2.5–12 days depending on the inhibitor;

Table 2. Comparative MAO-A-inhibiting potency of various selective and reversible MAO-A inhibitors

Drug	MAO-A inhibition ED_{50} (mg/kg p. o.)		Decrease in HVA ED_{50} (mg/kg p. o.)	Increase in 5-HT threshold dose (mg/kg p. o.)
	Liver	Brain		
Amiflamine	30	10	3	1
Brofaromine	1	1	3	10
Cimoxatone	1	1	1	1
Moclobemide	0.6	1.5	1	3
Perlindole	< 30 (80%)	< 30 (80%)	–	–
Toloxatone	≫100 (0%)	>100 (20%)	–	–

HVA, Homovanillic acid
In vivo estimates of the 5-HT deamination in rat liver and brain homogenates were done 2 h after pretreatment with oral doses of the drugs. (For methodological details see WALDMEIER et al. 1983)

Table 3. In vitro MAO-inhibiting potency of some selective MAO-A inhibitors

Drug	IC_{50} (μmol/l)		Ratio	Ref.
	5-HT	PEA		
Amiflamine	5	>1000	> 200	
Cimoxatone	0.003	0.2	66	DA PRADA et al. (1983)
Moclobemide	1	>1000	>1000	
Brofaromine	0.06	30	500	WALDMEIER et al. (1983)
Toloxatone	3.8	200	143	KAN et al. (1978)

Note: The in vitro estimates of the IC_{50} values from different studies are not strictly comparable with each other, due to differences in the assays.

MAITRE et al. 1976), the inhibition of MAO-A with selective MAO-A inhibitors is of rather short duration; recovery of enzymatic activity, as demonstrated by estimations of the kinetics of inhibition of 5-HT deamination after treatment with these drugs, occurs within less than 24 h (STROLIN-BENEDETTI et al. 1979; DA PRADA et al. 1982), or, in the case of brofaromine, 48 h (WALDMEIER et al. 1983 a, b). The short duration of action, indicative of reversible binding of these drugs to the enzyme active sites, has an important clinical consequence: lack of accumulation and maintenance of selectivity after chronic treatment. Irreversible selective drugs such as clorgyline (MAO-A selective) or pargyline (MAO-B preferential) do not, for instance, retain their substrate specificity and inhibit both MAO forms if given in sufficiently high doses and for a prolonged period of time (FOWLER 1982).

The reversibility and the competitive nature of their in vivo action is substantiated by the observation that the increase in the availability of the endogenous monoamines (5-HT, DA) resulting from tetrabenazine treatment antagonizes the MAO-A-inhibiting effects of these drugs. Under in vitro conditions, however, dif-

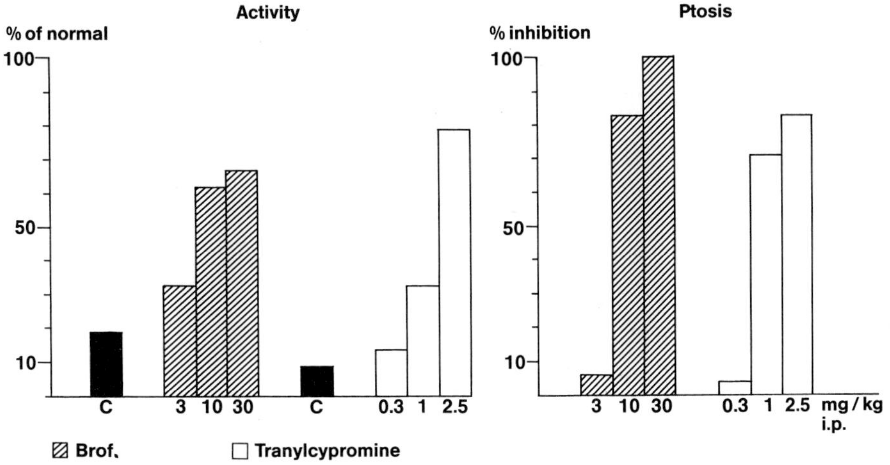

Fig. 1. Antogonism of tetrabenazine-induced behavioral depression in rats ($n=10$) by brofaromine (▨) and tranylcypromine (□). Each column represents the mean cumulative scores as percentages of the values before drug administration; *C*, activity after tetrabenazine alone. Motor activity and ptosis were evaluated on scales of 0–4 (0, no activity/no ptosis: 4, normal activity/maximal closure of the eyes). Drugs were given 30 min before tetrabenazine 10 mg/kg i.p. and the effects were rated intermittently for up to 1 h

ferences were observed in the ease with which these drugs could be dissociated from the enzyme by serial dilutions and dialysis. Although kinetics experiments in vitro confirm the reversibility of action of amiflamine and cimoxatone, the latter binds firmly to the enzyme (FOWLER and STROLIN BENEDETTI 1983) and, as was recently shown, even more so than brofaromine or moclobemide (WALDMEIER 1985). This apparently paradoxical behavior of these drugs under in vitro conditions has not yet been fully explained. However, as suggested by WALDMEIER (1985), the "degree of reversibility", e.g., the readiness with which these agents are displaced from the enzyme sites by endogenous or exogenous substrates, could be an important feature and is particularly relevant in regard to the therapeutic efficacy and tolerability of these drugs.

Pharmacological properties of selective MAO-A inhibitors reflect their biochemical mode of action. Like classical MAOIs these drugs antagonize various central depressant and autonomic effects of amine-depleting agents such as reserpine and tetrabenazine. The comparative effects of brofaromine and tranylcypromine in reversing the hypoactivity and ptosis induced by tetrabenazine in the rat are illustrated in Fig. 1. To some extent, however, selective MAO-A inhibitors could be differentiated from classical antidepressants in routine screening procedures. Table 4 shows comparative effects of selective MAO-A inhibitors and other respresentative antidepressants on reserpine- and apomorphine-induced hypothermia in mice. Apart from selective inhibitors of 5-HT uptake, other types of drugs and MAO-A inhibitors are consistently active in reversing the hypothermic effect of reserpine. Interestingly, however, they do not reverse efficiently the hypothermic effect of a high dose of apomorphine, which is suggested

Table 4. Reversal of reserpine- and apo-morphine-induced hypothermia in the mouse

Drug	Minimum effective dose for reversal of hypothermia (mg/kg, i. p./s. c.)	
	Reserpine (2 mg/kg s. c.)	Apomorphine (10 mg/kg s. c.)
Antidepressants		
Imipramine	0.3	2.5
Clomipramine	3	1
Fluoxetine	≫30[a]	10
D-Femoxetine	10	10
Citalopram	≫30	25
MAO-A Inhibitors		
Clorgyline	3	≫ 3
Amiflamine	< 5[a]	10
Brofaromine	10[a]	≫100[a]
Cimoxatone	< 0.25[a]	100
Moclobemide	1	≫ 25[a]
Other MAOIs		
Selegiline	30[a]	1
Tranylcypromine	3	≫ 30

[a] mg/kg p. o.; ≫, No effect at this dose.

to involve noradrenergic-serotoninergic mechanisms. In contrast, selegiline, which is an irreversible selective MAO-B inhibitor, antagonizes apomorphine hypothermia at a dose which is near to the dose inhibiting MAO-B by 50%. It reverses reserpine-induced hypothermia marginally only at doses 30 times higher. The reason for the different behavior of selective MAO-A and MAO-B inhibitors in these two tests is not clear. It is nevertheless interesting to note that MAO-A and MAO-B inhibitors affect 5-HTP- and tryptamine-induced excitation in mice and rats differently, suggesting that the substrate specificities of the two forms of the enzyme could be different in these two species (DELINI-STULA and RADEKE 1985).

On the other hand, in rats the selectivity of the MAO-inhibiting action, is exemplified by the differential effect of these drugs on the excitation syndrome induced by tryptamine and the stereotyped behavior induced by PEA. As illustrated in Table 5, tryptamine effects are clearly potentiated by selective MAO-A inhibitors, but those of PEA are not. Conversely, MAO-B inhibitors enhance PEA effects (ORTMANN et al. 1984, 1985) but are ineffective in the tryptamine test (DELINI-STULA and RADEKE 1985).

Moreover, selective MAO-A inhibitors, but not MAO-B inhibitors, increase the 5-HTP-induced effects and there is a good correlation between the extent of 5-HTP potentiation and the MAO-A-inhibiting potency (ORTMANN et al. 1980). Figure 2 illustrates the 5-HTP-potentiating effects of brofaromine, toloxatone, and tranylcypromine.

Table 5. Potentiation of tryptamine- and PEA-induced effects

Drug	ED_{50} (mg/kg)		MAO inhibition brain ED_{50} (mg/kg)	
	Tryptamine	PEA	A	B
MAO-A inhibitors				
Clorgyline	0.5	10	0.1	> 10 s.c.
Brofaromine	< 2.5	100	1.0	>100
Cimoxatone	0.5	100	1	–
Moclobemide	2.5	5	1.5	10 p.o.
MAO-B inhibitors				
Selegiline	25	0.1	10	0.09 s.c.
Pargyline	≫25	0.25	5	0.3 s.c.
Caroxazone	25	1	>100	>100 p.o.

>, Less than 50%.
≫, no effect at this dose.
From ORTMANN et al. (1985), WALDMEIER et al. (1983). DELINI-STULA and RADEKE (1985, and unpublished)

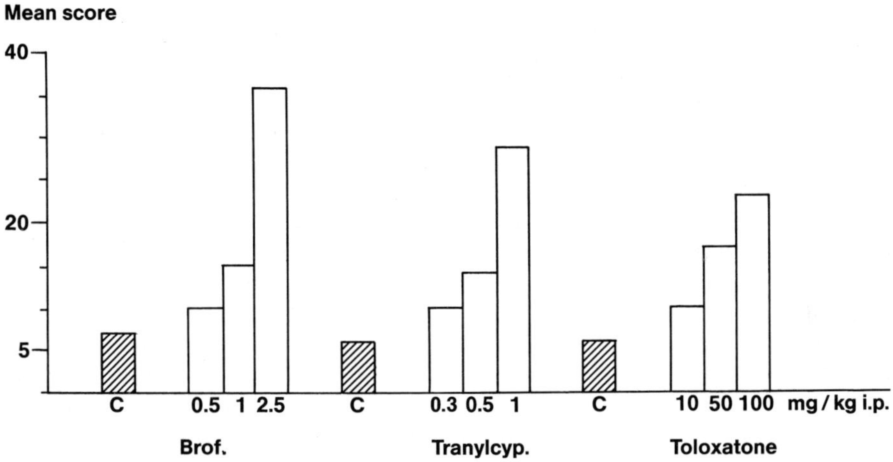

Fig. 2. Potentiation of the 5-HT-induced head twitch in the mouse by brofaromine (*Brof.*), tranylcypromine (*Tranylcyp.*), and toloxatone. Each column represents the mean cumulative score for head twitch of 20 mice. Drugs were given 30 min before L-5-HT, 100 mg/kg i.p. *C*, control

However, apart from the psychopharmacological properties suggesting the antidepressant potential of these drugs which are clearly related to their biochemical mode of action, their general effects on different types of behavior are rather poorly characterized. It is interesting that classical irreversible and nonselective MAOIs induce aggressive, rage reactions in rats if combined with L-dopa or with classical antidepressants (RANDRUP and MUNKVAD 1969), but in contrast suppress aggressive, belligerent attacks of pairs of mice subjected to stressful electric shocks ("fighting behavior"; TEDESCHI et al. 1969). A selective MAO-A inhibitor such as clorgyline was found to induce excessive excitation and motor hyperactivity in rats treated with L-dopa, but the combination of selegiline with L-dopa produced an opposite effect (MAITRE et al. 1976). Even though such interactions are conventionally ascribed to the inhibition of MAO, it is not explained why these behavioral effects showed a time-course different from the time-course and duration of MAO-A inhibition (MAITRE et al. 1976). Certain differences also appear to exist between the behavioral effects of classical antidepressants and MAOIs. Recently we found that brofaromine and imipramine influence the novelty-oriented exploratory responses (indicating neophobia) in the open field in a different manner after repeated administration in rats. Whereas brofaromine showed dose-dependent inhibition of open-field behavior after single dose administration, with tolerance to this inhibitory effect after multiple doses, the opposite was true for imipramine (DELINI-STULA and HUNN 1986). There are, however, no comparable studies with other selective and reversible MAO-A inhibitors.

3 Interaction with Tyramine and the Side-Effect Profile

The most important and clinically relevant property of MAOIs is their ability to enhance the effects of sympathomimetic amines, particularly tyramine, by virtue of their enzyme-inhibiting properties. The inhibition of tyramine deamination, leading to the elevation of its blood concentration, is believed to be the cause of the hypertensive crises which may have a fatal outcome. A number of animal and human studies were therefore devoted to investigation of the interaction of selective and reversible MAO-A inhibitors and tyramine.

Under in vitro conditions in an isolated vas deferens preparation, YOUDIM and FINBERG (1983) demonstrated that the enhancement and the duration of the contractile tyramine response, even by the reversible MAO-A inhibitors, is dependent on the affinity of the drugs for the enzyme active sites. Under in vivo conditions, however, besides the selectivity of action the competitive nature of the enzyme inhibition is the most important factor limiting the extent and duration of the interaction with tyramine.

Comparing the effect of graded doses of brofaromine, clorgyline, and tranylcypromine, administered daily for 5 days, on tyramine-induced (i.v.) hypertension in rats, WALDMEIER et al. (1983) found that brofaromine significantly potentiates high (300 μg/kg) but not low (50 μg/kg) doses of tyramine. This effect was observed at oral doses 10 to 30 times higher than the mean effective dose (ED_{50}) for MAO-A inhibition. With tranylcypromine significant and much larger increases in blood pressure were observed after treatment with 0.3 mg/kg, a dose which is approximately equal to the ED_{50} values for MAO-A and MAO-B inhibition in the liver and in the brain. Also, clorgyline produced greater and highly significant enhancement of the pressor effects of low and high tyramine doses. In a very elaborate investigation of the interaction of MAOIs with orally administered tyramine. DA PRADA et al. (1984) found that in freely moving rats moclobemide (100 mg/kg p.o.), caroxazone (100 mg/kg p.o.) and brofaromine (30 mg/kg p.o.) barely increased the blood pressure; if present, the effect was of short duration (not exceeding 10 min). Cimoxatone and amiflamine produced an increase in blood pressure of about the same order of magnitude, but with longer-lasting effects.

The results of animal experiments are largely corroborated by the studies of the interaction of selective and reversible MAO-A inhibitors with tyramine in man. DOLLERY et al. (1984) found, for instance, that subchronic treatment with toloxatone (5 × 200 mg daily for 1 week) does not appreciably influence the pressor effects of tyramine in healthy volunteers. In the same study cimoxatone showed a moderate enhancement of the effects of tyramine and its effectiveness appeared to be considerably lower than that of irreversible MAOIs. After increasing oral doses, up to 150 mg (KORN et al. 1984), and daily 150 mg doses given for 1 week (KORN et al. 1986), moclobemide produced no significant blood-pressure response to oral tyramine load (50 mg). It also failed to increase the effects of eating cheese and wine. In depressed patients treated with moclobemide for 4 weeks, the pressor response to i.v. tyramine was enhanced about 1.5-fold. In comparison it has been reported that the irreversible MAOIs may give up to a 100-fold increase in the sensitivity of tyramine (KORN et al. 1986).

In acute and subchronic treatment with brofaromine in the therapeutic and MAO-A-inhibiting range of doses in man (BIECK and ANTONIN 1982; BIECK et al. 1983–1985; HOLSBOER et al. 1984) brofaromine was also shown to induce only moderate enhancement of tyramine sensitivity. A remarkable finding was that brofaromine showed a ceiling of tyramine potentiation at doses of between 50 and 150 mg/day. In contrast, a highly significant and cumulative increase of the sensitivity to tyramine was induced by doses of tranylcypromine of 10–25 mg/day (BIECK and ANTONIN 1982). Moreover, there was a clear-cut difference in the duration of the tyramine potentiation induced by these two drugs. After discontinuation of the treatment with brofaromine the sensitivity to tyramine normalized within 8 days, whereas in the case of tranylcypromine the normalization was complete after about 3 weeks (BIECK et al. 1984; P. R. BIECK and K. H. ANTONIN, unpublished).

Like moclobemide, brofaromine enhanced the pressor effects of tyramine in depressed patients treated with 150 mg/day for 4 weeks. The increase of sensitivity, although significant, was however small and much less pronounced than after tranylcypromine (about 4-fold, according to HOLSBOER et al. 1984, unpublished).

It is obvious from all these studies that selective and reversible MAO-A inhibitors, although not completely devoid of tyramine-potentiating effects, are certainly much less effective in this respect than irreversible and nonselective MAOIs. The ceiling of the potentiating effect, as observed with brofaromine in man, combined with the short duration of the tyramine-induced blood pressure increase, as well as the rather rapid normalization of the sensitivity to tyramine, could also be interpreted as contributory safety factors in the prevention of fatal hypertensive crises.

Increased sensitivity to tyramine, although the most extensively discussed and certainly serious, is neither the most frequent nor the only clinically relevant side effect of MAOIs. Other not frequent but serious adverse effects such as hepatotoxicity have been reported after treatment with iproniazid, pheniprazine, phen-

Table 6. Side effects of classical MAOIs

Common but not serious	Serious
Hypotension	Toxic hepatitis
Insomnia	Hypertensive crisis
Impaired sexual function	Polyneuritis, also ophthalmic, due to antipyridoxine effects
Hyperphagia	Inhibition of many other enzymes
Weight gain	
Urinary retention	
Disinhibition syndrome	
Provocation or exacerbation of psychosis	
Edema	

elzine, tranylcypromine, and some other MAOIs. The nature of the hepatotoxic effect is not completely understood. It seemed to be related to the hydrazinic moiety of the MAOIs, although idiosyncratic response and activation of viral infections have also been incriminated. In any case, the hepatotoxic reactions do not appear to be related to either the dose or the duration of the treatment. At present, it is not possible to judge how safe the new MAOIs are in this respect, but chemically they are a distinctly different category of drugs and, moreover, their interaction with the enzymes is reversible.

The most common side effects of classical MAOIs, however, are related to their biochemical and pharmacological properties. They are listed in Table 6. Whereas insomnia and exacerbation or provocation of psychosis could also be expected to occur after selective and reversible MAO-A inhibitors, present clinical experience is insufficient to allow estimation of the incidence of other side effects (see also PARE 1985). In general, if one considers the side-effect profile of the MAOIs in comparison with the well known side-effect profile of the tricyclic antidepressants, the advantages of the MAOIs are evident.

4 Therapeutic Potential of New MAOIs

As stressed by PARE (1985) and reviewed by MURPHY et al. (1984), early clinical trials with classical MAOIs were in many respects inadequate and have led to erroneous conclusions that these drugs are weak antidepressants or suitable only for treatment of a particular type of depressed patient. On the other hand, more recent studies indicate that MAOIs could be considered as true antidepressants which are effective in depressive states of various etiologies, including endogenous depression. However, the general view is that the MAOIs are most effective in patients presenting a particular symptom profile which includes irritability, obsessive preoccupations, marked anxiety or panic episodes, and autonomic disturbances such as hypersomnia, lethargy and fatigue, weight gain and hyperphagia (NIES and ROBINSON 1982). There is also substantial evidence and agreement that MAOIs are effective antianxiety agents.

Clinical studies with new selective and reversible MAO-A inhibitors are still in progress and therefore little can be said at present about their true antidepressant activity, which, it should be borne in mind, is not necessarily solely dependent on their biochemical mode of action. Nevertheless, the results reported so far with moclobemide, toloxatone, and brofaromine, appear encouraging. They are in accordance with the predictions, in that they indicate that selective inhibition of MAO-A is an active therapeutic principle.

References

Bieck PR, Antonin KH (1982) Monoamine oxidase inhibition by tranylcypromine: assessment in human volunteers. Eur J Clin Pharmacol 22:301–308

Bieck PR, Antonin KH, Jedrychowski M (1983) Monoamine oxidase inhibition in healthy volunteers by CGP 11 305 A, a new specific inhibitor of MAO-A. Mod Probl Pharmacopsychiatry 19:53–62

Bieck PR, Antonin KH, Cremer G, Gleiter C (1984) Tyramine pressor effects of CGP 11 305 A in comparison to tranylcypromine after prolonged treatment of human volunteers. In: Tipton KF, Dostert R, Strolin Benedetti M (eds) Monoamine oxidase and disease. Academic, London, pp 503–513

Bieck PR, Schick Ch, Antonin KH, Reimann I, Moerike K (1985) Tyramine kinetics before and after MAO inhibition with the reversible MAO inhibitor brofaromine (CGP 11 305 A). In: Boulton AA, Bieck PR, Maitre L, Riederer P (eds) Neuropsychopharmacology of the trace amines. Humana, Clifton, pp 411–426

Brodie BB, Pletscher A, Shore PA (1956) Possible role of serotonin in brain function and in reserpine action. J Pharmacol Exp Ther 116:9–11

Da Prada M, Keller HH, Kettler R, Schaffner R, Pieri M, Burkhard WP, Korn A, Haefely WE (1982) Ro-11-1163, a specific and short-acting MAO inhibitor with antidepressant properties. In: Kamijo K, Usdin E, Nagatsu TC (eds) Monoamine oxidase, basic and clinical frontiers. Excerpta Medica, Amsterdam, pp 183–196

Da Prada M, Kettler R, Keller HH, Haefely WE (1983) Neurochemical effects in vitro and in vivo of the antidepressant Ro 11-1163, a specific and short-acting MAO-A inhibitor. Mod Probl Pharmacopsychiatry 19:231–245

Da Prada M, Kettler R, Burkhard WP, Haefely WE (1984) Moclobemide, an antidepressant with short-lasting MAO-A inhibition: brain catecholamines and tyramine effects in rats. In: Tipton KF, Dostert P, Strolin Benedetta M (eds) Monoamine oxidase and disease. Academic, New York, pp 137–154

Delini-Stula A, Hunn C (1986) Effects of imipramine and brofaromine, a selective and reversible MAO-A inhibitor, on novelty-oriented behavior in rats. Pharmacopsychiatry 19:245–246

Delini-Stula A, Radeke E (1985) Behavioral and pharmacological characterisation of tryptamine-induced excitation syndrome in rats. In: Boulton AA, Maitre L, Bieck PR, Riederer P (eds) Neuropsychopharmacology of the trace amines. Humana, Clifton, pp 125–140

Dollery CT, Brown MJ, Davies DS, Strolin Benedetti M (1984) Pressor amines and monoamine oxidase inhibitors. In: Tipton KF, Dostert P, Strolin Benedetti M (eds) Monoamine oxidase and disease. Academic, New York, pp 429–441

Fowler CJ (1982) Selective inhibitors of monoamine oxidase types A and B and their clinical usefulness. Drugs Future 12(7):501–517

Fowler CJ, Ross SB (1984) Selective inhibitors of monoamine oxidase A and B: biochemical, pharmacological and clinical properties. Med Res Rev 4:323–358

Fowler CJ, Strolin Benedetti M (1983) Cimoxatone is a reversible tight-binding inhibitor of the A form of rat brain monoamine oxidase. J Neurochem 40:510–513

Holsboer F, Gerken A, Steiger A, Benkert O (1984) Antidepressant effects of CGP 11 305 A a competitive, selective and short-acting MAO-A inhibitor. In: Tipton KF, Doster P, Strolin Benedetti M (eds) Monoamine oxidase and disease. Academic, New York, pp 662–625

Johnston JP (1968) Some observations upon a new inhibitor of monoamine oxidase in brain tissue. Biochem Pharmacol 17:1285–1287

Kaene PE, Kan JP, Sontag N, Strolin Benedetti M (1979) Monoamine oxidase inhibition and brain amine metabolism after oral treatment with toloxatone in the rat. J Pharm Pharmacol 31:752–754

Kan JP, Malone A, Strolin Benedetti M (1978) Monoamine oxidase inhibitory properties of 5-hydroxymethyl-3-m-tolyloxazolidin-2-one (toloxatone). J Pharm Pharmacol 30:190–192

Korn A, Gasic S, Jung M, Eichler HG, Raffesber W (1984) Influence of moclobemide (RO 11-1163) on the peripheral adrenergic system: interaction with tyramine and tricyclic antidepressants. In: Tipton KF, Dostert P, Strolin Benedetti M (eds) Monoamine oxidase and disease. Academic, New York, pp 487–496

Korn A, Eichler HG, Fischbach R, Gasic S (1986) Moclobemide, a new reversible MAO inhibitor – interaction with tyramine and tricyclic antidepressants in healthy volunteers and depressive patients. Psychopharmacology 88:153–157

Maitre L, Delini-Stula A, Waldmeier PC (1976) Relations between the degree of monoamine oxidase inhibition and some psychopharmacological responses to monoamine oxidase inhibitors in rats. Ciba Found Symp 39:247–270

Murphy D, Sunderland T, Cohen R (1984) Monoamine oxidase inhibiting antidepressants, a clinical update. Psychiatr Clin North Am 7:549–562

Nies A, Robinson MD (1982) Monoamine oxidase inhibitors. In: Paykel ES (ed) Handbook of affective disorders. Churchill Livingstone, Edinburgh

Ortmann R, Waldmeier PC, Radeke E, Felner A, Delini-Stula A (1980) The effects of 5-HT uptake- and MAO-inhibitors on L-5-HTP- induced excitation in rats. Naunyn-Schmiedebergs Arch Pharmacol 311:185–192

Ortmann R, Schaub M, Felner A, Lauber J, Christen P, Waldmeier PC (1985) Phenylethylamine-induced stereotypies in the rat: a behavioral test system for assessment of MAO-B inhibitors. Psychopharmacology 84:22–27

Ortmann R, Schaub M, Waldmeier PC (1985) Effect of psychoactive drugs on behavior induced by 2-phenylethylamine in rats. In: Boulton AA, Maitre L, Bieck PR, Riederer P (eds) Neuropsychopharmacology of the trace amines. Humana, Clifton, pp 63–74

Pare CMB (1985) The present status of monoamine oxidase inhibitors. Br J Psychiatry 146:576–584

Randrup A, Munkvad I (1969) Relation of brain catecholamines to aggressiveness and other forms of behavioural excitation. In: Garattini S, Sigg EB (eds) Aggressive behaviour. Excerpta Medica, Amsterdam, pp 228–235

Strolin Benedetti M, Kan JP, Keane PE (1979) A new specific reversible type A monoamine oxidase inhibitor: MD 780515. In: Singer TP, Von Korff RW, Murphy DL (eds) Monoamine oxidase; structure, function and altered functions. Academic, New York, pp 335–340

Strolin Benedetti M, Boucher T, Fowler CJ (1983) The deamination of noradrenaline and 5-hydroxytryptamine by rat brain and heart monoamine oxidase and their inhibition by cimoxatone, toloxatone and MD 770222. Naunyn-Schmiedebergs Arch Pharmacol 323:315–320

Tedeschi DH, Fowler PJ, Miller RB, Macko E (1969) Pharmacological analysis of footshock-induced fighting behavior. In: Garattini S, Sigg EB (eds) Aggressive behaviour. Excerpta Medica, Amsterdam, pp 245–252

Tipton KF, Fowler CJ, Houslay MD (1982) Specificities of the two forms of monoamine oxidase. In: Kamijo K, Usdin E, Nagatsu T (eds) Monoamine oxidase, basic and clinical frontiers. Excerpta Medica, Amsterdam, pp 87–99

Waldmeier PC (1985) On the reversibility of reversible MAO inhibitors. Naunyn-Schmiedebergs Arch Pharmacol 329:305–310

Waldmeier PC, Felner AE, Maitre L (1981) Long-term effects of selective MAO inhibitors on MAO activity and amine metabolism. In: Youdim MBH, Paykel ES (eds) Monoamine oxidase inhibitors – the state of the art. Wiley, Chichester, pp 87–102

Waldmeier PC, Baumann PA, Delini-Stula A, Bernasconi R, Sigg K, Buech O, Felner AE (1983a) Characterization of a new, short-acting and specific inhibitor of type A monoamine oxidase. Mod Probl Pharmacopsychiatry 19:31–52

Waldmeier PC, Feldtrauer JJ, Stoecklin K, Paul E (1983b) Reversibility of the interaction of CGP 11 305 A with MAO A in vivo. Eur J Pharmacol 94:101–108

Youdim MBH, Finber JPM (1983) Implications of MAO-A and MAO-B inhibition for antidepressant therapy. Mod Prob Pharmacopsychiatry 19:63–74

Unsolved Problems in the Pharmacotherapy of Depression

B. WOGGON

Abstract

Five unsolved problems in the pharmacotherapy of depression are discussed: (a) it is not possible to differentiate endogenous and nonendogenous depression; (b) a selective efficacy of serotonin and noradrenaline reuptake inhibitors cannot be demonstrated; (c) the relationship between plasma levels and antidepressant effect is still unclear: plasma levels are influenced by pharmacogenetic factors, age, route of application, and concomitant treatment with other drugs; (d) evidence is growing for the development of tolerance towards therapeutic effects of antidepressants; (e) no pretreatment variable allows prediction of treatment response: the best predictor is the initial response to treatment.

1 Introduction

Originally, the title of this paper was to be "Future treatment of depression." After intensive meditation on this topic, I came to the conclusion that the time for this subject is either too late or too early. Some years ago, it would have been much easier to give an outlook on the future treatment of depression. I would have drawn this sketchy picture: A depressed patient coming to see a doctor would have been examined with the following tests: (a) dexamethasone suppression test and sleep EEG for a biologically founded differential diagnosis of endogenous versus nonendogenous depression; (b) 24-h urine sampling and measuring of 3-methoxy-4-hydroxy-phenylglycol (MHPG) for differentiation between a serotonin or noradenaline deficiency; (c) application of a test dose and measuring of the plasma level for prediction of the right dose. Unfortunately, during the last few years the results of many studies have shown that this picture most probably will never become reality. Therefore, I decided to change the title of my paper to "Unsolved problems in the pharmacotherapy of depression." Because of the limited space, it is not possible to present a complete catalogue of all unsolved questions. The selection is based on personal experiences and expectations of a clinician engaged in treatment and research.

Psychiatric University Hospital, Research Department, Lenggstrasse 31, CH-8029 Zürich, Switzerland.

2 Endogenous and Nonendogenous Depression

In his first paper on the antidepressant efficacy of imipramine, KUHN (1957) wrote that he believed typical endogenous depressions to react especially positively to imipramine. Many studies have tried to confirm the different responsiveness of endogenous and nonendogenous depression to antidepressant drugs. The findings are controversial, and the discussion is still going on. The most crucial point is that up to now it has not been possible to find valid criteria for the differentiation of endogenous and nonendogenous depression, for example, psychopathological symptoms, life events, and course characteristics. The same is true for so-called biological markers of endogenous depression. Nonsuppression or early escape from suppression of cortisol secretion by dexamethasone was proposed as a sensitive (50%) and highly specific (95%) laboratory test for the diagnosis of melancholia (CARROLL et al. 1981; CARROLL 1982). A positive test result was even thought to give a clear indication for somatic antidepressant treatment. Since the first reports, several studies have shown that a considerable percentage of patients of various diagnostic groups are dexamethasone suppression test (DST) nonsuppressors. Furthermore, a number of intervening variables have been identified which influence the DST nonsuppressor rate, for example, weight loss, hospital admission (stress), withdrawal of psychotropic drugs or alcohol, and suicide attempts (VON ZERSSEN et al. 1986).

A shortened latency to REM sleep has been proposed to be another biological marker for endogenous depression (KUPFER 1978), but detailed studies could not reveal any specificity of shortened REM latency for endogenous depression (BERGER et al. 1982).

3 Noradrenaline and Serotonin Deficiency

The primary biochemical effects of tricyclic antidepressants and monoamine oxidase (MAO) inhibitors fit well into the catecholamine and serotonin hypothesis of depression (SCHILDKRAUT 1965; COPPEN 1967). Both types of antidepressant cause an increase of serotonin and noradrenaline in the synaptic cleft, either by inhibition of neuronal reuptake or by inhibition of MAO. Much effort has been invested in the question of whether reuptake inhibitors of serotonin have a different clinical profile to noradrenaline reuptake inhibitors. Even after the development of almost specific substances such as zimelidine and maprotiline, no differences could be found (NYSTROEM and HALLSTROEM 1985). This was the case not only for parallel group designs but also for crossover designs changing nonresponding patients to a substance with the opposite biochemical effect (EMRICH et al. 1985).

These negative findings concerning a selective action of reuptake inhibitors led to the following interpretation: depressive syndromes might be biochemically heterogeneous, and therefore the selective action of the different types of reuptake inhibitors could not be proven in biochemically unselected patients. Measuring of the main metabolite of noradrenaline MHPG in 24-h urine samples resulted in promising findings concerning the hypothesis of two biochemically different types of depression (SCHILDKRAUT et al. 1978). Furthermore, it could be shown that patients with low MHPG values responded better to noradrenaline reuptake inhibitors than to serotonin reuptake inhibitors (BECKMANN and GOODWIN 1975; COBBIN et al. 1979; MAAS et al. 1984; SCHATZBERG et al. 1981). Unfortunately, other studies could not reproduce these promising results (COPPEN et al. 1979; PUZYNSKI et al. 1984; SHARMA et al. 1986).

4 Pharmacokinetics

Plasma levels of antidepressants are closely related to the applied dose, but their correlation to clinical efficacy is still unclear. The great interindividual variability of plasma levels is partly due to genetically determined differences in the metabolism of antidepressants and to additional drug treatment (ALEXANDERSON et al. 1969). Two genetically controlled hydroxylation deficiencies have been described, the debrisoquine and mephenytoin polymorphism (DICK et al. 1982; KÜPFER et al. 1982). A simple test procedure allows one to classify patients as poor or extensive metabolizers for debrisoquine or mephenytoin. BERTILSSON and ÅBERG-WISTEDT (1983) showed that debrisoquine metabolic ratio and steady-state plasma concentrations of desipramine are closely and significantly correlated ($r_s = 0.92$, $n = 10$). This result was surprising because the debrisoquine metabolic ratio was measured 2–5 years after the determination of the desipramine plasma levels.

In a similar study with maprotiline-treated patients who were exposed to the debrisoquine test 10 years later, we found no significant correlation ($r_s = 0.48$, $n = 16$). In contrast to the sample of BERTILSSON and ÅBERG-WISTEDT, our patients were not drug-free before the debrisoquine test. NORDIN et al. (1985) have shown that the metabolic ratio for debrisoquine is significantly higher during than after treatment with nortriptyline. In 78 newly hospitalized depressed patients, we performed the debrisoquine and mephenytoin test before treatment with maprotiline (WOGGON et al. 1986). The metabolic ratio for debrisoquine and maprotiline plasma levels at day 10 showed a statistically significant but not very high correlation ($r_s = 0.44$, $n = 78$). This was not quite unexpected, as maprotiline is hydroxylated by several pathways, giving the possibility for compensation (BAUMANN et al. 1986). The clinical relevance of the hydroxylation capacity is still open to discussion. Some findings suggest that patients who do not efficiently hydroxylate antidepressants may have a lesser incidence of side effects with high concentrations of parent compounds (DEVANE et al. 1981; GARVEY et al. 1984).

The relationship between metabolites and parent drugs seems to influence efficacy and side effects. In addition to genetically determined metabolic differences, some other variables play an important role, for example, age, route of application (oral or parenteral), and combination with other drugs, especially neuroleptics (BOCK et al. 1983; FARAVELLI et al. 1983; KUTCHER et al. 1986; NELSON et al. 1982; VANDEL et al. 1986).

Another difficult question concerns the relationship between the time course of EEG effects and plasma levels. Nomifensine, for example, develops peak plasma levels in the 1st and 2nd h after intravenous or oral application, whereas the maximum EEG changes are seen 6 h after application (SIEGFRIED and TÄUBER 1984).

5 Tolerance

COHEN and BALDESSARINI (1985) have reported the development of tolerance to therapeutic effects of antidepressants despite stable plasma levels of tricyclic antidepressants and stable degree of inhibition of platelet MAO. This finding confirms the observation by MANN, who in 1983 described the loss of antidepressant effect with long-term MAO inhibitor treatment without loss of MAO inhibition in four patients.

6 Prediction of Treatment Response

Up to now, it has been impossible to predict treatment response on the basis of pretreatment variables. The best predictor for treatment response seems to be the patient's initial response to a given treatment. Although depressive symptomatology responds very similarly to different antidepressant treatments, responders always show an early onset of improvement within 7–10 days (SMALL et al. 1981; WOGGON 1980, 1983).

The greatest difficulty for the registration of early changes in psychopathological symptoms is the so-called time bias: doctor and patient both expect an improvement in response to a given treatment. Therefore, methods are needed which enable us to control time bias. Some trials have been made with ratings of randomly presented video recordings. Unfortunately, clothes, hairdressing, make-up, movements, and voice give important clues towards decoding the random presentation.

Speech analysis could be a possibility to overcome time bias. The information contained in human speech can be decomposed into a static component, representing the individual sound characteristics of a speaker (identity), and a dynamic component, reflecting reactive changes of voice due to the immediate environment (short-term fluctuations) or to the speaker's global affective state (long-term fluctuations).

In a pilot study, the speech of six hospitalized patients was registered six times over 2 weeks at 2-day-intervals under comparable experimental conditions for approximately 4 min. During the 1st week, the distribution of "energy per second" remained stable, with both the mean and standard deviation considerably smaller than the norm ($M = 20$, $SD = 10$). During the 2nd week, both parameters progressively took on values not very unlike those representative of the general population (STASSEN et al. 1987). The time course was well in accordance with the improvement of depressive symptoms documented with the Hamilton Rating Scale for Depression (HAMILTON 1960) and the system of the Arbeitsgemeinschaft für Methodik und Dokumentation in der Psychiatrie (AMDP 1979).

7 Outlook for the Future

The first two antidepressants were discovered 30 years ago. Since that time, we have been trying to understand why and how they act against depression. This task has not been successfully fulfilled. The search for new drugs has been fruitful concerning the reduction of side effects and expansion of the treatment possibilities for so-called therapy-resistant depression. Some of the new antidepressants, for example, mianserin and trimipramine, do not fit into the frame of long-believed and beloved hypotheses. Such disappointing findings demonstrate that the spirit of the age should not be narrow-minded, but open to any idea based on basic sciences or clinical observation. In the history of psychopharmacotherapy, clinical observation has been the first step towards new discoveries stimulating basic science research (KALINOWSKY 1980). Most of us expect future progress from combined efforts of basic scientists and clinicians.

References

Alexanderson B, Evans DAP, Sjöqvist F (1969) Steady-state plasma levels of nortriptyline in twins: influence of genetic factors and drug therapy. Br Med J 4:764–768

Arbeitsgemeinschaft für Methodik und Dokumentation in der Psychiatrie AMDP (ed) (1979) Das AMDP-System. Springer, Berlin Heidelberg New York

Baumann P, Gabris G, Jonzier-Perey M, Koeb L, Schöpf J, Woggon B (1986) Pharmacogenetics of antidepressive drugs. In: Shagass C, Josiassen RC, Bridger WH, Weiss KJ, Stoff D, Simpson GM (eds) Biological psychiatry. Proceedings of the IVth World Congress of Biological Psychiatry, Philadelphia. Elsevier, New York, pp 249–251

Beckmann H, Goodwin FK (1975) Antidepressant response to tricyclics and urinary MHPG in unipolar patients. Arch Gen Psychiatry 32:17–21

Berger M, Doerr P, Lund R, Bronisch T, von Zerssen D (1982) Neuroendocrinological and neurophysiological studies in major depressive disorders: Are there biological markers for the endogenous subtype? Biol Psychiatry 17:1217–1242

Bertilsson L, Åberg-Wistedt A (1983) The debrisoquine hydroxylation test predicts steady-state plasma levels of desipramine. Br J Clin Pharmacol 15:388–389

Bock JL, Nelson JC, Gray S, Jatlow PI (1983) Desipramine hydroxylation: Variability and effect of antipsychotic drugs. Clin Pharmacol Ther 33:322–328

Carroll BJ (1982) The dexamethasone suppression test for melancholia. Br J Psychiatry 140:292–304

Carroll BJ, Feinberg M, Greden JF, Tarika J, Albala AA, Haskett RF, James NM et al. (1981) A specific laboratory test for the diagnosis of melancholia. Arch Gen Psychiatry 38:15–22

Cobbin DM, Requin-Blow B, Williams LR, Williams WO (1979) Urinary MHPG levels and tricyclic antidepressant drug selection. Arch Gen Psychiatry 36:1111–1115

Cohen BM, Baldessarini RJ (1985) Tolerance to therapeutic effects of antidepressants. Am J Psychiatry 142:489–490

Coppen A (1967) The biochemistry of depression. Br J Psychiatry 113:1237–1264

Coppen A, Rao VAR, Rathven CRJ, Goodwin BL, Sandler M (1979) Urinary 4-hydroxy-3-methoxyphenylglycol is not a predictor for clinical response to amitriptyline in depressive illness. Psychopharmacology 64:95–97
Devane CL, Wolin RE, Rovere RA, Panahon NC, Sutfin TA, Jusko WJ (1981) Excessive plasma concentrations of tricyclic antidepressants resulting from usual doses: a report of six cases. J Clin Psychiatry 42:143–147
Dick B, Küpfer A, Molnar J, Braunschweig S, Preisig R (1982) Hydroxylierungsdefekt für Medikamente (Typus Debrisoquin) in einer Stichprobe der Schweizer Bevölkerung. Schweiz Med Wochenschr 112:1061–1067
Emrich HM, Berger H, von Zerssen D (1985) Differentialtherapie des depressiven Syndroms: Ergebnisse einer Therapiestudie mit Fluvoxamin vs. Oxaprotilin. In: Hippius H, Matussek N (eds) Differentialtherapie der Depression: Möglichkeiten und Grenzen. Karger, Basel, S. 66–73 (Advances in pharmacotherapy, vol 2)
Faravelli C, Broadhurst AD, Ambonetti A, Ballerini A, de Biase L, La Malfa G, Das M (1983) Double-blind trial with oral versus intravenous clomipramine in primary depression. Biol Psychiatry 18:696–706
Garvey MJ, Tuason VB, Johnson RA, Valentine RH, Cooper TB (1984) Elevated plasma tricyclic levels with therapeutic doses of imipramine. Am J Psychiatry 141:853–856
Hamilton M (1960) A rating scale for depression. J Neurol Neurosurg Psychiatry 23:56–62
Kalinowsky LB (1980) The discoveries of somatic treatments in psychiatry: Facts and myths. Compr Psychiatry 21:428–435
Küpfer A, Dick B, Preisig R (1982) A new drug hydroxylation polymorphism in man: the incidence of mephenytoin hydroxylation deficient phenotypes in an European population study. Naunyn Schmiedebergs Arch Pharmacol 321:R33
Kuhn R (1957) Über die Behandlung depressiver Zustände mit einem Iminodibenzylderivat (G 22355). Schweiz Med Wochenschr 87:1135–1140
Kupfer DJ (1978) Application of EEG sleep for the differential diagnosis and treatment of affective disorders. Pharmacopsychiatry 11:17–26
Kutcher SP, Reid K, Dubbin JD, Shulman KI (1986) Electrocardiogram changes and therapeutic desipramine and 2-hydroxy-desipramine concentrations in elderly depressives. Br J Psychiatry 148:676–679
Maas JW, Koslow SH, Katz MM, Bowden CL, Gibbons RL, Stokes PE, Robins E, Davis JM (1984) Pretreatment neurotransmitter metabolite levels and response to tricyclic antidepressant drugs. Am J Psychiatry 141:1159–1171
Mann JJ (1983) Loss of antidepressant effect with long-term monoamine oxidase inhibitor treatment without loss of monoamine oxidase inhibition. J Clin Psychopharmacol 3:363–366
Nelson JC, Jatlow PI, Bock J, Quinlan DM, Bowers MB (1982) Major adverse reactions during desipramine treatment. Arch Gen Psychiatry 39:1055–1061
Nordin C, Siwers B, Benitez J, Bertilsson L (1985) Plasma concentrations of nortriptyline and its 10-hydroxymetabolite in depressed patients – Relationship to the debrisoquine hydroxylation metabolic ratio. Br J Clin Pharmacol 19:832–835
Nystroem C, Hallstroem T (1985) Double-blind comparison between a serotonin and a noradrenaline reuptake blocker in the treatment of depressed outpatients. Acta Psychiatr Scand 72:6–15
Puzynski S, Rode A, Bidzinski A, Mrozek S, Zaluska M (1984) Failure to correlate urinary MHPG with clinical response to amitriptyline. Acta Psychiatr Scand 69:117–120
Schatzberg AF, Rosenbaum AH, Orsulak PJ, Rohde WA, Maruta T, Kruger ER, Cole JO, Schildkraut JJ (1981) Toward a biochemical classification of depressive disorders. III. Pretreatment urinary MHPG levels as predictors of response to treatment with maprotiline. Psychopharmacology 75:34–38
Schildkraut JJ (1965) The catecholamine hypothesis of affective disorders: A review of supporting evidence. Am J Psychiatry 122:509–522
Schildkraut JJ, Orsulak PJ, Schatzberg AF, Guderman JE, Cole JO, Rohde WA, LaBrie RA (1978) Toward a biochemical classification of depressive disorders. I. Differences in urinary MHPG and other catecholamine metabolites in clinically defined subtypes of depressions. Arch Gen Psychiatry 35:1427–1433

Sharma IJ, Venkitasubramanian TA, Agnihotri BR (1986) 3-MHPG as a non-predictor of antidepressant response to imipramine and electroconvulsive therapy. Acta Psychiatr Scand 74:252–254

Siegfried K, Täuber K (1984) Pharmacodynamics of nomifensine: A review of studies in healthy subjects. J Clin Psychiatry 45(4):33–38

Small JG, Milstein V, Kellams JJ, Small IF (1981) Comparative onset of improvement in depressive symptomatology with drug treatment, electroconvulsive therapy, and placebo. J Clin Psychopharmacol [Suppl] 1(6):62S–69S

Stassen HH, Angst J, Kuny S (1987) Affective state and voice: An investigation into the nonverbal information in human speech. A pilot study with 6 psychiatric patients. Arch Gen Psychiatry (submitted)

Vandel S, Sandoz M, Vandel B, Bonin B, Allers G, Volmat R (1986) Biotransformation of amitriptyline in man: interaction with phenothiazines. Neuropsychobiology 15:15–19

Von Zerssen D, Berger M, Doerr P, Lauer C, Krieg C, Pirke KM (1986) The role of the hypothalamus-pituitary-adrenocortical system in depression. In: Hippius H, Klerman GL, Matussek N (eds) New results in depression research. Springer, Berlin Heidelberg New York, pp 205–216

Woggon B (1980) Veränderungen der psychopathologischen Symptomatik während 20tägiger antidepressiver oder neuroleptischer Behandlung. Psychiatria Clin (Basel) 13:150–164

Woggon B (1983) Prognose der Psychopharmakotherapie. Enke, Stuttgart (Forum der Psychiatrie vol 68)

Woggon B, Bosshart P, Meyer JW, Gabris G, Baumann P, Küpfer A (1986) Correlations between metabolism, clinical efficacy and side-effects of antidepressants. In: Shagass C, Josiassen RC, Bridger WH, Weiss KJ, Stoff D, Simpson GM (eds) Biological Psychiatry. Proceedings of the IVth World Congress of Biological Psychiatry, Philadelphia. Elsevier, New York, pp 252–254

Anxiety, Dementia, and Other Special Topics

Long-Term Treatment of Anxiety: Benefits and Drawbacks

M. LADER

Abstract

Anxiety disorders are common conditions, often chronic, occurring in the general population with a prevalence of about 3%. Long-term use of tranquillizers varies from 0.5% of the total adult population in Sweden and 1.3% in Denmark to 3.1% in Great Britain and 5% in France. This use is tending to become more and more long-term. Long-term efficacy of benzodiazepine medication has not been established. Adverse effects include psychomotor and cognitive impairment, especially in the elderly; some, but not all, effects show tolerance. Some impairment can be demonstrated even after years of use. Rebound and withdrawal reactions after long-term use are common. Practical guidelines to minimize long-term use are suggested.

1 Introduction

Great concern has been voiced over the high rate of prescribing of anti-anxiety medication, mainly the benzodiazepines, in terms of both the extent of prescribing and the long-term nature of many of these treatments. The possibility of dependence and of psychological deficits has been raised, and doubts have been cast on the efficacy of the benzodiazepines used as anti-anxiety agents long-term. In this article, I will briefly review the long-term treatment of anxiety with respect to the benefit-risk ratio, and I shall also evaluate alternatives to the benzodiazepines, both drug and non-drug.

2 Epidemiology of Anxiety

It is important to establish the prevalence of anxiety states and also their natural history: are they common and are they chronic? Unfortunately, there are few studies which directly address these issues. After reviewing a wide variety of data, SARTORIUS (1980) concluded "that anxiety neurosis and phobia make up approximately 20% of all neuroses and thus occur in the general population with a prevalence of at least 2–3%.". Using rather wider criteria, REICH (1986) estimated the prevalence of generalized anxiety disorder to be 3%, with another 3% for panic disorder and 6% for agoraphobia.

The question of chronicity is even less satisfactorily answered. In 1973; ISAAC MARKS and I reviewed the data up to that point and found that about 50% of

Department of Psychiatry, Institute of Psychiatry, De Crespigny Park, London SE5 8AF, UK.

anxiety states had a satisfactory outcome at 1- to 20-year follow-up (MARKS and LADER 1973). However, total remissions were less common, and some patients seem merely to adapt to a tolerably low level of symptom severity. On the debit side is some increased morbidity from such conditions as peptic ulcer and hypertension and increased mortality from suicide and circulatory disease. We can conclude that anxiety states are common, often chronic or at the least recurrent, and carry risks of excess morbidity and mortality.

3 Use of Anti-anxiety Medication

The Institute for Research in Social Behavior, Oakland, California, in close collaboration with staff of the National Institute of Mental Health in Bethesda, Maryland, has carried out a series of community-based surveys of psychotropic drug use, locally, nationally and internationally. I shall present some data from the 1981 cross-national comparison of anti-anxiety/sedative drug use (BALTER et al. 1984). In this study, samples of 1500–2000 adults in ten European countries and the United States were asked about their use of anti-anxiety/sedative medications in the previous year. The past-year prevalences of such use varied from Belgium with 17.6%, through the United States with 12.9% and Denmark with 11.9%, to Sweden with 8.6% and the Netherlands with 7.4% (Table 1). Females consistently used these drugs at about twice the rate of males, and higher prevalence rates were found in the age-groups above 34 years.

The duration of drug use was examined. The proportion of adult population in each country who took these medications long-term, i.e. continuously for all of the previous 12 months, varied considerably from 5.8% in Belgium and 5% in France, through 3.1% in Great Britain and 1.8% in the United States, to 1.3% in Denmark and only 0.5% in Sweden. As a proportion of all users, long-term users ranged from 33.2% in Belgium to 10.9% in Denmark and 6.2% in Sweden (Table 1). Thus, some countries have high anti-anxiety drug use, which tends to be related to high long-term use; others are more sparing users and try to avoid long-term use.

Trends over time are more disturbing. MARKS (1983) calculated that in 1967–1968, 58% of all psychotropic prescriptions were for single short courses of treatment, and only 27% were long-term repeats. By 1977–1978, only 16% were for single courses, and repeat prescriptions made up 64% of the total. A survey of prescribing rates of different groups of general practitioners in the United Kingdom revealed a tenfold variation between different doctors in their rates of issuing repeat prescriptions without seeing the patient again; only 15% of all prescriptions are for psychotropics, but the bulk of repeats are for this group of drugs (FLEMING and CROSS 1984).

However, such prescribing must be set against the frequency and chronicity of anxiety disorders reviewed earlier. Data on the characteristics of long-term users in the United States were obtainable from a 1979 survey by the Insitute for Research in Social Behavior. In that sample of 3161 people, 11% had used anti-anxiety medication in the past 12 months, benzodiazepines accounting for 84% of use

Table 1. Long-term use of anti-anxiety/sedative drugs

	Belgium	Denmark	France	FRG	Great Britain	Italy	Nether-lands	Spain	Sweden	Switzer-land	USA
% adult population using drugs	17.6	12.6	15.9	11.2	11.6	11.5	7.7	15.1	9.2	15.5	13.5
<1/12 months	3.8	5.9	6.5	5.8	4.2	6.5	3.8	6.3	6.7	9.2	9.3
12/12 months	5.8	1.3	5.0	1.6	3.1	1.6	1.7	3.8	0.5	1.2	1.8
% users	21.8	49.1	40.7	52.9	37.2	56.4	50.5	44.3	76.9	63.1	71.7
<1/12 months											
12/12 months	33.2	10.9	31.5	14.1	27.4	14.2	22.5	26.5	6.2	8.4	14.2

(MELLINGER et al. 1984). Of this 11% of adults, 15% were long-term users, i.e. for 12 months or more. This 15% could be divided into 3% who had taken anti-anxiety medication regularly for 1–3 years, another 6% who had taken it for 3–7 years and the remaining 6% who had taken it regularly for over 7 years. Thus, 0.66% of the adult American population – over a million people – are very long-term users indeed. In this survey, long-term users were older than short-term users and nonusers: 71% vs 48% vs 34% respectively were over the age of 50. However, women constituted 61% of long-term users, as against 71% of short-term users. Long-term users were no more likely than short-term users to have psychic distress but did tend to suffer more from both anxiety and depression. What did distinguish the long-term users was their high rate of somatic ill health: 75% reported two or more health problems, as compared with 60% of short-term users and 28% of nonusers. Cardiovascular conditions headed the list, followed by arthritis.

4 Long-term Efficacy

The benzodiazepines are by far the most widely used anti-anxiety drugs, and their efficacy, at least in the short-term, is well established. A meta-analysis of standard controlled short-term trials of benzodiazepines suggested that the average improvement on rating scales with these drugs was about twice that of placebo medication (Quality Assurance Project 1985). In terms of numbers, about two-thirds of patients improve adequately in overall clinical terms.

The appropriate length for a course of benzodiazepine treatment is unclear. RICKELS et al. (1982) recorded a high relapse rate within 6 months of discontinuing benzodiazepines in chronically anxious patients. However, in another study, almost half of patients switched to placebo after 6 weeks' treatment remained well (RICKELS et al. 1983). A 1-year follow-up of 131 chronically anxious patients treated for 6 months with diazepam showed 37% to have remained well. A further 20% remained well for over 3 months after treatment (RICKELS et al. 1986). The authors strongly recommend intermittent rather than continuous therapy for these patients.

The long-term anxiolytic efficacy of benzodiazepines has been questioned (Committee on the Review of Medicines 1980). Although individual case reports claim continuing efficacy, few systematic studies have examined this issue. RICKELS et al. (1984) produced data that suggested no waning of diazepam's efficacy in 22 weeks of treatment. The data do not tell us whether these patients would have done just as well with only 6 weeks of treatment. Only one predictor of patients who respond to short-term benzodiazepine therapy with an extended period of wellbeing has been identified, namely, absence of previous anxiety episodes (RICKELS et al. 1985).

One problem in evaluating long-term efficacy is the possible supervention of dependence and withdrawal problems. Thus, recrudescence of anxiety following discontinuation of medication may reflect rebound or withdrawal anxiety rather than relapse of the original condition.

5 Adverse Effects

The short-term unwanted effects of the benzodiazepines are mainly those of oversedation, such as sleepiness and lassitude. In the medium term, accumulation may occur, especially with those benzodiazepines, such as diazepam and chlordiazepoxide, which are long-acting and/or have persistent active metabolites. With long-term use, accumulation reaches a plateau, and tolerance effects become important. Clinical experience suggests that patients become tolerant of any sedative side effects of the benzodiazepines, or at the least, they stop complaining of them. Clinical anecdotes also suggest that some patients suffer excessive sedation with impaired psychomotor performance, poor memory and concentration, motor incoordination with ataxia, dysarthria and diplopia, and muscle weakness and vertigo (Ashton 1986). Such effects are most marked in the elderly, in whom drowsiness, impaired coordination and ataxia, leading to falls and fractures, poor memory and even acute confusional episodes with hospital admissions for investigation of "dementia", may follow the use of quite modest doses. The impairment of psychomotor function has been implicated as a cause of traffic accidents (Skegg et al. 1979). Interactions with alcohol are particularly dangerous.

The performance of 43 long-term benzodiazepine users was examined on a battery of behavioural and cognitive tests and subjective mood-rating scales (Lucki et al. 1986). The performance of such users did not differ from that of anxious non-users matched for age and sex, except that critical flicker fusion (CFF) thresholds were lower. A test dose of their routine medication was given to about half of the chronic users, and they were retested. Some impairment was then noted in CFF thresholds and short-term memory, suggesting lack of tolerance to the drug. However, psychomotor and subjective effects did seem to show tolerance.

Our own interest in the long-term effects of benzodiazepines on psychological performance was stimulated by a pilot study of 22 patients withdrawing from normal-dose, long-term benzodiazepine treatment; their data were compared with those of two control groups, one recruited from research and technical staff, the other from the community. Patients and controls were assessed repeatedly on the Digit Symbol Substitution Test, Symbol Copying Test, Cancellation Task, Auditory Reaction Time and Key-tapping Rate. A substantial and prolonged practice effect was found on all the tests except reaction time and key-tapping. Prior to withdrawal, the patients did not show the performance decrement on the cancellation task, reaction time and key-tapping customarily associated with the initial phases of benzodiazepine therapy. A rebound performance increment was observed on tapping rate during the withdrawal. Patients demonstrated impaired performance on tasks requiring the combined use of sensory and fine motor skills (Petursson et al. 1983).

In a more extensive study, 145 subjects were tested (Golombok et al. 1988). They comprised three groups: (a) 50 patients who had taken benzodiazepines for at least a year and were currently taking them, (b) 61 subjects who had never taken benzodiazepines or who had taken them for less than a year and (c) 34 subjects who had been chronic users but had not taken them for at least 6 months. No clear differences were found between the groups with respect to a wide range of psychomotor and cognitive tests. However, when the total benzodiazepine intake (dose versus duration) of the current users was correlated with test performance, some relationships emerged: these were significant with respect to some measures of visual perceptual analysis and new learning. These relationships were not due to current benzodiazepine intake or to anxiety levels.

Affective reactions have been described with benzodiazepine use. Both depression and affective dulling have been noted (LADER and PETURSSON 1981). Conversely, benzodiazepines can provoke exaggerated reactions, particularly hostility and aggression. Patients on low chronic doses sometimes commit uncharacteristic antisocial acts, such as shoplifting or sexual offences (LADER and PETURSSON 1981). Higher doses may be associated with outbursts of rage and violent behaviour and have been suggested as a contributory cause of baby-battering (BOND and LADER 1984).

Possible neurotoxic effects have been investigated. In the first report, marginal computerized axial tomography (CAT) scan abnormalities were noted in chronic users as compared with placebo. These users had higher ventricle/brain ratios than controls, although less than alcoholics (LADER et al. 1984). Clearer abnormalities have been described in patients who have abused benzodiazepines (SCHMAUSS and KRIEG 1987).

5.1 Tolerance, Dependence and Withdrawal

Acute tolerance is seen at its most dramatic following benzodiazepine overdose, when the psychotropic effects wane rapidly despite persisting high plasma concentrations (GREENBLATT et al. 1978). Another clinical example concerns the dose of intravenous diazepam needed for preoperative sedation, which was higher in patients taking anxiolytics or hypnotics regularly than in non-users (COOK et al. 1984). In normal volunteers, tolerance to some, but by no means all, benzodiazepine effects can be demonstrated (FILE and LISTER 1983; ARANKO et al. 1983; HIGGITT et al. 1988).

In patients who had been taking normal therapeutic doses of benzodiazepines for at least 6 months, tolerance was assessed by administering test doses of diazepam, and various responses were compared with those of a normal group (PETURSSON and LADER 1984). In the patients, the expected increase in plasma growth hormone concentrations in response to diazepam was almost entirely suppressed, indicating marked tolerance. Subjective sedation was attenuated, suggesting partial tolerance, but EEG fast-wave responses showed no tolerance. In patients taking high doses of benzodiazepines for at least a year, marked tolerance was seen to the psychomotor effects of a test dose of lorazepam (ARANKO et al. 1985). Tolerance may persist to some extent for months after benzodiazepine withdrawal (HIGGITT et al. 1988).

Dependence is a hypothetical construct for the state induced by the compensatory adaptive changes which occur in the central nervous system as a result of drug administration (HAEFELY 1986). Evidence for physical dependence comes from rebound and withdrawal on discontinuation of the medication. To date, rebound and withdrawal have been distinguished in the clinical literature, but this is a spurious dichotomy (LADER and FILE 1987). Rebound can be defined as the increase in severity of the initial symptoms beyond pretreatment or placebo-treated levels after short- or long-term drug administration. Rebound insomnia after the use of benzodiazepine hypnotics is well documented (KALES et al. 1983; LADER and LAWSON 1987). Rebound symptoms have been described following short-term benzodiazepine treatment (PECKNOLD et al. 1982; POWER et al. 1985). The importance of the rate of termination is shown by a study in which rebound was prevented by tapering the dosage of the benzodiazepine (FONTAINE et al. 1984).

Withdrawal from high (supratherapeutic, abuse) doses of benzodiazepines has been known for a long time to be attended by a variety of symptoms including seizures and paranoid reactions (PETURSSON and LADER 1984). Initially, withdrawal after therapeutic dosage was indicated only by sporadic case reports (e.g. KHAN et al. 1980), but it has now been confirmed in both laboratory and clinical studies (HALLSTROM and LADER 1981; TYRER et al. 1981; PETURSSON and LADER 1981). Even with therapeutic doses, there is some evidence that a withdrawal syndrome is found more frequently the longer the treatment, e.g. 6 compared with 22 weeks (RICKELS et al. 1983, 1984).

Withdrawal symptoms, summarized by LADEWIG (1984), fall roughly into three categories: (a) psychological symptoms of anxiety, such as apprehension, irritability, insomnia and dysphoria; (b) bodily symptoms of anxiety, particularly tremor, palpitations, vertigo, sweating and severe muscle spasms; and (c) perceptual disturbances, such as hypersensitivity to light, sound and touch, pains, depersonalization, feeling of motion, metallic taste. It is difficult to distinguish this syndrome from that described as rebound, except perhaps for the third group of symptoms.

The first two categories may resemble the original anxiety, but as with rebound, the symptoms are more severe (LADEWIG 1984). Most commonly, these symptoms subside in 5–15 days, which is not consistent with a reemergence of the original anxiety (TYRER et al. 1983). The fact that they are part of a withdrawal response is also indicated by their presence in patients who have been taking benzodiazepines in therapeutic doses for 6 months or more for a nonpsychiatric reason, e.g., chronic muscle spasm following a sports injury (LADER, personal observation).

Gradual withdrawal may be followed by a milder, yet specific, syndrome, which is the same whether the dose was high or low (HALLSTROM and LADER 1981). However, even with gradual withdrawal from low doses, prolonged and bizarre responses have been described (ASHTON 1984). ASHTON emphasizes how physically ill the patients felt. Agoraphobic, panic and depressive syndromes may occur (OLAJIDE and LADER 1984).

The frequency of withdrawal reactions is difficult to estimate. Often, the sample is selected from repeated attenders at psychiatric outpatient clinics or general practice surgeries, or self-selected at patient mutual help groups. But perhaps 15%–30% of long-term (longer than a year) users will encounter problems trying to discontinue medication. Of these, perhaps a third will develop severe and/or protracted withdrawal syndromes.

5.2 Benefit-Risk Ratio of Long-Term Anxiolytic Use

MARKS (1985) has suggested three stages of investigation required before the overall benefit-risk ratio of chronic anti-anxiety medication can be determined: (a) measurement of medical benefit/risk, (b) evaluation of social and moral issues and (c) estimation of economic aspects. The evidence reviewed above suggests that efficacy beyond a few months is insufficient to warrant continuous use in view of the problems of neuropsychological deficits and the risk of dependence. No social, moral or economic considerations can outweigh such an adverse benefit-risk ratio.

6 Practical Guidelines

Nevertheless, there are many patients who suffer chronic anxiety symptoms, and attention has focussed on how best to treat them. DRURY (1985), a United Kingdom general practitioner, has urged that patients should be told that there is no place for continuous long-term medication. Instead, intermittent courses of therapy should be the mainstay of drug treatment. Patients already on long-term medication should be urged to taper and then discontinue their drugs. The adjunctive use of non-drug measures, such as relaxation therapy, biofeedback, counselling and supportive psychotherapy, is regarded as an important part of therapy both for the chronic user withdrawing and for the patient with a chronic unremitting anxiety state (NASDAHL et al. 1985).

The importance of vigorous treatment cannot be overemphasized. Chronic anxiety can become a serious condition in terms of its toll on normal personal, occupational and social functioning, and the full gamut of alternative therapies must be explored (Quality Assurance Project 1985). Furthermore, prevention of long-term anxiolytic use is preferable to attempts to reverse such use. Benzodiazepines should be reserved for short-term use (LADER and PETURSSON 1983).

6.1 Alternatives

Alternative therapies fall into two groups, drug and non-drug. A wide range of drugs have been used to treat anxiety and include barbiturates, meprobamate, antihistamines, antidepressants, antipsychotics and β-adrenergic blocking agents (BALLENGER 1984, LADER 1984). Considerations of space preclude a full discussion, but the following summary points are apposite:

1. The barbiturates and meprobamate have worse benefit-risk ratios than the benzodiazepines and should never be used to treat anxiety.
2. Antihistamines are generally ineffective anxiolytics.
3. Antidepressants are useful, especially when there is an admixture of depression, but compliance is often poor.
4. Antipsychotic drugs in low dosage may have a place in treating the anxious patient previously dependent on benzodiazepines, barbiturates or alcohol.

5. β-blockers may be quite effective for patients whose prime symptoms of anxiety are palpitations, gastrointestinal upset or tremor.

A recent development in the area of anxiolytic drugs has been that of new compounds which are chemically and pharmacologically dissimilar to the benzodiazepines (WILLIAMS 1983). The former may or may not act on the benzodiazepine-γ-aminobutyric acid (GABA) receptor complex. If such a compound does act there, it may be found to be less sedative than its predecessors, but its dependence liability is probably still substantial. Newer anti-anxiety compounds which do not act on GABA mechanisms have been developed. The most advanced is buspirone, which is becoming available in several countries, including the Federal Republic of Germany and the United States. It is novel chemically and pharmacologically (GOA and WARD 1986). Its introduction into clinical practice will result in a total reappraisal of the benefit-risk ratio of long-term use, as all the indications to date suggest that it has little or no dependence potential. Indeed, its lack of cross-tolerance to the benzodiazepines may give rise to practical clinical problems (SCHWEIZER et al. 1986).

The main alternatives to drug treatment involve relaxation, counselling, supportive psychotherapy, hyperventilation training, and cognitive therapy, among a whole range of psychological methods (GELDER 1986). As psychologists become more involved in general practice psychiatry, such techniques will become more widely available.

7 Conclusions

The whole topic of the long-term drug treatment of anxiety has excited much attention over the past decade. Attitudes to the benzodiazepines have changed quite markedly, and these drugs are no longer regarded as panaceas (CLINTHORNE et al. 1986). The pendulum may have swung too far with respect to short-term anti-anxiety medication: these drugs are still invaluable for acute anxiety reactions. Their use in the long-term is not justified, except in a few patients who have failed to respond to all forms of appropriate treatment, drug and non-drug. Unfortunately, too often what has been instituted as a short-term interventional course of anti-anxiety medication slips insidiously into a long-term treatment, often because rebound and then withdrawal reactions preclude easy discontinuation. The advent of new, non-dependence-inducing medications may yet allow us to manage acutely anxious patients without the fear of chronic use and to treat chronically anxious patients with intermittent drug therapy.

References

Aranko K, Mattila MJ, Seppala T (1983) Development of tolerance and cross-tolerance to the psychomotor actions of lorazepam and diazepam in man. Br J Clin Pharmacol 15:545–552
Aranko K, Mattila MJ, Nuutila A, Pellinen J (1985) Benzodiazepines, but not antidepressant or neuroleptics, induce dose-dependent development of tolerance to lorazepam in psychiatric patients. Acta Psychiatr Scand 72:436–446
Ashton H (1984) Benzodiazepine withdrawal: an unfinished story. Br Med J 288:1135–1140
Ashton H (1986) Adverse effects of prolonged benzodiazepine use. Adv Drug Reaction Bull 118:440–443
Ballenger JC (1984) Psychopharmacology of the anxiety disorders. Psychiatr Clin North Am 7:757–771
Balter MB, Mannheimer DI, Mellinger GD, Uhlenhuth EH (1984) A cross-national comparison of anti-anxiety/sedative drug use. Curr Med Res Opin 8 Suppl. 4:5–20
Bond A, Lader M (1984) The psychopharmacology of aggression. In: Gaind RN et al. (eds) Current themes in psychiatry, vol 3. Spectrum, Jamaica, pp 123–159
Clinthorne JK, Cisin IH, Balter MB, Mellinger GD, Uhlenthuth EH (1986) Changes in popular attitudes and beliefs about tranquilizers. Arch Gen Psychiatry 43:527–532
Committee on the Review of Medicines (1980) Systematic review of the benzodiazepines. Br Med J 282:719–720
Cook PJ, Flangan R, James IM (1984) Diazepam tolerance: effect of age, regular sedation, and alcohol. Br Med J 289:351–353
Drury VWM (1985) Benzodiazepines – a challenge to rational prescribing. JR Coll Gen Pract 35:86–88
File SE, Lister RG (1983) Does tolerance to lorazepam develop with once weekly dosing? Br J Clin Pharmacol 16:645–650
Fleming DM, Cross KW (1984) Psychotropic drug prescribing. JR Coll Gen Pract 34:216–220
Fontaine R, Chouinard G, Annable L (1984) Rebound anxiety in anxious patients after abrupt withdrawal of benzodiazepine treatment. Am J Psychiatry 141:848–852
Gelder MG (1986) Psychological treatment for anxiety disorders: a review. JR Soc Med 79:230–233
Goa KL, Ward A (1986) Busprione. A preliminary review of its pharmacological properties and therapeutic efficacy as an anxiolytic. Drugs 32:114–129
Golombok S, Moodley P, Lader M (1988) Cognitive impairment in long-term benzodiazepine users. Psychol Med (in press)
Greenblatt DJ, Woo E, Allen MD, Orsulak PJ, Shader RI (1978) Rapid recovery from massive diazepam overdose. JAMA 240:1872–1874
Haefely W (1986) Biological basis of drug-induced tolerance, rebound, and dependence. Pharmacopsychiatry 19:353–361
Hallstrom C, Lader M (1981) Benzodiazepine withdrawal phenomena. Int Pharmacopsychiatry 16:235–244
Higgitt A, Fonagy P, Lader M (1988) The development of tolerance to the benzodiazepines and its long-term persistence. Psychol Med Monogr [Suppl] (in press)
Kales A, Soldatos CR, Bixler EO, Kales JD (1983) Rebound insomnia and rebound anxiety: a review. Pharmacology 26:121–137
Khan A, Joyce P, Jones AV (1980) Benzodiazepine withdrawal syndromes. NZ Med J 92:94–96
Lader M (1984) Anxiety drugs. In: Karasu TB (ed) The somatic therapies. American Psychiatric Association, Washington, pp 53–83
Lader MH, File S (1987) The biological basis of benzodiazepine dependence. Psychol Med 17:539–547
Lader MH, Lawson C (1987) Sleep studies and rebound insomnia: methodological problems, laboratory findings and clinical implications. Clin Neuropharmacol 10:291–312
Lader MH, Petursson H (1981) Benzodiazepine derivatives – side effects and dangers. Biol Psychiatr 16:1195–1121
Lader MH, Petursson H (1983) Rational use of anxiolytic/sedative drugs. N Ethicals 20:49–77

Lader MH, Ron M, Petursson H (1984) Computed axial brain tomography in long-term benzodiazepine users. Psychol Med 14:203–206
Ladewig D (1984) Dependence liability of the benzodiazepines. Drug Alcohol Depend 13:139–149
Lucki I, Rickels K, Geller AM (1986) Chronic use of benzodiazepines and psychomotor and cognitive test performance. Psychopharmacology 88:426–433
Marks IM, Lader M (1973) Anxiety states (anxiety neurosis): a review. J Nerv Ment Dis 156:3–18
Marks J (1983) The benzodiazepines – for good or evil. Neuropsychobiology 12:115–126
Marks J (1985) Chronic anxiolytic treatment: benefit and risk. In: Kemali D, Racagni G (eds) Chronic treatments in neuropsychiatry. Raven, New York, pp 173–183
Mellinger GD, Balter MB, Uhlenhuth EH (1984) Prevalence and correlates of the long-term regular use of anxiolytics. JAMA 251:375–379
Nasdahl CS, Johnston JA, Coleman JH, May C, Drugg JH (1985) Protocols for the use of psychoactive drugs – Part IV: protocol for the treatment of anxiety disorders. J Clin Psychiatr 46:128–132
Olajide D, Lader M (1984) Depression following withdrawal from long-term benzodiazepine use: a report of four cases. Psychol Med 14:937–940
Pecknold JC, McClure DJ, Fleuri D, Chang H (1982) Benzodiazepine withdrawal effects. Prog Neuropsychopharmacol Biol Psychiatry 6:517–522
Petursson H, Lader M (1981) Withdrawal from long-term benzodiazepine treatment. Br Med J 283:643–645
Petursson H, Lader M (1984) Dependence on tranquillizers. Oxford University Press, Oxford (Maudsley monograph, no 28)
Petursson H, Gudjonsson GH, Lader MH (1983) Psychometric performance during withdrawal from long-term benzodiazepine treatment. Psychopharmacology 81:345–349
Power KG, Jerrom DWA, Simpson RJ, Mitchell M (1985) Controlled study of withdrawal symptoms and rebound anxiety after six week course of diazepam for generalised anxiety. Br Med J 29:1246–1248
Quality Assurance Project (1985) Treatment outlines for the management of anxiety states. Aust NZ J Psychiatry 19:138–151
Reich J (1986) The epidemiology of anxiety. J Nerv Ment Dis 174:129–136
Rickels K, Case GW, Downing RW (1982) Issues in long-term treatment with diazepam. Psychopharmacol Bull 18:38–41
Rickels K, Case WG, Downing RW, Winokur A (1983) Long-term diazepam therapy and clinical outcome. JAMA 250:767–771
Rickels K, Case WG, Winokur A, Swenson C (1984) Long-term benzodiazepine therapy: benefits and risks. Psychopharmacol Bull 4:608–615
Rickels K, Case WG, Downing RW, Winokur A (1985) Indications and contraindications for chronic anxiolytic treatment: is there tolerance to the anxiolytic effect. In: Kemali D, Racagni G (eds) Chronic treatments in neuropsychiatry. Raven, New York
Rickels K, Case WG, Downing RW, Fridman R (1986) One-year follow-up of anxious patients treated with diazepam. J Clin Psychopharmacol 6:32–36
Sartorius N (1980) Epidemiology of anxiety. Pharmacopsychiatry 13:249–253
Schmauss C, Krieg JC (1987) Enlargement of cerebrospinal fluid spaces in the long-term benzodiazepine abusers. Psychol Med 17:869–873
Schweizer E, Rickels K, Lucki I (1986) Resistance to the antianxiety effect of buspirone in patients with a history of benzodiazepine use. N Engl J Med 314:719–720
Skegg DCG, Richards SM, Doll R (1979) Minor tranquillizers and road accidents. Br Med J 1:917–919
Tyrer P, Rutherford D, Huggett T (1981) Benzodiazepine withdrawal symptoms and propranolol. Lancet I:520–522
Tyrer P, Owen R, Dawling S (1983) Gradual withdrawal of diazepam after long-term therapy. Lancet I:1402–1406
Williams M (1983) Anxioselective anxiolytics. J Med Chem 26:620–628

Future Directions in Anxiety Research

C. BRÆSTRUP and E. B. NIELSEN

Abstract

More than 3.5 million patients suffer from anxiety in the United States of America alone. While our knowledge of the basic biological mechanisms of anxiety is very poor, we have a good understanding of the mechanism of action of various anxiolytic drugs at the molecular level. Their mechanism of action often relates to the inhibitory neurotransmitter GABA and it might be speculated that GABA has a role in anxiety. Future research will concentrate on designing better anxiolytic drugs, based for example on the discovery of partial benzodiazepine receptor agonists, and also on GABA uptake inhibitors as enhancers of GABAergic function. Furthermore, scientific studies will focus on a search for putative biological defects related to anxiety, such as defects in the GABA/benzodiazepine receptor chloride channel complex.

1 Introduction

Anxiety is often regarded as "minor" – minor in relation to the "major" affective disorders, schizophrenia, depression, and mania. The incidence of anxiety, however, is not minor; it has been estimated that 3.5 million patients in the United States of America suffer from anxiety and the figures for benzodiazepine sales in Denmark, for example, suggest that 8% of the population daily uses a benzodiazepine to counteract anxiety, insomnia, and so on. Furthermore, attacks of anxiety can have serious consequences, such as severe impairment of normal social and cognitive functions, sometimes to the point of complete inability to cope with normal life tasks.

Real insight into the biology of anxiety must await a solution to the mind–brain problem. How is a biological process, presumably electrical activity in neurons, transcribed into conscious experiences and emotions, in this context fear, apprehension, inner tension, restlessness, excitability, and hostility? All we can say at present is that anxiety occurs when, in the brain, there is a certain activity pattern in certain neurons that are firing in a certain spatial and temporal pattern, and that this structurally complex activity is anxiety. Such a concept, unspecific though it is, at least justifies further biological research.

There is no certain abnormality in anxiety. In schizophrenia, increased numbers of brain dopamine receptors in the basal ganglia have been reported; in depressed patients, reduced CSF concentrations of 5-hydroxyindoleacetic acid and lower numbers of serotonin uptake sites in blood platelets (and brain?) have

Pharmaceuticals R&D, NOVO Industrial A/S, DK-2880 Bagsværd, Denmark.

been noted; in Parkinson's disease, the concentration of dopamine in the basal ganglia is reduced; in Huntington's chorea, the levels of the inhibitory neurotransmitter γ-aminobutyric acid (GABA) and its enzyme marker, glutamate decarboxylase, are reduced while in Alzheimer-type dementia, the levels of acetylcholine and other neurotransmitters are reduced. Similar changes in neurotransmitters have not been reported in anxiety states. This may not be surprising, since anxiety is part of a biologically useful reaction to danger, i.e., the preparation of the organism for flight or fight or, in less severe cases, enhancement of cardiac output and alertness. Normal anxiety is a prerequisite for a well-functioning individual, and no abnormality should be sought. Pathological anxiety may represent simply a marginal "overreaction" in otherwise normal neuronal circuits, and there may be little measurable deviation from normality. Nevertheless, several physiological indices of anxiety are related to neurotransmitter function, i.e. increased pulse rate, increased forearm blood flow, augmented sweat gland activity, reduced salivation, and much increased muscle activity. Such changes reflect altered autonomic activity – mainly an increase in sympathetic discharge, particularly in the β-adrenergic system – and are probably not related to the pathology of anxiety but reflect the secondary physiological expression of the condition. Consequently, β-adrenergic blockers can relieve symptoms of anxiety but not the underlying driving force, except in rare cases where the symptoms, in a vicious circle, worsen the anxiety.

2 A GABA Theory of Anxiety?

The dopamine theory of schizophrenia was originally founded on the fact that neuroleptic drugs block dopamine receptors while dopamine "enhancers" (such as amphetamine) precipitate schizophrenia-like symptoms (MUNKVAD et al. 1980). A GABA hypothesis of anxiety is possible on similar grounds. Figure 1 shows a schematic representation of a GABAergic synapse. About 30% of the brain's synapses use GABA as their inhibitory neurotransmitter. GABAergic neurotransmission can be enhanced in a number of different ways and it is remarkable that anxiety relief is observed, apparently irrespective of which is used to enhance GABA function.

Benzodiazepines bind with high affinity to the benzodiazepine receptor (Fig. 1, site 5; BRÆSTRUP and NIELSEN 1983). When binding has occurred (within minutes), the conformation of the benzodiazepine receptor changes, thereby enhancing GABA receptor function indirectly. This means that the "gain" of the GABA molecule produces stronger inhibition on the postsynaptic neurone than in the absence of a benzodiazepine. Thus, an anxiolytic effect is produced by indirect (allosteric) enhancement of GABA.

GABA receptor function (Fig. 1, site 4; FALCH et al. 1984) can also be increased by directly acting GABA receptor agonists. Only two compounds have been available for clinical studies, muscimol and THIP; they may relieve anxiety in man, and they produce an anticonvulsant effect. Convulsions and anxiety often have commonality at the biological/pharmacological level.

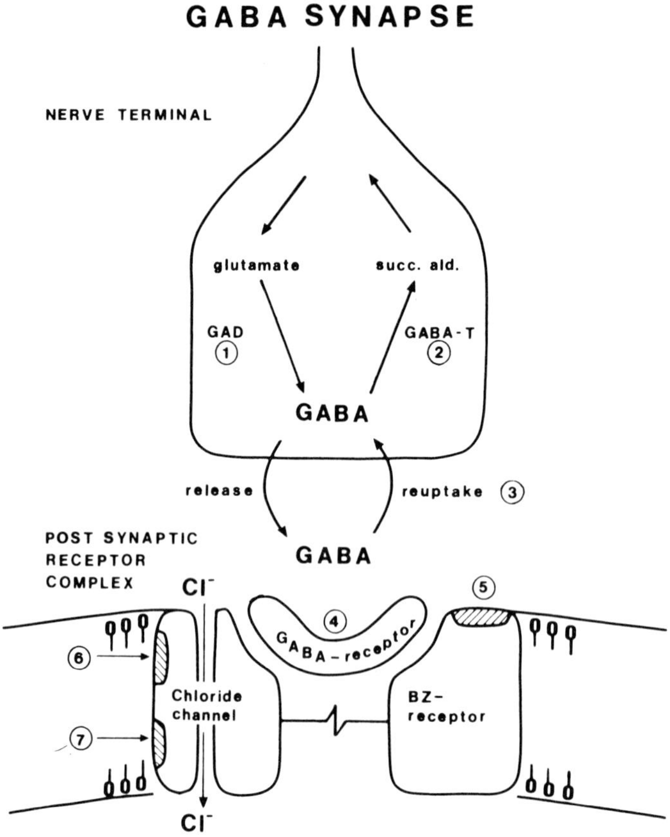

Fig. 1. Highly schematic representation of a GABAergic synapse. Seven specific sites are shown (enzymes, channels, or receptors) which are targets for drugs producing anxiolytic, anticonvulsant, anxiogenic, and/or convulsant effects. *BZ,* Benzodiazepine; *GABA-T,* GABA transaminase; *GAD,* glutamic acid decarboxylase; *succ. ald.,* succinic aldehyde

The inhibitory effect of GABA is mediated by chloride channels. Occupation of GABA receptors by GABA causes chloride channels to open. When a chloride diffuses from the outside of the cell to the inside through this channel, the inside becomes more negatively charged and the electrical activity of the cell is then inhibited. The chloride channel, which may well consist of more than one protein molecule (possibly even the GABA receptor and the benzodiazepine receptor molecules), is endowed with two further binding sites (Fig. 1, sites 6 and 7; see OLSEN 1981). Some barbiturates, notably of the hypnotic type (e.g., pentobarbital), act on one of these sites and thereby increase the opening time for chloride channels. This, in turn, means that GABAergic neurotransmission is enhanced. This effect of the barbiturates is probably responsible for their anxiolytic effect. Another class of compounds, represented by the pyrazolopyridines (e.g., etazolate), also acts on chloride channels and thereby indirectly enhances GABAergic function. Preliminary clinical trials have demonstrated that such compounds have anxiolytic properties (COLLINS et al. 1976) but their toxicity has precluded their further development.

GABAergic neurotransmission can also be enhanced by reducing the presynaptic metabolism of GABA via the GABA-degredating enzyme, GABA-transaminase (Fig. 1, site 2). γ-vinyl-GABA (GVG) is an irreversible inhibitor of GABA-transaminase, and shows potent anticonvulsant effects both in animals and man (see HAMMOND and WILDER 1985). Investigations of the anxiolytic potential of GVG have not yet been conducted.

Finally, GABAergic transmission can be enhanced by forcing GABA to stay longer in the synapse before it is removed. The removal mechanism for GABA is reuptake, either into the synaptic terminal or into glial cells. Compounds which inhibit GABA reuptake (Fig. 1, site 3) will be discussed in further detail below.

Just as anxiety can be reduced by enhancing GABAergic neurotransmission, it can be increased by reducing GABAergic neurotransmission. This latter mechanism has been demonstrated using a number of compounds; most notable is the inverse agonist at benzodiazepine receptors, FG 7142. When FG 7142 binds to benzodiazepine receptors it fails to produce the anxiolytic and anticonvulsant effects which are normally elicited by benzodiazepines; rather, severe anxiety is elicited (DOROW et al. 1983). FG 7142 acts by reducing GABAergic neurotransmission. Another compound, pentylenetetrazol (PTZ), which was previously used for convulsive "therapy," produces fits of anxiety prior to the occurrence of convulsions (RODIN 1958). PTZ has recently been shown to act directly on the chloride channel of the GABA/benzodiazepine chloride channel complex.

3 Future Research on the Role of GABA in Anxiety

Detailed knowledge of the various components of GABAergic neurotransmission offers several interesting approaches to research on anxiety. It cannot be excluded that patients with pathological anxiety suffer from defects in specific components of the postsynaptic GABA receptor complex. At present, methods are available for detecting defects in subunits of the GABA receptor complex (e.g., the benzodiazepine receptor or certain aspects of chloride channel function). These biochemical methods can also reveal defects in the functional couplings among the various components of the receptor complex. The biochemical methods, however, have not yet been developed to a level of sophistication allowing investigation of the living human brain. However, with the development of positron emission tomography techniques, such investigations will be possible. Conventional biochemical investigations of post-mortem human brain tissue are not yet available; thus the actual state of the GABAergic neurotransmission system in anxiety is unknown. The role of GABA in the epileptic human brain is also unknown; however, GABAergic defects have been demonstrated in animal strains with genetic susceptibility to seizures.

Present knowledge of how the benzodiazepine receptor recognizes various types of receptor ligands opens new approaches to research on pharmacotherapy of anxiety. The benzodiazepine receptor responds to a continuum of receptor li-

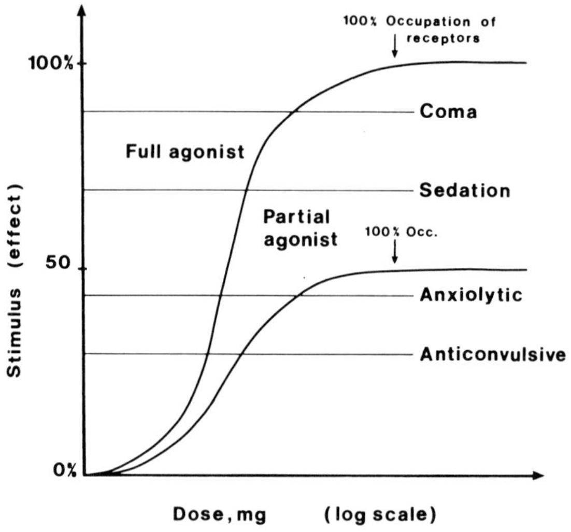

Fig. 2. Diagrammatic representation of the dose–response curve for a full benzodiazepine agonist (e.g., diazepam) and a partial agonist (e.g., ZK 91296). The partial agonist produces the "full" stimulus at the receptor, even after a high dose, which occupies all BZ receptors. Thus, a partial agonist fails to elicit effects which require high stimulus, e.g., sedation and loss of consciousness

gands (BRÆSTRUP et al. 1984), ranging from benzodiazepines with full agonist activity, to receptor antagonists which antagonize benzodiazepines (and also inverse agonists), and agents such as FG 7142 which produce severe anxiety in man. This situation implies that agents exist with effects in between the agonist and the antagonist action, i.e., so-called partial agonists. Thus, these compounds possess some of the effects of the benzodiazepines but not others. Figure 2 illustrates that a partial agonist with, for example, 50% efficacy may produce anxiolytic and anticonvulsant effects, but not sedation. A partial agonist binds to the receptor in such a way that it does not produce the full "stimulus" even when all receptors are occupied; a partial agonist causes the receptor to change less than does a full agonist. Animal experiments suggest that partial agonists may not readily produce tolerance, a major problem with the benzodiazepines. Partial agonists have been synthesized (e.g., ZK 91296 and CGS 9896), but clinical experience with these awaits the results of further studies.

Future research on the pharmacotherapy of anxiety should furthermore focus on alternative ways to enhance GABAergic neurotransmission. Inhibition of reuptake, a mechanism which retains the normal physiological regulatory properties (the effect of the drug is only observed when the nerve releases its neurotransmitter), is a mechanism which has proved highly effective and useful in other neurotransmitter systems, most notably noradrenaline and serotonin. However, it has not yet been available for the GABA system. Recently, however, YOUNGER et al. (1984) observed that well-known GABA uptake inhibitors with amino acid structure, e.g. nipecotic acid, guvacine and hydroxynipecotic acid (Fig. 3), cross the blood–brain barrier when coupled to a lipophilic "anchor." The lipo-

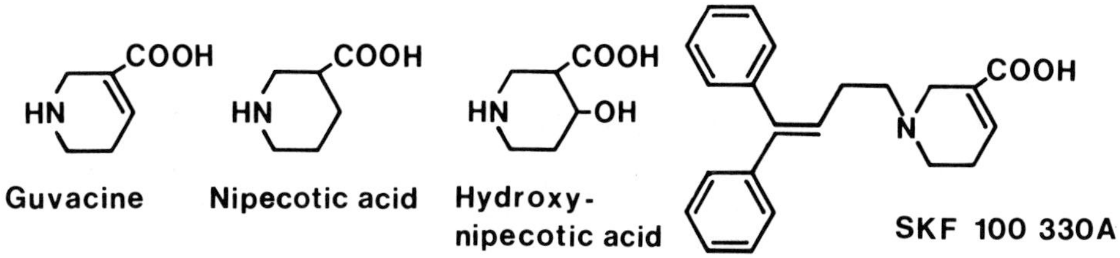

Fig. 3. Chemical structures of representative GABA uptake inhibitors

Table 1. The effect of GABA uptake inhibitors on seizure and anxiety reactions

Compound	GABA uptake IC_{50} (μM)[a]	DBA/2 seizures (mg/kg)[b]	Water lick conflict MED (mg/kg)[c]
Guvacine	2.3	>30	–
SKF 100330A	0.39	4	20
Diazepam	>100	0.2	3
Valproate	>100	30	400

[a] Uptake of [^{3}H]-GABA in a rat cortical synaptosomal preparation.
[b] ED_{50} value, mg/kg; i.p. 30 min before exposure to 113 dB sound level.
[c] Minimal effective dose; unpublished; methods as described in PETERSEN and LASSEN (1981).

philic tail carries the amino acid through the blood–brain barrier and through lipid membranes. In addition, the anchor enhances the affinity of the amino acid for the uptake site and makes these new types of uptake inhibitors sufficiently potent for therapeutic applications. The GABA uptake inhibitors are potent anticonvulsants, in particular in a mouse strain (DBA/2), where seizures are elicited by high-intensity sound. In this model, SKF 100 330A, a representative GABA-uptake inhibitor, is very potent (Table 1).

To find out whether GABA uptake inhibitors may afford protection against anxiety, we have investigated the effect of the potent GABA-uptake inhibitor, SKF 100 330 A, for anxiolytic effects in an animal model – the water lick conflict test. In this paradigm, SKF 100 330A was as potent and as effective as diazepam (Table 1). This result indicates that GABA uptake inhibitors may have anxiolytic potential; research in the late 1980s will reveal whether this indirect potentiation of GABA neurotransmission is superior to current therapies.

4 Concluding Remarks

The involvement of GABA in the mechanism of anxiolytic drug action dates to the mid-1970s (HAEFELY et al. 1975; COSTA et al. 1975). At present, the molecular biology of anxiolytics is well understood at the cellular level; further research will be aimed at detecting basic defects in the GABA system in anxiety, and at applying the new knowledge to the development of better drugs. Besides the GABA system, there will be continued interest in mapping the significance of the locus coeruleus noradrenaline system in anxiety (REDMOND 1986) and in the mechanisms of lactate-induced anxiety. In addition, research will be directed at establishing the role, if any, of other neurotransmitters in anxiety. In this connection, it has recently been demonstrated that certain glutamate antagonists have anxiolytic efficacy in animal models (BENNETT and AMRICK 1986), and buspirone, a nonbenzodiazepine with anxiolytic activity, has a high affinity for a 5-HT_{1A} receptor, thus implicating 5-HT mechanisms as other targets for new anxiolytic drugs (RIBLET et al. 1982).

References

Bennett DA, Amrick CL (1986) 2-Amino-7-phosphonoheptanoic acid (AP7) produces discriminative stimuli and anticonflict effects similar to diazepam. Life Sci 39:2455–2461

Bræstrup C, Nielsen M (1983) Benzodiazepine receptors. In: Iversen L, Iversen DS, Snyder SH (eds) Handbook of psychopharmacology, vol 17. Plenum, New York, pp 285–384

Bræstrup C, Honorè T, Nielsen M, Petersen EN, Jensen LH (1984) Ligands for benzodiazepine receptors with positive and negative efficacy. Biochem Pharmacol 33:859–862

Collins P, Sakalis G, Minn FL (1976) Clinical response to a potential non sedative anxiolytic. Curr Ther Res 19:512–515

Costa E, Guidotti A, Mao CC, Suria A (1975) New concepts on the mechanism of action of benzodiazepines. Life Sci 17:167–186

Dorow R, Horowski R, Paschelke G, Asmis M, Braestrup C (1983) Severe anxiety induced by FG 7142, a β-carboline ligand for benzodiazepine receptors. Lancet II:98–99

Falch E, Christensen V, Jacobsen P, Bybjerg J, Krogsgaard-Larsen P (1984) *Amanita muscaria* in medicinal chemistry. I. Muscimol and related GABA agonists with anticonvulsant and central non-opioid analgesic effects. In: Krogsgaard-Larsen P, Christensen SB, Kofod H (eds) Natural products and drug development. Munksgaard, Copenhagen, pp 504–524

Haefely W, Kulcsár A, Moehler H, Pieri L, Polc P, Schaffner R (1975) Possible involvement of GABA in the central actions of benzodiazepines. In: Costa E, Greengard P (eds) Mechanism of action of benzodiazepines. Raven, New York, pp 131–151

Hammond EJ, Wilder BJ (1985) Gamma-vinyl GABA. Gen Pharmacol 16:441–447

Munkvad I, Randrup A, Fog R (1980) Amphetamines and psychosis. In: de Wied D, Nam Keep PA (eds) Hormones and the brain. MTP Press, Lancester, pp 221–229

Olsen RW (1981) GABAbenzodiazepine-barbiturate receptor interactions. J Neurochem 37:1–13

Petersen EN, Lassen JB (1981) A water lick conflict paradigm using drug experienced rats. Psychopharmacology 75:236–239

Redmond DE Jr (1986) The possible role of *locus coeruleus* noradrenergic activity in anxiety-panic. Clin Neuropharmacol 9:40–42

Riblet LA, Taylor DP, Eison MS, Stanton HC (1982) Pharmacology and neurochemistry of buspirone. J Clin Psychiatry 43:11–16

Rodin E (1958) Metrazol tolerance in a "normal" volunteer population. Electroencephalogr Clin Neurophysiol 10:433–446

Younger LM, Fowler PJ, Zarevics P, Setler PE (1984) Novel inhibitors of γ-aminobutyric acid (GABA) uptake: anticonvulsant actions in rats. J Pharmacol Exp Ther 228:109–115

Dementia: Classification and Aspects of Treatment

C. G. GOTTFRIES

Abstract

The syndrome dementia is defined by evidence of a decline in memory, thinking, and emotional functions. In this article, dementia is delimited only by its symptoms; the etiology, the course, and the extensiveness of the disorder are not used as criteria of a dementia syndrome. In the descriptive diagnoses of dementia disorders, however, different aspects of the disorders are used. Descriptive diagnoses are (a) benign senile forgetfulness, (b) primary degenerative disorders, (c) secondary dementias, (d) cerebrovascular disorders with dementia, (e) reversible dementias, and (f) dementias with unknown etiology. Primary degenerative disorders include the subgroups (a) senile dementia of Alzheimer type (SDAT), (b) Alzheimer's disease (AD), (c) Pick's disease, and (d) Huntington's chorea. The question whether SDAT and AD should be included in one group is discussed. Very interesting and stimulating treatment research is going on in the field of dementias. Although there has still been no real breakthrough, some results indicate that dementia symptoms may be influenced by treatment. At present, treatment strategies go along the following lines: (a) pharmacological treatment, (b) control of sleep apneas and circulatory disturbances, (c) brain tissue transplantation, and (d) psychotherapy and mental activation. The pharmacological manipulation of dementia disorders focuses on substituting failing neurotransmitter systems. The use of nootropic drugs and gangliosides is still at an experimental level. Findings of vitamin B_{12} deficiency in late-onset dementia make vitamin B_{12} substitution relevant. White matter disturbances such as incomplete infarctions are reported in brains from demented patients. Coincident findings of increased sleep apneas with severe hypoxemia make studies of circulatory disturbances of interest. Transplantation of brain tissue has already left the animal experimental level and been applied to patients with parkinsonism. In some investigations, it is shown that mental activation causes not only a mental improvement but also changes in cerebrospinal fluid indicating the stimulation of trophic factors.

1 Introduction

Before trying to classify different dementia disorders, the concept of dementia has to be defined. One definition of dementia is that it is a syndrome where there is evidence of a decline in memory and thinking which is of a degree sufficient to impair functioning in daily living. Deterioration of emotional functions may also be included as a criterion. Sometimes it is added that this syndrome should be present in a setting of clear consciousness for a confident diagnosis to be established. If this aspect of the diagnosis is used, then pseudodementias or other groups of syndromes causing mental impairment must be defined. Examples of other syndromes are delirium or clouding of mind, which include symptoms of

Department of Psychiatry and Neurochemistry, St. Jörgen's Hospital, Gothenburg University, S-42203 Hisings Backa, Sweden.

temporary decline in memory and thinking. Functional disorders such as severe depressions with inhibition also cause a decline in thinking and emotional behavior.

In some textbooks, dementia is also defined as a disorder which is long-standing (at least 6 months) or irreversible. If the course of the disorder is used in the definition of the illness, then one must separate temporary or reversible from irreversible mental impairment, which may be difficult or sometimes impossible.

Dementia may also be defined as a syndrome which is global, although memory and thinking are given the heaviest weight. If the extent of the disorder is used in the definition of the concept, then amnesic syndromes must also be separated from the concept of dementia.

The classification of dementias used in this article is based upon the definition of the dementia syndrome as a decline in intellectual and emotional functions independent of the etiology, the course, or the extensiveness of the disorder. Descriptive diagnoses are used, and the names of different forms of dementia are often based on compromises between different aspects of the disorder, such as symptomatology, etiology, course, and extensiveness. The classification is shown in Fig. 1.

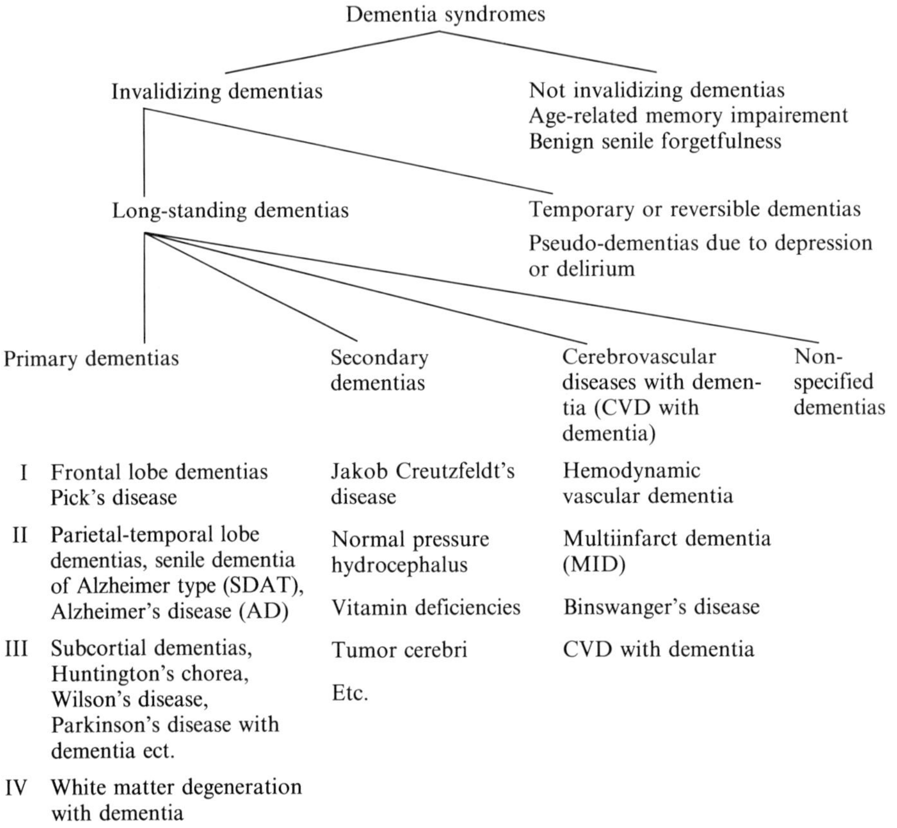

Fig. 1. Classification of dementia syndroms

2 Classification of Dementia

2.1 Normal Aging or Benign Senile Forgetfulness

We are still uncertain whether mental impairment in old age is a quantitative disorder in which the normal aging processes are exaggerated and accelerated and dementia appears when reserves are exhausted and compensatory mechanisms fail. At present, there are data indicating that above the age of 65 years, there is an involution process in the brain causing atrophy, reduced enzyme activities, and reduced concentrations of neurotransmitters and their metabolites. It is also evident that especially in the higher age-group, there is a strong correlation between aging and mental impairment (GOTTFRIES 1986). Thus, it must be accepted that in the very high age-group, there may be a dementia syndrome which is due to normal aging factors, to which syndrome the name "benign senile forgetfulness" is given.

2.2 Reversible Dementias

As the syndrome dementia is defined only by its symptomatology, the concept of reversible dementias must be used for those with a rather short duration. In the elderly, deliriums or confusional states are often seen to cause severe mental impairment. Deliriums have an abrupt onset and a short duration. These conditions may be secondary to somatic disases or environmental factors temporarily causing an insufficiency of the brain. In the elderly functional psychoses with depression and inhibition may also go together with mental impairment, sometimes so severe that they can hardly be differentiated from a primary demential illness. These conditions are often named "pseudodementias."

2.3 Primary Degenerative Dementia Disorders

This group includes patients where a pathological degeneration of the neurons is assumed to take place. The group includes disorders such as senile dementia of Alzheimer type (SDAT) Alzheimer's disease (AD), Pick's disease, and Huntington's chorea. In SDAT, the symptomatology and the course of the disorder are taken into consideration. The disorder has an insidious onset, which occurs above the age of 65, and it progresses slowly. The diagnosis can, however, only be confirmed by postmortem investigations, as structural changes in the form of senile plaques and fibrillary tangles must be present.

AD is a dementia disorder very similar to SDAT; however, it has a somewhat more malignant course. The onset of the disorder occurs before 65, which distinguishes it from SDAT. In AD, the diagnosis must also be confirmed postmortem by histological investigation of brain tissue, where senile plaques and fibrillary tangles are present. Especially in the United States, the two disorders are brought together into one group, the Alzheimer type dementia (AD/SDAT). In Europe, however, the disorders are still kept apart. The AD group is considered to be rather homogenous, although subgroups can be defined (MAYEUX et al. 1985). The SDAT group, however, is assumed to be a rather heterogenous group.

Investigations in Scandinavia (SJÖGREN et al. 1952; SOURANDER and SJÖGREN 1970) showed that in family studies, AD and SDAT behave like two separate disorders. There are also biochemical findings indicating that the early- and late-onset types of Alzheimer dementia should be kept apart (GOTTFRIES et al. 1983; ROSSOR et al. 1984).

2.4 Secondary Dementias

It is obvious somatic disorders of the brain may cause a mental impairment, which may sometimes be difficult to differentiate from dementia of primary type. Tumors of the brain, infections, and hydrocephalus are examples of such disorders. Jakob-Creutzfeldt dementia used to be assigned to the primary dementias, but as it is now evident that this disorder is due to virus infections, it is assigned to the group of secondary dementias.

2.5 Cerebrovascular Disorders

It is obvious that brain lesions caused by several infarctions may cause not only neurological symptoms but also a mental impairment, defined as dementia. This disorder has an abrupt onset and a step-by-step course. The infarctions can be assumed to cause the behavioral changes; therefore, the disorder is named "multi-infarction dementia" (MID). There may, however, be other forms of dementia due to disorders of the brain vessels. At our institute, we have investigated a group of nine patients with infarctions of the brain diagnosed at the postmortem investigation (WALLIN and GOTTFRIES, in preparation). However, in this group of patients there was no abrupt onset, and there seemed to be no causal relationship between the amount and/or localization of the brain infarctions and the dementia syndrome. Although only few and limited infarctions were found, the patients had a global dementia. Interestingly, a rather general biochemical damage was found, in the form of reduced concentrations of 5-hydroxyindoleacetic acid (5-HIAA) and choline acetyltransferase (CAT). In these brains, no Alzheimer lesions were found, and no microinfarctions either. The frontal cortex and hippocampus were investigated histologically. One may assume a disorder of the small vessels, which can be named "cerebrovascular disorder" (CVD) with dementia."

It is obvious that not all dementias found in the high age-groups can be classified as SDAT or MID. The concept of senile dementia (SD) is used in different ways: sometimes the diagnosis SD includes all dementias seen in patients above the age of 65 independent of etiology; sometimes this concept is restricted to dementia with onset above the age of 65 where no etiology for the demential illness is found. In the classification of dementias, the concept of SD is not of very much use. If it is not used, a group of dementias with unknown etiology must be formed.

3 Treatment Aspects

At present, the following strategies are used in the treatment of dementias:

1. Pharmacological treatment
   Substitution of neurotransmitters
   Nootropic drugs
   Gangliosides
   Vitamin B_{12} substitution
2. Treatment of sleep apnea and circulatory disturbances
3. Brain tissue transplantation
4. Psychotherapy and mental activation

3.1 Pharmacological Treatment

Interesting biochemical research during the last two decades has shown that in patients with dementia disorders, especially those with AD/SDAT, there are disturbances of neurotransmitter functioning. Reduced activity of CAT indicates rather severe damage to the acetylcholine (ACh) system. It seems, however, that monoamines and neuropeptides are also to some extent disturbed in brains from patients with AD/SDAT. The multiple lesions found in these brains indicate that there may be some more fundamental disturbance in the brains of these patients, the nature of which we do not know. Although the disturbed neurotransmitter functioning has no etiological importance, the disturbances can be of pathogenetic importance. In fact, it has been shown that the monoamine metabolites homovanillic acid (HVA), 5-HIAA, and 3-methoxy-4-hydroxyphenylglycol (HMPG) in the cerebrospinal fluid (CSF) can be correlated to behavioral changes in the patients (G. Bråne, G.C. Gottfries, I. Karlsson, L. Parnetti, L. Svennerholm, unpublished observations). Based on these findings, pharmacological strategies have been formulated. Rather extensive research has been carried out in order to manipulate the ACh system. Drugs that influence presynaptic, synaptic, and postsynaptic ACh function have been tried. Choline and lecithine precursors have been given, but the result is rather negative. Inhibitors of acetylcholine esterase, physostigmine, and tetrahydroaminoacridine (THA) have also been given. Psychological tests confirm an improved memory when patients are treated with physostigmine, but the clinical value of this improvement is marginal. Physostigmine has a very rapid half-life and is therefore also very impractical in clinial use. THA, however, has a longer half-life and is therefore more suitable for clinical practice. However, there have been very few investigations with this drug, and further trials are needed to confirm the effect of THA. In one investigation, a rather positive effect was found (Summers et al. 1986). Postsynaptic cholinergic agonists can also be considered in trials for activating cholinergic function. Arecoline and spiropiperidyl (RS86) have been used in some trials, but the effect found hitherto is rather marginal. In summary, the effect of cholinergic drugs has not been as promising as was expected.

From the pathogenetic point of view, it is assumed that disturbances of the ACh system may explain some of the intellectual symptoms seen in AD/SDAT.

However, the parkinsonlike motor functional disturbances seen in AD (PEARCE 1974) must be related to disturbances in dopamine (DA) metabolism (GOTTFRIES et al. 1983). It is also logical to relate emotional disturbances, for instance, symptoms of lowered mood, to disturbances in the metabolism of noradrenaline (NA) and 5-hydroxytryptamine (5-HT). Irritability, anxiety, and reduced sexual activity, which are also seen in AD/SDAT, may also be related to disturbances of the monoamine metabolism.

The monoamine neurotransmitter systems can be activated by drug treatment at a presynaptic, synaptic, or postsynaptic level. In several studies, attempts have been made to substitute or to activate the DA system. When using dopaminergic drugs, target symptoms should be not only motor function disturbance but also symptoms of intellectual impairment according to some studies (NYBERG et al. 1983; G. BRÅNE, C.G. GOTTFRIES, I. KARLSSON, L. PARNETTI, and L. SVENNERHOLM, unpublished observations). Some of the studies in which L-dopa was used have reported marginal clinical effects in patients with dementia, but many of these studies have been negative. Investigations with dopaminergic agonists such as lisuride and bromocriptine have so far also been negative (GOTTFRIES 1983).

One group of symptoms in the dementia syndrome reflects depressed mood. Trials have been made to treat these symptoms with antidepressants. The tricyclic antidepressants have an anticholinergic effect, however, and usually give rise to side effects of such an extent that such drugs cannot be used in demented patients. A new type of antidepressant with a more selective effect on monoamines has been introduced. Examples of such drugs are zimelidine, alaproclate, citalopram, femoxetine, and fluoxetine. In our institute, we have investigated the effect of alaproclate and citalopram. In pilot studies, improvements have been seen in symptoms of mood disturbances. It is not only the mood level that has been influenced: symptoms of irritability and aggressiveness have also been positively influenced. Studies have shown that after citalopram treatment lasting 4 weeks, the levels of 5-HIAA and HMPG are decreased in the cerebrospinal fluid. The postdexamethasone cortisol levels have also been normalized after treatment with citalopram (BALLDIN et al., in preparation). Further investigation of the effect of selective 5-HT reuptake blockers in the treatment of AD/SDAT and possibly also CVD with dementia would seem to be of value. Treatment with tryptophane has been used in a few studies, but no consistent result is reported.

In dementia disorders, ADOLFSSON et al. (1980) have reported increased activity of monoamine oxidase (MAO)-B in old age and a still higher increase in patients with AD/SDAT. The biological importance of this increased enzyme activity is uncertain; still, it would be of interest to try MAO inhibitors in the treatment of AD and SDAT. Selective MAO inhibitors are available, and these would reduce the risk of the treatment.

Some biochemical studies of brains from patients with AD/SDAT have shown signs of not only a neuron loss but also chemical lesions of the remaining neurons (CARLSSON 1986). The rather disappointing results in pharmacological trials to substitute neurotransmitters may be explained by a dysfunction of the neurons. In normal aging, however, it seems that the remaining neurons can respond to feedback systems. Perhaps it would theefore be more rewarding to treat patients with normal aging or benign senile forgetfulness with these types of drugs instead of AD/SDAT patients.

"Nootropics" is the name of drugs that activate the metabolism of the neurons not only by increasing the cerebral blood flow. In animal experiments, piracetam (2-osopyrrolidine-1-acetamide) has been shown to improve memory functions and to protect against hypoxia. Several investigations have been made in man to examine its effect on disturbed cerebral brain functioning. The results are contradictory as regards its effect on dementia disorders (GOTTFRIES 1983). At present, there are also some piracetamanalogues, pramiracetam and oxiracetam. Only preliminary investigations have been made with these analogues, and valid conclusions are not possible (ITIL et al. 1982; BRANCONNIER et al. 1983).

Hydergine (ergoloid mesylates) is a drug which has several effects on brain function. In the treatment of organic brain syndromes, the clinical effect may be due not to the effect of the drug on cerebral blood flow, as was previously suggested, but to the effect on neuronal metabolism. In terms of neurotransmitter activity, the drug induces mainly blockade of central α-adrenergic receptor sites and stimulation of both dopaminergic and serotoninergic receptor sites (LOEW et al. 1978). Investigations in AD/SDAT and also in patients with normal aging have shown clinical improvements, and this drug is among those most commonly used for institutionalized populations (ZAWADSKI et al. 1978).

At present, several neurotransmitters or neuromodulators of neuropeptide type are characterized. Some of these or analogues such as adrenocorticotropic hormone (ACTH) derivatives, ORG2766, vasopressin, deamino-D-arginine vasopressin (DDAVP), naloxone, and cholecystokinin (CCK) have been used in the treatment of dementia syndromes. The effect has not as yet been very promising. The central effect registered by some of the drugs may take the form of modulating arousal.

The gangliosides seem to be of importance for the propagation of the impulse at the synapse level. In one study (GOTTFRIES et al. 1983), it was shown that the gangliosides in the caudate nucleus in brains from patients with AD/SDAT are reduced. In fact, other membrane components such as myelin also seem to be disturbed in patients with AD/SDAT (SVENNERHOLM et al. 1987). As treatment with gangliosides (GM_1) has been successful for peripheral neuron lesions, it would seem interesting to test the gangliosides also in dementia disorders. The gangliosides have a trophic effect and influence the sprouting of axons. Such an investigation is at present in progress at our institute.

In a careful investigation of dementia disorders (REGLAND et al. 1988) it was found that no less than 23% of patients diagnosed as SDAT cases had such low vitamin B_{12} levels in serum that a B_{12} deficiency had to be suspected. In this group of patients, it was also found that there were low pepsinogen concentrations in serum. This indicates an atrophic gastritis. According to this finding, it must be suspected that in old age a deficiency of the mucous membranes of the gut may be present, possibly due to senile changes. Essential nutrients such as vitamin B_{12} and perhaps others (zinc, amino acids) are absorbed insufficiently, which may have pathogenetic importance for the dysfunction of the brain. Vitamin B_{12} substitution may therefore be a relevant treatment in subgroups of dementias with late onset.

3.2 Treatment of Sleep Apnea and Circulatory Disturbances

Investigations by SOURANDER et al. (1985) have shown that in patients with dementia, there are sleep disturbances in the form of sleep apneas. They also showed that these apneas were rather severe and caused hypoxia. BRUN and GUSTAFSON showed as far back as 1976 that there were white matter changes in patients with AD/SDAT and CVD with dementia. This was confirmed biochemically at out institute (GOTTFRIES et al. 1985). Neuropathologically these changes are described as incomplete infarctions, which can be interpreted as changes caused by hypoxemia. Due to these findings, it may be relevant to study sleep disorders, arhythmias, and circulatory disturbances in patients with dementia syndromes.

3.3 Brain Tissue Transplantation

Brain tissue transplantation is a rather interesting field of research, which has already left the level of animal experiments and been applied to patients with parkinsonism. This treatment strategy may of course be of interest as regards disorders due to selective disturbances of brain tissue. It has been assumed that in AD/SDAT, there are selective disturbances of some neurotransmitter systems, but recent data indicate rather multiple lesions in the brains of these patients. This treatment strategy will therefore be difficult to apply to AD/SDAT.

3.4 Psychotherapy and Mental Activation

Psychotherapy and mental activation are of great importance in the treatment of dementia disorders. Certainly, the brain is influenced by trophic and atrophic factors. A stimulating environment induces trophic factors to dominate in the brain. In an investigation by KARLSSON et al. (1985), it was shown that in patients with dementia disorders who were intensively stimulated, levels of somatostatin and HVA in CSF increased. It can be assumed that the opposite takes place if elderly and demented people are brought to institutions with a nonstimulating milieu. BRÅANE (1986) has also shown that a dementia disorder influences not only the individual patient but also the whole family. A supporting psychotherapy directed not only to the patient but also to the family concerned is therefore of great importance.

Acknowledgements. This research was supported by grants from the Swedish Medical Research Council, The Pfannenstill Foundation, The Lundbeck Foundation, Greta and Johan Kock's Foundations, and The Foundation for Old Servants.

References

Adolfsson R, Gottfries CG, Oreland L, Wiberg Å, Winblad B (1980) Increased activity of brain and platelet monoamine oxidase in dementia of Alzheimer type. Life Sci 27:1029–1034

Branconnier RJ, Cole JO, Dessain EC, Spera KF, Ghazvinian S, DeVitt D (1983) The therapeutic efficacy of pramiracetam in Alzheimer's disease: Preliminary observations. Psychopharmacol Bull 19:276

Bråne G (1986) Normal aging and dementia disorders – coping and crisis in the family. Prog Neuropsychopharmacol Biol Psychiatry 10:287–295
Brun A, Gustafson L (1976) Distribution of cerebral degeneration in Alzheimer's disease. A clinico-pathological study. Arch Psychiatr Nervenkr 223:15–33
Carlsson A (1986) Neurotransmitters in old age and dementia. In: Hafner H, Moschel G, Sartorius N (eds) Mental health in the elderly: A review of the present state of research. Springer, Berlin Heidelberg New York
Gottfries CG (1983) Dementia. In: Hippius H, Winokur G (eds) Clinical psychopharmacology. Excerpta Medica, Amsterdam, pp 271–285 (Psychopharmacology, vol 1/2)
Gottfries CG (1986) Nosological aspects of differential typology of dementia of Alzheimer type. In: Bergener M (ed) Dimensions in aging. Academic, London, pp 207–219
Gottfries CG, Adolfsson R, Aquilonius SM, Carlsson A, Eckernäs SE, Nordberg A, Oreland L, et al. (1983) Biochemical changes in dementia disorders of Alzheimer type (AD/SDAT). Neurobiol Aging 4:261–271
Gottfries CG, Karlsson I, Svennerholm L (1985) Senile dementia – A white matter disease? In: Gottfries CG (ed) Normal aging, Alzheimer's disease and senile dementia. Aspects on etiology, pathogenesis, diagnosis and treatment. Éditions de L'Université de Bruxelles, Bruxelles, pp 111–118
Itil TM, Menon GN, Bozak M, Songar A (1982) The effects of oxiracetam (ISF 2522) in patients with organic brain syndrome (a double-blind controlled study with piracetam). Drug Dev Res 2:448
Karlsson I, Widerlöv E, Melin EV, Nyth AL, Bråne GAM, Rybo E, Rehfeld JF, Bissette G, Nemeroff CB (1985) Changes of CSF neuropeptides after environmental stimulation in dementia. Nord Psykiatr Tidsskr [Suppl 11] 49:75–81
Loew DM, van Deusen EB, Meier-Ruge W (1978) Effect on the central nervous system. In: Berde B, Schild HO (eds) Ergot alkaloids and related compounds. Springer, Berlin Heidelberg New York, pp 421–531 (Handbook of experimental pharmacology, vol 49)
Mayeux R, Stern Y, Spanton S (1985) Heterogeneity in dementia of the Alzheimer type. Evidence of subgroups. Neurology (NY) 35:453–461
Nyberg P, Nordberg A, Wester P, Winblad B (1983) Dopaminergic deficiency is more pronounced in putamen than in nucleus candatus in Parkinson's disease. Neurochem Pathol 1:193–202
Pearce J (1974) Mental changes in parkinsonism (letter). Br Med J 1:445
Regland B, Gottfries CG, Oreland L, Svennerholm L (1988) Low B12 levels related to high activity of platelet MAO in patients with dementia disorders. A retrospective study. Acta Psychiatr Scand (Accepted for publication)
Rossor MN, Iversen LL, Reynolds GP, Mountjoy CQ, Roth M (1984) Neurochemical characteristics of early and late onset types of Alzheimer's disease. Br Med J 288:961–964
Sjögren T, Sjögren H, Lindgren AGH (1952) Morbus Alzheimer and morbus Pick. A genetic clinical and patho-anatomical study. Acta Psychiatr Neurol Sand [Suppl] 82
Sourander P, Sjögren H (1970) The concept of Alzheimer's disease and its clinical implications. In: Wolstenholme GEW, O'Connor M (eds) Alzheimer's disease and related conditions. Churchill, London, pp 11–36
Sourander L, Polo O, Alihanka J (1985) Sleep apnea and hypoxia in patients with senile dementia. Nordic Psychiatric Congress, 29 May–1 June
Summers WK, Majovski LV, Marsh GM, Tachiki K, Kling A (1986) Oral tetrahydroaminoacridine in long-term treatment of senile dementia, Alzheimer type. N Engl J Med 315:1241–1245
Svennerholm L, Gottfries CG, Karlsson I (1987) Neurochemical changes in white matter of patients with Alzheimer's disease. In: NATO Conference on multidisciplinary approach to myeline diseases. (In press)
Zawadski RT, Glazer GB, Lurie E (1978) Psychotropic drug use among institutionalized and non-institutionalized medicaid aged in California. J Gerontol 33:825–834

Test Models and New Directions in Dementia Research

L. L. IVERSEN

Abstract

Psychopharmacology research in the dementia field is particularly difficult because there are no effective treatments on which to base models. Much effort is devoted to attempts to replace defective brain chemical transmitters or neuropeptides, with particular emphasis on the cholinergic system. There is also interest in noradrenaline, serotonin and somatostatin deficits. New directions include the study of glutamate-related excitotoxins such as quinolinic acid as possible causative agents for cerebral degeneration in dementia. Glutamate receptor antagonists, e.g. MK-801, may have the potential to limit or slow down neurodegenerative processes. Neurotrophic factors, e.g. nerve growth factor, may also possess the ability to protect neurons from irreversible loss.

1 Introduction

Psychopharmacology research in the dementia area has a high priority because of the urgency of the problem. It is a particularly difficult area, however, because the approaches used in the past have been singularly unsuccessful, so far, in providing treatments that have any important therapeutic efficacy. Thus, models based on attempts to improve cerebral perfusion, or to enhance cerebral metabolism do not appear likely to prove fruitful avenues for future research efforts. In this chapter three alternative strands of research strategy will be briefly reviewed.

2 Replacement Therapy Strategies

2.1 Cholinergic

The successful development of L-dopa as a neurotransmitter replacement therapy in Parkinson's disease, together with the discovery that the forebrain cholinergic system is severely damaged in patients dying with Alzheimer's dementia, has made cholinergic replacement therapy an attractive strategy (for review see BARTUS et al. 1986; PERRY 1986). It is now generally agreed that administration of pre-

Merck Sharp and Dohme Research Laboratories, Neuroscience Research Centre, Terlings Park, Harlow, UK.

cursors such as choline or lecithin is not a successful approach – and indeed it is difficult to see how this could be effective as the enzymic machinery needed to convert choline to acetylcholine is lacking in the Alzheimer brain. The most successful attempts to use the cholinergic approach have been those which employed acetylcholinesterase inhibitors, and a number of clinical studies have demonstrated definite, albeit modest and transient, beneficial effects in Alzheimer's patients treated with physostigmine (HOLLANDER et al. 1986). Similar improvements in memory and cognitive performance have been reported in elderly monkeys treated with physostigmine (BARTUS et al. 1980), and the elderly primate has emerged as a valuable animal model for testing novel agents of possible use in dementia. A remarkably high rate of success was recently reported in a clinical trial of the cholinesterase inhibitor tacrine (1,2,3,4-tetrahydro-9-aminoacridine) (SUMMERS et al. 1986). An obvious problem with cholinesterase inhibitors or other cholinomimetic agents is that such compounds have numerous adverse effects on the peripheral system. Compounds presently available also have only a limited ability to penetrate into CNS and a poor duration of action. It remains to be seen whether the cholinergic replacement approach can become a useful means of offering palliative relief. The rationale for this approach remains strong.

2.2 Other Monoamines

Studies of postmortem brain have shown that damage is not confined to the cholinergic pathways in Alzheimer's dementia. There is also evidence for varying degrees of loss of other monoaminergic projection pathways to cerebral cortex and hippocampus, notably those containing noradrenaline and 5-hydroxytryptamine (5-HT) (WINBLAD et al. 1985; ROSSOR and IVERSEN 1986). ARNSTEN and GOLDMAN-RAKIC (1985) also observed a decrase in noradrenaline content in various areas of cerebral cortex in the aging monkey brain, and postulated that this might play a key role in the cognitive deficits exhibited by such animals. They showed that the α_2-agonist clonidine was able to restore normal performance in aged monkeys tested on delayed response tasks, and suggested that such agents might play a useful role in therapy. Clinical experience with clonidine, however, has suggested that it may impair cognitive performance rather than enhance it, and at least one report has failed to replicate the beneficial effects claimed in the elderly nonhuman primate (DAVIS et al. 1987). Nevertheless, this work has opened a possible new avenue for psychopharmacology research which deserves further study.

Rather little is known about the effects of 5-HT-related agents on higher brain functions. The 5-HT uptake inhibitors zimelidine and alaproclate, however, have been reported to have beneficial effects on memory performance in animals and in man. Alaproclate was also reported to be able to enhance behavioral responses to centrally acting cholinergic stimulants suggesting a potentially interesting interaction with central cholinergic mechanisms (for review see ALTMAN and NORMILE 1986).

2.3 Neuropeptides

The selective changes which occur in cerebral cortex peptides in Alzheimer's dementia suggest that there is considerable selectivity in cortical neurodegenerative changes. Thus, no changes have been observed in cholecystokinin, vasoactive intestinal polypeptide, enkephalins, neurotensin or neuropeptide Y (Rossor and Iversen 1986). On the other hand, a consistent reduction in somatostatin has been found, particularly in frontal and temporal cortex (Rossor and Iversen 1986). A marked reduction in cortical levels of corticotropin-releasing factor (CRF) has also been reported in Alzheimer's patients, although surprisingly this was most severe in occipital cortex, an area not normally associated with the most marked neuropathological changes (De Souza et al. 1986). Attempts to replace neuropeptides are inherently difficult, because of the inability of these substance to penetrate into CNS from the circulation. A pilot study with the stable somatostatin analogue L-363,586 administered i.v. to Alzheimer's patients failed to yield any consistent improvements in cognitive performance (Cutler et al. 1985).

3 The Excitotoxin Hypothesis

3.1 Excitotoxins

The neurotoxic actions of L-glutamate and related compounds which act on excitatory amino acid receptors in brain are well documented (for review see Coyle 1982). The powerful glutamate-like excitants kainic acid and ibotenic acid have been widely used as research tools in recent years. They cause local destruction of neurons in the vicinity of a micro-injection site in brain – without damaging non-neural elements or nerve fibres or terminals arising away from the injection site. The idea that similar endogenous or exogenous excitotoxins may be responsible for the loss of neurons in a variety of neurodegenerative diseases has gained ground in recent years. Endogeneous toxins of this type might include L-glutamate and L-aspartate, released in excessively large amounts – in response, for example, to cerebral ischaemia or hypoglycaemia (Schwarcz and Meldrum 1985). Other endogenous excitotoxins, however, might arise from the abnormal metabolism of other amino acids. In particular, the substance quinolinic acid is an intermediate formed during the metabolic degradation of L-tryptophan. Quinolinic acid is a glutamate-like excitatory agent and causes neurotoxic changes when administered into CNS. It has been suggested that the formation of abnormally large amounts of quinolinic acid in the aging brain might contribute to the onset of degenerative changes in certain neuronal populations (Schwarcz et al. 1984). Although quinolinic acid can be detected in animal and human brain, however, the amounts are relatively small, and so far no changes have been observed in patients with Alzheimer's dementia (Moroni et al. 1986). Competitive antagonists which act at glutamate receptors, particularly those of the *N*-methyl-D-aspartate (NMDA) type, can protect against excitotoxic damage in animal models, but these compounds do not penetrate well into CNS and have generally required intracranial administration (Schwarcz and Meldrum 1985).

3.2 MK-801: A Novel Glutamate Antagonist

MK-801 {(+)-5-methyl-10,11-dihydro-5H-dibenzo[a,d]cyclohepten-5,10-imine maleate} was shown by CLINESCHMIDT et al. (1982) to be a potent orally active anticonvulsant agent with anxiolytic and sympathomimetic properties. We have recently discovered that MK-801 is a potent antagonist of NMDA receptors (WONG et al. 1986). We found that [^{3}H]MK-801 binds to a specific population of receptor sites in rat brain and these appear to be associated with glutamate receptors of the NMDA type. Thus MK-801 antagonises the depolarising actions of NMDA in rat cerebral cortex in vitro and leaves responses to other selective glutamate-like agonists unchanged (quisqualic acid, kainic acid). The antagonism is noncompetitive and agonist dependent in character. [^{3}H]MK-801 binding was displaced by structural analogues of MK-801 and by the dissociative anaesthetics phencyclidine (PCP), ketamine and the sigma ligand (±) SKF 10047. Unlike PCP, MK-801 was a very weak displacer of binding to sigma sites labelled with SKF 10047. A study of the regional distribution of [^{3}H]MK-801 binding using quantitative autoradiographic techniques revealed an uneven distribution of sites in rat brain (BOWERY and HUDSON 1986). The highest concentrations of [^{3}H]MK-801 binding sites were detected in the hippocampus, particularly the CA1 region, the molecular layer of the dentate gyrus and superficial layers of the cerebral cortex. Moderate levels were observed in the caudate putamen and thalamic medial and lateral geniculate nuclei. Very low levels were present in the cerebellum, substantia nigra, corpus callosum, superior colliculus and medulla pons. This pattern concurs with that previously reported for the NMDA sites labelled with [^{3}H]-glutamate (MONAGHAN and COTMAN 1985).

3.3 Neuroprotective Effects of MK-801

Systemically administered MK-801 protects against neuronal degeneration caused by intracerebral injections of NMDA agonists (FOSTER et al. 1986, 1987). Stereotaxic injections of NMDA, kainic acid or quinolinic acid (in 1 μl), pH 7.4, were made into the right striatum or dorsal hippocampus of rats under equithesin anaesthesia. MK-801 (dissolved in 0.9% saline) was administered i.p. and saline-injected animals served as controls. For histological analyses, animals were perfused with fixative after 7 days and microtome sections stained with cresyl violet. For neurochemical measurements, animals were killed after 7 days, the striatum or hippocampus dissected and assayed for choline acetyltransferase (CAT) or glutamate decarboxylase (GAD) activity, respectively.

Unilateral injection of quinolinic acid or NMDA into the striatum (60–300 nmol) or dorsal hippocampus in the control group ($n=4$) resulted in an area of neuronal degeneration extending for several millimetres around the injection site. Treatment with 10 mg/kg MK-801 1 h prior to NMDA or quinolinic acid injection ($n=4$) caused almost complete protection, with only a few necrotic neurons in the immediate vicinity of the injection site. A quantitative assessment of the neuroprotective effects of MK-801 was made by measuring the activity of marker enzymes for intrinsic neuronal populations. MK-801 given i.p. at 10 mg/

kg 1 h before NMDA or quinolinic acid injection caused a complete protection of these effects in both striatum and hippocampus. The specificity of MK-801 for NMDA-induced neurodegeneration was indicated by the finding that kainate-induced CAT decrements in the striatum were not protected by MK-801 up to 10 mg/kg. MK-801 remained effective as a neuroprotective even when given 1–3 h after neurotoxin injections. It is possible that MK-801 or a related NMDA receptor antagonist may offer the possibility of testing the "excitotoxin" hypothesis of Alzheimer's dementia, although clinical trials will inevitably be difficult to design and to perform.

4 Neurotrophic Factors

4.1 Nerve Growth Factor

The mouse salivary gland protein "nerve growth factor" (NGF) was discovered more than 30 years ago. It has long been known as a selective stimulator of the growth and differentiation of certain sensory neurons and of adrenergic cells in the sympathetic nervous system (for review see LEVI-MONTALCINI 1982). Because initial attempts to test NGF in the CNS focused on adrenergic neurons, on which it is largely ineffective, it was thought until recently that NGF did not have any central actions. However, this can now be seen to be incorrect, as CNS cholinergic neurons particularly in the forebrain do indeed respond to NGF. Increased synthesis of the cholinergic marker enzyme CAT can be observed when CNS cholinergic neurons are exposed to NGF either in tissue culture or after NGF injections into CSF in young animals (MOBLEY et al. 1985; HEFTI et al. 1985). Furthermore, intracranial administration of NGF promotes the survival of septohippocampal neurons in rat brain after surgical lesion of their axons in adult animals which normally leads to cell death (KROMER 1987; HEFTI 1986). HENDRY and IVERSEN (1973) first suggested that NGF might act as a "retrograde trophic factor", secreted by target tissues and picked up by adrenergic fibres that made successful synaptic contact with such targets. NGF may act as a growth-promoting factor during development, but may continue to be needed for neuronal survival throughout the life of the neuron. New data on the NGF system in brain suggests that it may act similarly there as a retrograde trophic factor for forebrain cholinergic projections. Thus, NGF appears to be synthesised not in the cholinergic neurons in rat brain, but by their targets in cerebral cortex. NGF injected exogenously into brain is selectively accumulated by cholinergic neurons and retrogradely transported back to their cell bodies (SEILER and SCHWAB 1984). A simple explanation for the selective degeneration of cholinergic pathways to forebrain in Alzheimer's dementia might thus be that this occurred as the result of a primary loss of the cortical target normally innervated by these fibres or their failure to synthesise adequate amounts of NGF (HEFTI 1983). Preliminary data on postmortem brain from patients dying with Alzheimer's dementia, however, have failed to detect any abnormality in NGF mRNA content (GOEDERT et al. 1986). Nevertheless, the delivery of exogenous NGF (or an NGF-like substance) might represent a means of slowing or preventing the degeneration of CNS cholinergic projections in Alzheimer's patients. The problems of drug delivery, however, are considerable and not easily overcome.

4.2 Other Neurotrophic Factors

NGF is by no means the only growth factor in the nervous system, although it remains the most fully characterised and the only one available in sufficient amounts as a pure molecule to allow its neuropharmacological potential to be evaluated. In recent years other factors have been described which promote the survival and growth of particular groups of neurons. These include materials which act specifically on sensory neurons, parasympathetic cholinergic neurons and spinal cord cells (Thoenen and Edgar 1985; Crutcher 1986). NGF may not be the only factor capable of acting on forebrain cholinergic neurons, Bostwick et al. (1986) described a low-molecular weight material in rat brain extracts which promotes the survival of rat septohippocampal neurons in culture; this activity was not destroyed by exposure to NGF antibodies.

More research is needed to understand more fully the range of neurotrophic factors that exists in CNS and the roles which these substances play in the maintenance of neuronal survival in the adult and especially the aging brain. At the moment, because most are poorly characterised in molecular terms and available only in minute amounts, they offer a very difficult but challenging area of pharmacology.

5 Conclusions

Dementia research will continue to be a priority area for many years to come. A new wave of research during the past decade has revealed a great deal of information about the precise nature of the neurodegenerative changes which occur in the brain in Alzheimer's dementia – and this knowledge has already prompted a number of new lines of research aimed at restoring some degree of normality to the chemical imbalances thus revealed. At a more fundamental level, however, we continue to have little understanding of why these characteristic degenerative changes occur in Alzheimer's dementia – nor do we know which research strategies may ultimately allow us to arrest the inexorable course of the disease. This must remain a goal for the next century rather than the present one.

References

Altman H, Normile HJ (1986) Serotonin, learning and memory: implications for the treatment of dementia. In: Crook T, Bartus RT, Ferris S, Gershon S (eds) Treatment development strategies for Alzheimer's disease. Powley, Conn, pp 361–384

Arnsten AFT, Goldman-Rakic PS (1985) Catecholamines and cognitive decline in aged nonhuman primates. Ann NY Acad Sci 444:218–234

Bartus RT, Dean RL, Beer B (1980) Memory deficits in aged Cebus monkeys and facilitation with central cholinomimetics. Neurobiol Aging 1:145–152

Bartus RT, Dean RL, Fisher SK (1986) Cholinergic treatment for age-related memory disturbances. In: Crook T, Bartus RT, Ferris S, Gershon S (eds) Treatment development strategies for Alzheimer's disease. Powley, Conn, pp 421–450

Bostwick JR, Lander D, Perez-Polo JR, Appel SH (1986) A brain trophic factor and nerve growth factor enhance cholinergic properties in explants of the medial septal nucleus. Soc Neurosci Abstracts 12:586

Bowery NG, Hudson AL (1986) The distribution of ^{3}H-MK-801 binding sites in rat brain determined by in vitro receptor autoradiography. Br J Pharmacol 89:775

Clineschmidt BV, Martin GE, Bunting PR (1982) Anticonvulsant activity of (+)-5-methyl-10,11-dihydro-5H-dibenzo[a,b]cyclohepten-5-,10-imine (MK-801), a substance with potent anticonvulsant, central sympathomimetic and apparent anxiolytic properties. Drug Dev Res 2:123–134

Coyle JT (1982) Excitatory amino acid neurotoxins. In: Iversen LL, Iversen SD, Snyder SH (eds) Handbook of psychopharmacology, vol 15. Plenum, New York, pp 237–270

Crutcher KA (1986) The role of growth factors in neuronal development and plasticity. CRC Crit Rev Clin Neurobiol 2:297–333

Cutler NR, Haxby JV, Narang PK, May C, Burg C, Reines SA (1985) Evaluation of an analogue of somatostatin (L-363,586) in Alzheimer's disease. N Engl J Med 312:725

Davis RE, Callahan MJ, Downs DA (1987) Clonidine disrupts aged-monkey delayed response performance. In: Wurtman R, Corkin SH, Growdon JH (eds) Alzheimer's disease: advances in basic research and therapies. Center for Brain Sciences and Metablism, Cambridge MA

De Souza EB, Whitehouse PJ, Kuhar MJ, Price DL, Vale WW (1986) Reciprocal changes in corticotropin-releasing factor (CRF)-like immunoreactivity and CRF receptors in cerebral cortex of Alzheimer's disease. Nature 319:593–595

Foster AC, Gill R, Kemp JA (1986) Protection of N-methyl-D-aspartate-induced neuronal degeneration by systemic administration of MK-801. Br J Pharmacol 89:870P

Foster AC, Gill R, Woodruff GN (1987) MK-801 prevents degeneration of striatal neurones caused by intrastriatal injection of quinolinic acid. Br J Pharmacol 90:7P

Goedert M, Fine A, Hunt SP, Ullrich A (1986) Nerve growth factor mRNA in peripheral and central rat tissues and in the human central nervous system: lesion effects in the rat brain and levels in Alzheimer's disease. Mol Brain Res 1:85–92

Hefti F (1983) Alzheimer's disease caused by a lack of nerve growth factor? Ann Neurol 13:109–110

Hefti F (1986) Nerve growth factor (NGF) promotes survival of septal cholinergic neurons after fimbrial transsections. J Neurosci 6:2155–2162

Hefti F, Hartikka J, Eckenstein F, Gnahn H, Heumann R, Schwab M (1985) Nerve growth factor (NGF) increase choline acetyltransferase but not survival or fiber growth of cultured septal cholinergic neurons. Neuroscience 14:55–68

Hendry IA, Iversen LL (1973) Reduction in the concentration of nerve growth factor in mice after sialectomy and castration. Nature 243:500–504

Hollander E, Mohs RC, Davis KL (1986) Cholinergic approaches to the treatment of Alzheimer's disease. Br Med Bull 42:97–100

Kromer LF (1987) Nerve growth factor treatment after brain injury prevents neuronal death. Science 235:214–216

Levi-Montalcini R (1982) Developmental neurobiology and the natural history of nerve growth factor. Annu Rev Neurosci 5:341–362

Mobley WC, Rutkowski JL, Tennekoon GI, Buchanan K, Johnston MV (1985) Choline acetyltransferase activity in striatum of neonatal rats increased by nerve growth factor. Science 229:284–286
Monaghan DT, Cotman CW (1985) Distribution of N-methyl-D-aspartate-sensitive L-[^{3}H]-glutamate binding sites in rat brain. J Neurosci 5:2909–2919
Moroni F, Lombardi G, Robitaille Y, Etienne P (1986) Senile dementia and Alzheimer's disease: lack of changes of the cortical content of quinolinic acid. Neurobiol Aging 7:249–253
Perry EK (1986) The cholinergic hypothesis – ten years on. Br Med Bull 42:63–69
Rossor M, Iversen LL (1986) Non-cholinergic neurotransmitter abnormalities in Alzheimer's disease. Br Med Bull 42:70–74
Schwarcz R, Meldrum B (1985) Excitatory amino acid antagonists provide a therapeutic approach to neurological disorders. Lancet II:140–143
Schwarcz R, Foster AC, French ED, Whetsell WO, Kohler C (1984) Excitotoxic models for neurodegenerative disorders. Life Sci 35:19–32
Seiler M, Schwab ME (1984) Specific retrograde transport of nerve growth factor (NGF) from neocortex to nucleus basalis in the rat. Brain Res 300:33–36
Summers WK, Majovski LV, Marsh GM, Tachiki K, Kling A (1986) Oral tetrahydroaminoacridine in long term treatment of senile dementia, Alzheimer type. N Engl J Med 315:1241–1245
Thoenen H, Edgar D (1985) Neurotrophic factors. Science 229:238–242
Winblad B, Hardy J, Backman L, Nilsson L-G (1985) Memory function and brain biochemistry in normal aging and in senile dementia. Ann NY Acad Sci 444:255–268
Wong EH, Kemp JA, Priestley T, Knight AR, Woodruff GN, Iversen LL (1986) The anticonvulsant MK-801 is a potent *N*-methyl-D-aspartate antagonist. Proc Natl Acad Sci USA 83:7104–7108

On Current Research in Affective Disorders

R. Fog

To give a short review of all the excellent papers of the current research in affective disorders in this volume is not an easy task. A lot of new data have emerged since I gave a similar review 3 years ago (Fog 1985).

It has, however, been clearly demonstrated that we still have to deal with many problems: there is still no general consensus as to the definition and classification of depressions. How do we distinguish between endogenous and non-endogenous depression? How do we define "atypical depression" (in which monoamine oxidase inhibitors, MAOIs, seem to be an adequate treatment)? Will we be able to develop tests for endogenous depression (dexamethasone suppression, sleep EEG, etc.)? We also have problems in controlling the treatment (compliance, tolerance, plasma concentrations, etc.), and it is difficult to define "adequate" doses of cyclic antidepressants. We know very little about the interaction between environment and biology, which also influences our knowledge of the effect of maintenance therapy. How do we translate animal data to clinial facts? This problem also influences our concepts of "selective" drugs and of "second" and "third" generations of cyclic antidepressants.

In spite of all the difficulties promising research results are emerging: CSF adrenaline has been found to be reduced in endogenous as well as in non-endogenous depressions, and vasoactive intestinal peptide (VIP) is decreased in non-endogenous depressions. We know more about the relation between adequate treatment and the rates of suicide and mortality. We have learned that in unipolar depression recurrence seems to be the rule rather than the exception. Only few (5%) unipolar depressions develop into bipolar cases. About lithium we now know that treatment is effective in both unipolar and bipolar depressions; and lithium is safe provided that the guidelines are followed.

In the future we hope to get hold of biological markers for various types of depression. CSF adrenaline and peptides are possible candidates. New kinds of treatment may also emerge: the value of infusion therapy is still under discussion; other types of drug treatment (carbamazepine, valproic acid) may be useful in acute and prophylactive treatment; and there may be a place for selective and reversible MAOIs. Psychosurgery is still performed in some cases of prolonged depression, but most psychiatrists would nowadays be very hesitant about using these irreversible interventions, remembering the sad results from the "lobotomy era" in schizophrenia in the 1950s.

Laboratory of Psychopharmacology, St. Hans Hospital, DK-4000 Roskilde, Denmark.

We still know very little about the aetiology of affective disorders. The involvement of biogenic amines in antidepressant effects is still the most established fact. The same could, however, be said of a whole range of neuropsychiatric disorders such as schizophrenia, parkinsonism, Huntington's chorea and Tourette's syndrome (Fog and Regeur 1986). This is perhaps not very surprising since aminergic (especially dopaminergic) areas are an output system for many brain functions.

It has been suggested that instead of seeking for root causes of disorders, psychiatrists should search for maximally effective interventions (Beahrs 1986). It has also been argued that psychotherapy should have a more dominant place in the treatment of depressions, but we should remember that our remarkable ignorance concerning the actual effectiveness of psychoanalysis and psychotherapy is persisting well into the last decades of this century (Clare 1984).

One logical way for future research into the aetiology and pathogenesis of depressions has been suggested by Mogens Schou (Fog 1985): we should look for common neurobiological mechanisms in different effective treatments (cyclic antidepressants, MAOIs, ECT, lithium, etc.).

References

Beahrs JO (1986) Limits of scientific psychiatry. Brunner-Mazel, New York

Clare AW (1984) Psychotherapy. In: Duncan R, Weston-Smith M (eds) The encyclopedia of medical ignorance. Pergamon, Oxford, pp 1–7

Fog R (1985) An overview of neurobiological factors in antidepressant treatment. Acta Pharmacol Toxicol 56 [Suppl 1]:212–214

Fog R, Regeur L (1986) Neuropharmacology of tics. Rev Neurol (Paris) 124:856–859

Subject Index